Congenital Heart Disease

A symposium presented at the Washington meeting of the American Association for the Advancement of Science, December 29–30, 1958

Edited by

ALLAN D. BASS and GORDON K. MOE

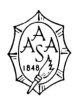

Publication No. 63 of the
American Association for the Advancement of Science
Washington D.C. • 1960

Preface

The last few years have brought spectacular advances in the field of cardiovascular surgery, advances which have been made possible by equally noteworthy progress in the study of pathological physiology of the human heart, and which have forced the development of improved techniques for diagnosis and for operative intervention. Now that much of the pioneer work has been done, it seemed appropriate to take stock of the present status of congenital heart disease, and to emphasize the interdependence of developmental morphology, pathology, physiology, diagnosis, and treatment. Accordingly, a symposium was arranged by the Section on Medicine of the AAAS for the meeting of the Association in Washington, D. C., in December 1958. With one exception, the papers presented at the meeting are included in this symposium volume.

When the symposium was planned, it was hoped that Dr. Bradley M. Patten could be one of the participants. Unfortunately, Dr. Patten had already agreed to serve as a guest professor at the Medical School of the University of Buenos Aires and was unable to accept the invitation. Because of his outstanding contributions to the developmental anatomy of the heart, his name would have been missed in any program on congenital heart disease. We are happy, therefore, that he consented to write the introductory chapter for this record of the transactions of the meeting.

We are grateful to many friends of the AAAS for their support and advice in arranging and publicizing the program, to the National Heart Institute for financial support, to the American Heart Association and the the American College of Cardiology for their endorsement, to Dr. André Cournand and Dr. Alfred Blalock, who kindly served as session chairmen, and particularly to the contributors who gave so generously of their time and efforts and enthusiasm. We wish to acknowledge also the work of Dr. Sue C. Hardman Ivie in preparing the Index.

ALLAN D. BASS, *Secretary*
GORDON K. MOE, *Chairman*
Section N

iii

134050

Contributors

FORREST H. ADAMS, Department of Pediatrics, School of Medicine, University of California, Los Angeles, California

ALEXANDER BARRY, The University of Michigan Medical School, Ann Arbor, Michigan

S. GILBERT BLOUNT, JR., University of Colorado Medical Center, Denver, Colorado

EUGENE BRAUNWALD, Clinic of Surgery, National Heart Institute, Bethesda, Maryland

JAMES R. BROWN, JR., United States Air Development Center, Johnsville, Pennsylvania

HOWARD B. BURCHELL, Section of Medicine, Mayo Clinic and Mayo Foundation, Rochester, Minnesota

DENTON A. COOLEY, Cora and Webb Mading Department of Surgery, Baylor University College of Medicine, and Surgical Services Baylor Affiliated Hospitals, Houston, Texas

G. S. DAWES, The Nuffield Institute for Medical Research, Oxford, England

GEORGE W. DEITZ, Division of Cardiology, Philadelphia General Hospital, Philadelphia, Pennsylvania

LEWIS DEXTER, Peter Bent Brigham Hospital, Boston, Massachusetts

JESSE E. EDWARDS, Section of Pathologic Anatomy, Mayo Clinic and Mayo Foundation, Rochester, Minnesota

SAMI A. KHALIL, Division of Cardiology, Philadelphia General Hospital, Philadelphia, Pennsylvania

JOHN W. KIRKLIN, Section of Surgery, Mayo Clinic and Mayo Foundation, Rochester, Minnesota

MAURICE LEV, Congenital Heart Disease Research and Training Center, Hektoen Institute, and the Department of Pathology, Northwestern University School of Medicine, Chicago, Illinois

DAVID H. LEWIS, Division of Cardiology, Philadelphia General Hospital, Philadelphia, Pennsylvania

C. WALTON LILLEHEI, Department of Surgery and Variety Club Heart Hospital, University of Minnesota Medical School, Minneapolis, Minnesota

JOHN LIND, Karolinska Sjukhuset and the Wenner-Gren Cardiovascular Research Laboratory, Stockholm, Sweden

ROBERT T. L. LONG, Clinic of Surgery, National Heart Institute, Bethesda, Maryland

ABDOL-NABI MOGHADAM, Division of Cardiology, Philadelphia General Hospital, Philadelphia, Pennsylvania

ANDREW G. MORROW, Clinic of Surgery, National Heart Institute, Bethesda, Maryland

BRADLEY M. PATTEN (Emeritus), The University of Michigan Medical School, Ann Arbor, Michigan

S. R. M. REYNOLDS, Department of Anatomy, University of Illinois, College of Medicine, Chicago, Illinois

RICHARD J. SANDERS, Clinic of Surgery, National Heart Institute, Bethesda, Maryland

MARC SAVARD, Mayo Clinic and Mayo Foundation, Rochester, Minnesota

F. MASON SONES, JR., Cardiac Laboratory, Cleveland Clinic Foundation, Cleveland, Ohio

HENRY SWAN, Department of Surgery, University of Colorado Medical Center, Denver, Colorado

H. J. C. SWAN, Mayo Clinic and Mayo Foundation, Rochester, Minnesota

JOHN D. WALLACE, United States Naval Air Development Station, Johnsville, Pennsylvania

JOSEF WARKANY, College of Medicine, University of Cincinnati, Cincinnati, Ohio

JAMES G. WILSON, Department of Anatomy, College of Medicine, University of Florida, Gainesville, Florida

EARL H. WOOD, Section of Physiology, Mayo Clinic and Mayo Foundation, Rochester, Minnesota

Contents

III DIAGNOSIS

IV SURGICAL THERAPY

Congenital Defects of the Heart: Retrospect and Prospect

BRADLEY M. PATTEN

University of Michigan Medical School, Ann Arbor, Michigan

The holding of a symposium such as this is a gratifying indication that the field of congenital defects of the heart is finally coming into its scientific maturity. The work of those contributing to it has involved the careful culling of previous studies, the integration of current findings with the work of the past that has stood the test of time, and above all the correlation of information from a variety of different disciplines. How great an advance this represents will be most keenly appreciated by the older workers in the field.

In the early years of this century anyone attempting to do research work on congenital defects of the heart was, perforce, a solitary investigator. The general attitude expressed by my clinical friends when I first tried to interest them in more accurate diagnosis of such cases was, with minor variations, "Why? They are hopeless accidents of defective development, with a dismal present and no future. I should not take the time from cases that I can really do something about."

Some of us, however, were stubborn plodders—and we needed to be. Without the interest of a large group of workers, there were no review articles to help us through the accumulation of four centuries of haphazardly growing literature. The very numbers of the references, in many languages and scattered through a wide range of journals, was discouraging. I still remember painfully wading through more than 300 articles just on defects at the foramen ovale.

There were, nevertheless, compensations in the first hand study of the old literature that would have been missed if references had been covered only in the form of the predigested concentrate of a review

1

article. Among other things was the chastening warning of the way the reputation of an investigator could make his mistakes particularly damaging. Botallo in 1565, for example, seized on cases exhibiting abnormal openings in the valvula foraminis ovalis as offering an improvement on Galen's idea that the blood entered the left side of the heart from the right by way of spaces between the trabeculae of the interventricular septum. The weight of Botallo's name behind this erroneous conception delayed for many years the acceptance of Servetus' contention that the passage of blood from right to left "does not take place through the median wall of the heart as commonly believed; but, by a grand device, the refined blood is driven from the right ventricle of the heart, in a long course through the lungs." The language in which Servetus elaborated his ideas well indicates the curious mixture of keen observation and dogma that pervaded the work of this period. "By the lungs it [the blood] is prepared, assuming a bright color. It is mingled with the inspired air and purged of its fulginous matter by expiration and so at length the left ventricle of the heart attracts by its diastole the whole mixture, a suitable ... material that ... may become vital spirit" (translation from reference 1).

Then too there were amazing examples of serious discussions based on unchecked hearsay, and the startling extent to which naïve speculations found their way into print. Cheever (2, p. 220) tells of the gardener of Tronningholm who was reputed to be able to stay under water for sixteen hours at a depth of 19 yards. When in due course of time this man died, it was revealed at autopsy that a wide open foremen ovale had provided him with an amphibian type of heart, which explained his remarkable ability to live under water. Although Cheever himself was evidently somewhat skeptical as to the authenticity of the story, he relates it as if it were familiar to, and credited by, his scientific contemporaries.

But perusal of the older literature should do more than afford amusing examples to bolster our smug satisfaction in having progressed so far. It should bring, also, a feeling of humbleness from the thoughtful reading of some of the truly remarkable work that has been done with little in the way of equipment, and the incisive thinking that was sometimes generations ahead of contemporary information.

Enough of retrospect. What is going on in the field currently, what are the immediate needs, and what may be expected in the years to come? As to the current situation, the papers presented in this symposium constitute the best possible summary. Most impressive is the sweep of the fields represented. They run the gamut from basic embryology, pathology, and experimental teratology through the modern refinements of diagnostic procedures, to techniques for setting up an extracorporeal circulation and the new surgical procedures thereby made feasible. A mere twenty years ago only a very few of the special fields discussed in this symposium had even begun to develop. Now many of them have attained compelling importance. I wish it were possible to say that the growth of embryological information had played the provocative role in these rapid advances. Such, however, is not the case. The impetus has come primarily from surgery. When, in 1938, Gross and Hubbard performed the first successful operation for ligation of a patent ductus arteriosus, it brought the realization that accurate diagnosis of congenital cardiac defects had become imperative because certain properly selected cases could now be helped by surgery. The dramatic operation for supplementing the blood going to the lungs in cases of congenital pulmonary stenosis, first reported by Blalock and Taussig in 1945, gave tremendous added momentum in this field. Only then did clinicians become really interested in what the embryologist could tell them about these defects, and bring him in as a consulting colleague.

As cardiac surgery has progressed, the need for accurate diagnosis has become increasingly urgent. The challenge is being splendidly met by angiocardiography, catheterization, and gas analyses of blood samples from critical sites in the circulation. The whole matter of the clinical handling of cases of congenital defects of the heart is currently one of the most dramatically progressive in the entire medical field.

And what of the future? He would be rash indeed who would attempt to predict too specifically. The greater freedom and safety in open cardiac surgery made possible by constantly improving pumping and aerating mechanisms for bypassing the heart is already clearly apparent. Operative procedures that have hitherto been precariously carried out with urgent haste within the blood-filled and beating heart, will be performed with a full view of the operative field and with due deliberation. The progress that will inevitably come in the developing of new surgical procedures for dealing with hitherto inoperable defects can be confidently predicted for the immediate future.

Looking farther ahead, certain trends are beginning to be apparent. At the moment the clinical handling of congenital defects of the heart is at a relatively better level than our knowledge of their etiology. But there are encouraging signs on the horizon. With the increasing effectiveness of methods of immunization and the availability of antibiotics, many of the former major causes of death have been brought under control. As this has happened, deaths resulting from congenital defects have become progressively more conspicuous in our public health statistics. Currently, in the United States they have moved up among the top ten causes of death. This has stimulated the interest of both basic scientists and clinicians, and we are seeing a tremendous increase in the amount of investigative work in the field. In the background is the hope that sometime—still much too far in the future—a better knowledge of how congenital defects arise may make it possible to lessen their incidence.

Progress, albeit slow, is being made in a number of directions. There is a growing awareness of the importance of timing in development. In the embryo each formative process has a normal schedule. There is a time at which it commences, a period in which it proceeds at maximum rate, and a phase in which the rate of growth diminishes and the differentiation of histological details becomes dominant. Embryologists are gradually working out the basic information from which "developmental timetables" may be constructed, but especially for a structure with a development as intricate as that of the heart, the information needs to be much more detailed and accurate than that which is now available. Moreover, it must be based on the study of sufficient numbers of embryos to minimize the distorting effect of individual variability. Such knowledge is important in dealing with problems of causation. Developing structures are most vulnerable at the time of their most rapid growth, and become rapidly more resistant to disturbing factors as they go into the slower moving processes of differentiation. With these critical times worked out more precisely and the information properly disseminated will come the realization that clinical histories that do not begin until the third or fourth month of gestation are of little help in assessing possible causative factors in malformations that have their genesis in the first and second months. Much of importance can be learned by the correlative study of specific instances of malformations in the light of properly documented disturbing factors during pregnancy, but the chronology of development for each of the organ systems must be worked out in more detail specifically for human embryos, and clinical histories must be started much earlier than is now customary.

Another indication of progress is the increasing attention beginning to be given to the great variety of the developmental mechanisms which may be involved in the genesis of congenital anomalies. Until recently most of the emphasis in discussing the etiology of anomalies was placed on the so-called developmental arrest concept. This is, in essence, the idea that a congenital defect represents the failure of completion of some normal developmental processes. Unqualified acceptance of this point of view leads to searching for causative factors only of an inhibiting nature. Such an outlook is too narrow. Some disturbing factors are certainly inhibitory in their action, but there are many developmental mechanisms other than "arrests" that are involved in the genesis of malformations. For example, an incompetent valve at the foramen ovale may be the result of too much resorption of septum primum in the formation of ostium secundum. Functionally similar defects arise by resorption occurring in areas not normally so involved. Chiaris' net, in contrast, is the result of too little resorption in the secondary molding of septum spurium. Premature closure of the foramen ovale is the result of too much growth of septum secundum. One of the types of stenosis involving the pulmonary outlet follows unequal division of the truncus arteriosus as a sequel to the truncoconal ridges developing off-center. In this instance the growth process is normal in character, but displaced in its relations. Examples of developmental disturbances that are not in the nature of arrests could be multiplied, but those cited are enough to emphasize that the developmental mechanisms involved in the genesis of abnormalities are many and varied, and that concentrating on possible inhibiting factors is far too limited an approach.

Again emphasizing the variety of factors involved, it is highly significant that the same defect can be produced in experimental animals by many different disturbing agents. Cleft palate, for instance, can result from the inbreeding of genetically susceptible strains, and also can be caused by such things as vitamin lack in the maternal diet, hypoxia in pregnant females, and by the injection of too much cortisone into the maternal organism. It can also follow irradiation of parental gonads before the pregnancy is initiated, and result from direct irradiation of the fetuses *in utero.* The implication of these findings for future work on the etiology of congenital defects seems quite clear. With the variety of developmental mechanism that may be involved, and the number of agents that may cause a given defect, any search for blanket causes is futile. Normal development is an exceedingly intricate complex of delicately balanced and closely integrated processes. Any one of the component processes can be suppressed or exaggerated, or can be displaced spatially in its relations to other growing parts. Furthermore, a particular growth process may be thrown out of timing so that it fails to synchronize with related growth processes in adjacent structures.

What we really need to know is more, much more, about the regulatory factors in normal development. How much of the development of a particular tissue or organ depends on the inherent developmental potentialities genetically within the cells and how much depends on the influence of its immediate environment? There is abundant evidence from tissue transplantation and organ culture that the relative importance of these two factors is radically different in different organs. Why is this so, and what are the controlling factors in the differences? Is the organ in which the inherent potencies are particularly strong especially vulnerable to genetic disturbances? Conversely, is the organ in which the molding effect of surrounding structures plays an important part more likely to be distorted by subtle changes in the biochemistry of adjacent tissues? What is it that slows growth at a given phase of development and accelerates differentiation? The cancer problem must certainly be closely linked to the factors regulating growth rate and differentiation. Progress in this territory might well be doubly rewarding.

From all angles the field of congenital malformations is a challenging one in which we are impatient to progress. We are rapidly becoming well grounded in our knowledge of the normal sequence of developmental processes, their timing, and their functional interdependences. Building on this basic information, we are in a position to take advantage of the assistance of the electron microscope and of the advances in the biochemistry. As biochemistry is pushed into cellular levels it will become ever more helpful in experimental embryology and teratology. Diligent utilization of the means now at our disposal and those opening before us should give us a steadily increasing insight into some of the intricate mechanisms and the controlling factors in normal development.

These approaches alone do not cover all aspects of the problem. We need to know also much more about genetics. We speak glibly about the fertilized ovum containing our entire hereditary endowment, but we have as yet practically no knowledge of how the genetic qualities are handed on from cell to cell in the countless mitoses involved in the growth of the embryo, and then finally distributed to the various differentiating organs. How, from the gene content of the zygote, are determining factors distributed so that the cells that finally form the iris produce a brown pigment such as there was in the eyes of the mother? Through what incredible series of cell divisions must the determining material have been selectively distributed to the cells of the tooth buds so that Johnny has the same sort of white, sound, and well-shaped teeth as his father?

To some of these questions we think we are beginning to see the glimmer of an answer. With many of the others we have as yet made little progress. But the route that we must travel is becoming increasingly clear, and we can not unreasonably hope that eventually some of the ways in which normal development is distorted will be well enough understood to let us move into the field of prevention.

REFERENCES

1. Dalton, J. D. *Doctrines of the Circulation*. Lea's Son and Co., Philadelphia, Pa., 1884, p. 115.
2. Cheever, C. A. A remarkable case of malformation of the heart in a boy aged thirteen years and six months. *New Engl. J. Med. Surg.* **10**:217–221 (1821).

I

DEVELOPMENT OF THE HEART
AND THE ORIGINS OF CONGENITAL
HEART DISEASE

Developmental Processes Involved in Cardiogenesis*

ALEXANDER BARRY

The University of Michigan Medical School, Ann Arbor, Michigan

If we regard the developing embryo as the resultant of the co-ordinated activity of its component cells, then it seems that we should attempt to analyze development in terms of cellular activity. This is especially pertinent from the point of view of the study of congenital malformations. Although the field of teratology is still in its infancy, I believe that there is general agreement that the various factors which affect development do so at the biochemical level. Admittedly our understanding of the underlying biochemistry of development is at present too rudimentary to make it possible for us to arrive at a complete biochemical understanding of congenital malformations, although in a few instances this goal has nearly been achieved. Nevertheless, it seems to me that this is the direction in which we are moving. This point of view almost forces us to analyze development in terms of cellular processes and functions. It is helpful to be able to say that in one anomaly the atrioventricular canal cushions have failed to fuse, and that in another there was excessive resorption of the inter-atrial septum primum. It is, however, more meaningful if we can analyze development, whether normal or abnormal, in terms of the sorts of functions which cells perform. From the study of morphogenesis it should be possible to make a start in this direction.

I propose to consider certain aspects of the development of the heart of the human embryo during approximately the second month of gestation. There are several reasons for emphasizing this period of cardiogenesis. It is during this time that the simple tubular heart

* This work was supported in part by a grant from the Michigan Heart Association.

11

becomes partitioned into four chambers, and there is strong reason to believe that the heart during this phase of its development is extremely prone to diverge from normal. It is unnecessary to enumerate to this audience what a variety of cardiac anomalies can result from faulty partitioning of the atria, the ventricles, and the truncus arteriosus. Additional confirmation as to the importance of this period of cardiogenesis has been dramatically shown by the experiments in teratogenesis, which indicate that it is during this period that an environmental insult is most likely to affect cardiac development.

I would like to begin with a very brief summary of some of the morphological changes exhibited by the heart during its partitioning. Somewhat more detailed descriptions can be found in the publications of Davis (2), Patten (6), Kramer (4), and Streeter (7). The simple tubular heart of the human embryo of ten somites (three weeks) enlarges and loops until by the fourth week of development its ventricular portion lies caudal to the atria and sinus venosus. At its cephalic end, this ventricular loop tapers to form the conus, which ejects blood into an unpaired truncus arteriosus. During the fourth and fifth weeks of development paired spiral ridges develop in the conotruncal region. These ridges gradually enlarge until they meet and fuse to form a spiral septum which divides the truncus arteriosus into an ascending aorta and a pulmonary trunk.

During the fifth week the single atrioventricular canal becomes divided into paired channels. This is brought about by the formation of the dorsal and ventral cushions of the atrioventricular canal, which partition it into right and left atrioventricular ostia. During this same time the atrial region also is being partitioned. The first step in this process is the formation of a thin septum which develops from the dorsal and cephalic wall of the atrium in approximately the mid-saggital plane. This septum is called septum I, since a second interatrial septum will develop subsequently. Septum I has the form of a crescent, and is so oriented that its two horns meet and are continuous with the atrioventricular canal cushions. Thus there is delimited an interatrial foramen, ostium I, which is bounded by the atrioventricular canal cushions and the free edge of septum primum. Septum I grows progressively toward the atrioventricular cushions until during the sixth week it fuses with them and obliterates ostium I.

Before this occurs, however, small perforations appear in septum I near its attachment to the dorsal wall of the atrium. These perforations enlarge, coalesce, and form the interatrial foramen secundum (ostium II).

Subsequently a second, relatively massive, muscular septum develops (septum II) to the right of septum I. This septum never forms a complete partition. Its free edge bounds an oval opening, the foramen ovale, which is so oriented with respect to septum I that the latter acts as a flap valve, permitting blood to pass from the right atrium to the left, but preventing flow in the reverse direction. For this reason septum I comes to be called the valve of the foramen ovale.

From this brief summary it is apparent that during the second month of gestation the heart has exhibited two striking phenomena, the fushion of originally separate parts and the development of perforations in an originally intact septum. Let us first consider the phenomenon of fushion in terms of cellular function.

At the end of the third week of gestation, the heart consists of a sleeve of embryonic myocardium within which lies a tube of endothelium. Between these two cellular layers is a layer of gelatinous material which Davis (1) called the cardiac jelly. Although this material has not been analyzed in human embryos, it has been shown in the hearts of chick embryos of comparable developmental ages that the cardiac jelly contains mucopolysaccharide acids with aldehyde groups (8). Since the cardiac jelly loses its metachromatic staining reaction after treatment with hyaluronidase, one can assume that this mucopolysaccharide is hyaluronic acid.

If one follows the histological differentiation of the conotruncal region, one sees the endothelial lining undergoing mitotic divisions. The cells thus formed migrate into the underlying cardiac jelly and acquire the typical stellate configuration of mesenchymal cells (6). Some investigators believe that certain cells of the myocardium also contribute to this embryonic endocardial tissue. This tissue has been called "endocardial cushion tissue" because it also forms the endocardial cushions of the atrioventricular canal. Streeter used the term "gelatinous reticulum." I would prefer to call it cardiac mesenchyme, since it has all the essential characteristics of mesenchyme. It consists of a reticulum of stellate mesodermal cells supported by a ground substance containing a mucopolysaccharide, and in its future development it will differentiate into fibroelastic connective tissue.

During the fourth and fifth weeks of development a pair of opposed ridges of this cardiac mesenchyme develop into the truncoconal ridges. These ridges increase in size until they come into contact and fuse across the lumen of the truncus and divide it into ascending aorta and pulmonary trunk. It seems to me that the growth of these masses of cardiac mesenchyme involves three distinct developmental processes. First, there is an increase in the number of cells, apparently due to mitotic activity of both the endothelial cells and the mesenchymal cells themselves. The second process is that of cell migration, whereby daughter cells move apart to form the loose cellular reticulum typical of mesenchyme. The third process is the continuing elaboration of ground substance. It is not possible to state with certainty which cells are concerned with this synthesis of mucopolysaccharides. It is generally felt that mesenchymal cells have this synthetic capacity. In view of the fact that metachromatically staining vacuoles have been seen in the endothelial lining in chick hearts of this age, it may be that the endothelial cells also take part in the formation of ground substance.

A similar process of partitioning takes place during the fifth week in the region of the atrioventricular canal. Masses of cardiac mesenchyme form on the dorsal and ventral walls of this channel. These dorsal and ventral cushions increase in size until they touch and fuse to divide the original atrioventricular canal into right and left channels. As far as can be determined, these cushions develop precisely as do the conotruncal ridges. The process of fusion was described by Streeter (7) who stated that at the time these masses come into contact "the endothelium is disappearing, which results in the fusion of the supporting gelatinous reticulum." He did not describe the way in which the endothelium disappeared, nor do I think that a study of fixed embryos can give us a detailed understanding of the process involved. Nevertheless, in studying such areas of fusion in the heart, I have never been able to see any trace of degenerating or pyknotic cells. Neither are there "epithelial rests" analogous to those found along the plane of fusion of the lateral palatine shelves. For this reason I believe that the endothelial cells are not destroyed or encarcerated.

It seems more likely that they either migrate out of the zone of contact, or differentiate into stellate mesenchymal cells. This latter process would not be as radical as it might seem, if one analyzes the character of the endothelial cells that line the lumen of the embryonic heart at this stage. These cells are called endothelial since they form the epithelial lining of the lumen of a vascular channel. Unfortunately, we tend to be conditioned by adult histology and tend to visualize an endothelium as a simple squamous epithelium which is separated from the underlying connective tissue by a delicate basement membrane. This pattern is not an accurate description of the endothelium covering the masses of cardiac mesenchyme which we have been discussing. Some of the cells appear to be unquestionably flat squamous endothelial cells. Others, however, although flat on their luminal surface, have processes that extend into the ground substance and anastomose with the stellate cells of the cardiac mesenchyme. We must wait for further study of these cells with the electron microscope before this relationship is understood. However, according to our present understanding, it seems that many of the cells forming the endothelial lining of the heart are not strikingly different from mesenchymal cells. From this point of view it is not surprising to find that when two such layers are brought into intimate firm contact, as in the fusion of the truncus ridges or the atrioventricular canal cushions, the endothelial cells become indistinguishable from the mesenchymal cells forming what Streeter called the "underlying gelatinous reticulum."

Another morphological change that takes place during the second month of development is the closure of the interventricular foramen. During the first part of this month the crest of the interventricular septum is capped by a mass of cardiac mesenchyme which is continuous dorsally with that of the atrioventricular canal cushions, and cephalically with that forming the ventricular edge of the conus septum. Thus the interventricular foramen is bounded on all sides by cardiac mesenchyme. This tissue increases in volume and gradually reduces the size of the interventricular foramen. During the seventh week the cardiac mesenchyme fuses to form a solid mass which plugs the foramen and completes the separation of right from left ventricle.

The last area of fusion I should like to discuss involves the inter-

atrial septum I. It is commonly stated that one finds cardiac mesenchyme only in the "primary heart tube," i.e., only in the atrioventricular canal, ventricles, conus, and truncus arteriosus. This is not
completely true. If one studies the histological structure of the interatrial septum I, it is seen to consist of a sheet of embryonic myocardium
embedded in ground substance. Between this lamina and the endothelial covering there is a thin distinct layer of cardiac mesenchyme.
At the free edge of septum I this mesenchymal layer is relatively massive. Thus, the interatrial foramen I, like the interventricular foramen,
is bounded by a continuous layer of cardiac mesenchyme. As septum
I grows, its free edge approaches the cardiac mesenchyme of the
atrioventricular canal partition and progressively reduces the size of
ostium I. Finally, during the sixth week ostium I is obliterated by a
fusion of the mesenchymal tissue bounding it. The histological changes
undergone by the tissues at this area of fusion resemble in all respects those seen in the fusion of the atrioventricular canal cushions
themselves.

To summarize, one may say that all these processes of fusion are
essentially similar. Fundamentally they involve growth, both of the
embryonic myocardium and of cardiac mesenchyme. This mesenchymal growth can be considered as involving at least three different,
although intimately related, processes: cell division, cell migration
and reorientation, and the synthesis by cells of a mucopolysaccharide
ground substance.

An apparently different phenomenon that must be considered in
discussing the development of the heart is that of the formation of
the interatrial foramen II (ostium II). This can be summarized by
stating that just prior to the fusion of septum I with the atrioventricular cushion masses one finds several small perforations in septum I
near its attachment to the dorsal wall of the atrium. This process has
been referred to as "resorption," a term which carries connotations of
cellular destruction and death. There is no question but that resorption involving cellular destruction does play a role in embryogenesis, as, for example, in the modeling of the wing of the embryonic
chick. If this sort of resorption takes place in the morphogenesis of
the heart, it is important that it be recognized, if only because one

would expect it to be regulated by factors quite different from those affecting cell growth, migration, and synthetic activity.

It is next to impossible to determine with certainty from a study of fixed embryos the precise growth mechanisms involved in the formation of ostium II. Nevertheless, I would like to present what I believe to be pertinent morphological evidence that makes me question the concept of cellular destruction in the perforation of septum I. In the University of Michigan Embryological Collection there were fourteen human embryos suitable for study of the histology of septum I immediately before and after the formation of ostium II. All these specimens were sectioned serially. In this material I was unable to find any evidence of cellular destruction. In no case could I find a single pyknotic cell or nucleus in septum I. Admittedly, this is negative evidence, but I feel it is sufficient to make us question whether cell resorption normally plays a role in the formation of ostium II. I would suggest that these perforations can be readily explained on the basis of a widening of the interstices between the myocardial fibers, followed by either a realignment of existing endothelial cells, or the establishment of a new endothelial channnel through septum I by differentiation of mesenchymal cells. It would be premature to regard this subject as closed. I do feel, however, that we should recognize the possibility that the perforation of septum I can be regarded as another instance of cellular reorientation and differentiation.

I should like to point out one pertinent fact concerning the development of the heart during the second month of development. We know from the evidence of morphogenesis, as well as the direct evidence of experimental teratogenesis, that it is during this period that the heart is very prone to depart from its normal course of development. The processes of cell division, migration, and synthesis would appear to be readily distorted. In several other organs it has been found that development is distorted as a consequence of abnormalities of the vascular supply. It should be recognized that there is no capillary bed in the embryonic heart during the period we have been discussing. The interatrial septum I, for example, depends for its nutrition on the atrial blood that bathes it on either side. The factors affecting cellular division, migration, and synthetic activity would seem necessarily to act directly on these cells. From the point of view of both normal and abnormal development this area would seem to be as simple a system as it is possible to find in the developing embryo for the analysis of primary developmental processes and the factors affecting them.

In order that this discussion may not be totally unbalanced, I should emphasize the fact that there are many developmental processes that are not confined to the period of embryogenesis. This period is generally taken to be the time when the basic patterns of the organ systems are being established. Streeter took as an end point the embryo of about 30 mm crown rump length (Horizon XXIII). Estimates as to the age of such an embryo vary between seven and eight weeks. For the purpose of this discussion it is sufficiently accurate to think of the period of embryogenesis as the first two months of gestation, and to speak of fetal development as occupying the remainder of gestation.

As an example of the fact that developmental processes are by no means restricted to the embryonic period, we can consider the differentiation of the myocardium. This is differentiated from splanchnic mesoderm, acquires its relationship as a part of the primitive tubular heart, and by the third week acquires the property of pulsating rhythmically. If we are correct in assuming that the human heart follows the general pattern that is seen in the hearts of other vertebrates (3), we can say that during the fourth week of development the myocardium of the atrium, and shortly thereafter, the myocardium of the sinus venosus differentiates similarly. It should be pointed out that although the myocardium of these chambers exhibits a cephalocaudal gradient as to its rate of inherent rhythmicity, no morphological characteristics have been found to correlate with this. During the second month it is possible to identify morphologically the beginnings of the atrioventricular conduction system. However, it is during the fetal period, and even postnatally, that it is possible to follow the final differentiation of nodal fibers, Purkinje fibers, and "typical" cardiac muscle fibers.

During the latter part of the embryonic period the cardiac mesenchyme begins to differentiate into fibroelastic connective tissue. In such areas as the developing valves and the future cardiac skeleton, one begins to see fine fibers within the ground substance. These presumably are either reticular fibers or small collagenous fibers, since they stain distinctively with such dyes as analine blue. It is during the fetal period, however, that one sees the striking differentiation of such morphological characteristics as the massive collagenous fibers of the cardiac skeleton, the multilayered fenestrated elastic membranes of the ascending aorta and pulmonary trunk, and the elastic and fibrous laminae of the cardiac valves. Certainly these developmental processes are of profound importance in both normal and abnormal development. Such a defect as primary endocardial sclerosis (endocardial fibroelastosis) emphasizes the fact that developmental processes of the fetal period can and do depart from their normal course to give rise to congenital malformations.

It is interesting to see the scope of the papers presented at this symposium. The majority are concerned with the fetal period. I believe that this is symptomatic of a general increase of interest in the functioning of the fetus. This is inevitable and proper. If future investigations into the physiology of the fetus follow the pattern seen in similar studies on the adult, we shall find that an understanding of function goes hand in hand with a knowledge of structure, especially of microscopic structure. The field of histogenesis presents a real challenge to the embryologist of the present and future. This is one of the major areas in which much work must and will be done, since as yet only the scantiest beginnings have been made toward a systematic study of the differentiating cells and tissues of the fetus. Without such a foundation we can never fully understand the complex development of fetal physiology.

REFERENCES

1. Davis, C. L. The cardiac jelly of the chick embryo. *Anat. Record* **27**:201–202 (1924).
2. Davis,, C. L. Development of the human heart from its first appearance to the stage found in embryos of twenty paired somites. *Carnegie Contribs. Embryol.* **19**:245–284 (1927).
3. Goss, C. M. The first contraction of the heart in rat embryos. *Anat. Record* **70**:505–524 (1938).
4. Kramer, T. C. The partitioning of the conus and truncus and the formation of the membranous portion of the interventricular septum in the human heart. *Am. J. Anat.* **71**:343–370 (1942).
5. Patten, B. M., Kramer, T. C., and Barry, A. Valvular action in the

embryonic chick heart by localized apposition of endocardial masses. *Anat. Record* **102**:299–312 (1948).

6. Patten, B. M. *Human Embryology*, 2nd ed., Section on Heart, pp. 656–691. Blakiston Publishing Division, McGraw-Hill, New York, 1953.

7. Streeter, G. L. Developmental Horizons in Human Embryos—Age Groups XI–XXIII. *Carnegie Contribs. Embryol.* **32**:133–203 (1948).

8. Ortiz, E. C. Estudio histoquimico de la gelatina cardiaca en el embrion de pollo. *Arch. inst. cardiol. Méx.* **28**:244–262 (1958).

Fetal Cardiovascular Homeostasis*

S. R. M. REYNOLDS

*Department of Anatomy, University of Illinois, College of Medicine
Chicago, Illinois*

The history of man's study of fetal cardiovascular phenomena is ancient, and bears the stamp of famous biologists, from Aristotle to Fallopius, Vesalius, and Hunter. It was not until Cohnstein and Zuntz in 1884 employed techniques that rendered these functions subject to quantitative measurement that men began to think in terms of heart rate, arterial blood pressure, and venous blood pressure. Since then, there has been a succession of studies directed toward an understanding of the physiological factors which serve to regulate these aspects of the circulation. It is an oversimplification, but not too much so, to say that only fetal electrocardiography, flowmeters, respiratory metabolism, and cineangiographic techniques have been brought to bear on problems of fetal cardiovascular physiology in addition to those of recording blood pressures and determining heart rate either from the pressure records, by auscultation, or palpation. Other conventional techniques employed by modern physiologists to aid them in a complementary fashion while recording cardiovascular functions have been the use of appropriate nerve section, nerve stimulation, and the use of drugs which act upon one or another part of the autonomic system. These procedures are frequently applied against a background of what is supposed to be the normal, basic physiologic state and under differing degrees of hypoxia or some other stressful stimulus.

Some consideration must be given to what is referred to above as the supposedly normal or basic physiologic state of the fetus. One may

* Original studies reported here were supported by USPHS Grant RG-4728, awarded by the National Advisory Health Council.

question, what is normal when one intrudes upon a given anatomical situation for the purposes of an experiment.

It has been found that anesthetics, some more than others, affect the fetus; it has been found that the duration of a period of observation may, under certain conditions, affect the basic physiologic state of the fetus.

It has likewise been found that even placing a pregnant ewe in a given position, as on her back, her side, or standing erect, affects the "basic functional state" of the fetus with respect to the gaseous content of its blood, and so almost certainly with respect to the character of its cardiovascular activity. We must remember, therefore, that a given experimental maneuver may elicit a fetal cardiovascular response which must be interpreted against a resting physiological state which is normal only for the conditions of the experiment. The variations of the several resting basic states must, I believe, reflect the several levels of homeostatic adjustment of which a fetus is capable, and these capabilities will vary according to the degrees of fetal development at the time.

To review these aspects of an extensive, interesting, and valuable segment of recent physiological literature would take more time than is permitted me. In order to convince oneself of this, one only needs to study three basic books dealing with the fetus, published within the past eighteen years. One, by Windle (18), entitled *Physiology of the Fetus*, surveys in two chapters the principal work of the past relative to fetal heart rates, the circulation of blood, and the development of neural control. Barcroft (3) in his *Researches on Pre-Natal Life*, provides a rich store of reasoned evidence that has done so much to shape our conception of how the circulation of the fetus develops, varies, and is controlled. The third book, *The Fetal Circulation*, by Barclay, Franklin, and Prichard (2), marked a turning point in our knowledge of fetal cardiovascular physiology and the changes which it undergoes at birth.

In essence, a few generalizations may be gleaned from such sources as these and the literature on which they are based. The heart rate is perhaps the most studied feature of fetal physiology because it can be measured in various ways, some of which are quite reliable. In general it is held, as Barcroft maintains, that the pulse rate diminishes as a fetus becomes older. However, if, as a result of a given experimental procedure, vagal control (which, he maintains, gains dominance as pregnancy advances) ceases, heart rate becomes very rapid. In the sheep, this may occur quite easily until about the 120th day of pregnancy. Afterwards, the fetus is able to maintain vagal tone quite well, for Barcroft says that the fetus "toughens" at this time (Fig. 1). This conclusion is a "reasonable" or a rationale one. It purports to show that the sheep fetus *in utero* gradually develops a postnatal and even an adult type of nervous control over the heart. Bauer has indeed shown this to be so in the neonatal rabbit, to which Barcroft likens the sheep fetus at a certain stage of its intrauterine existence. Thus Bauer has shown that depressor reflexes develop as early as the thirteenth day of life when rabbit pups are stressed, and by the forty-second day of life they operate under conditions of rest. In each case the level of blood pressure which acts as a stimulus is

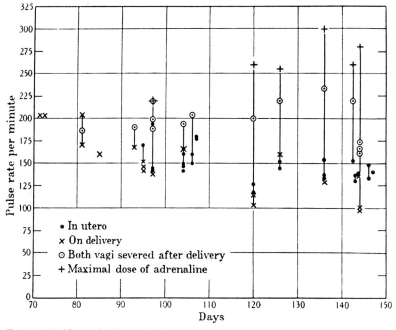

Fig. 1.   Evidence by Barcroft that the lamb fetus "toughens" in the latter part of pregnancy by development of vasomotor tone. Note slowing of resting heart rate (3).

the same. Similarly, with the carotid sinus threshold; it is demonstrable under stress about the fortieth day of life, but about eleven days later it operates under conditions of rest. In both cases, the blood pressures are equal (1) (Fig. 2).

Clearly the pathways for these reflexes exist in the rabbit at a time prior to their normal use but they are silent unless the animal be stressed. Barcroft implies that there is a similar type of mechanism when the lamb is *in utero*. This, however, apparently is contrary to what one sees in the chick, rat, and man (Table I). In my own work with sheep fetuses *in utero* I find a degree of confirmation of what Barcroft has shown (Fig. 3). However, I find much greater variation in blood pressure and heart rate because these, especially the latter, are subject to such a variety of physiological stimuli that a "normal" level is normal only for the conditions of the moment as we shall see.

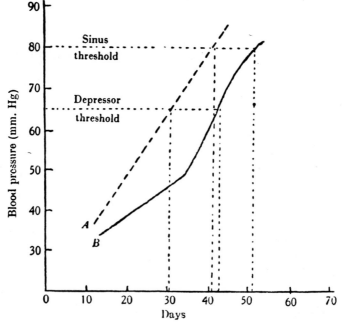

Fig. 2. Graph showing that in the newborn rabbit, vagus, and carotid sinus mechanisms are capable of functioning prior to the time they commence to function in a homeostatic sense. Normal functioning of these reflexes depends upon attainment of critical levels of blood pressure (1). *A*, after stress; *B*, normal.

TABLE I.   Heart rate in fetal, newborn, and adult animals (18)

	Early Fetus	Late Fetus	Newborn	Adult
Hen	120–170	220–264	295	320
Rat	96–114	123–248		184–280
Goat		120–246	145–240	
Ox		161	141	50
Dog		120–170	160	100
Monkey		100–180		140–240
Man	156	130–150	112	70

We record umbilical artery and venous pressures and heart rates *in utero* with the fetal membranes intact (17). The small catheters lie in a tributary of each vessel and are passed just to the point of their origin at the main umbilical vessels through which the blood flows uninterruptedly.

In our work, we use an intravenous anesthetic and the ewe lies on her side. Both of these conditions, according to Barcroft, should serve to abolish the vagal reflexes and so render our observations of limited value. I would agree with this were it not for the fact that the fetus under these conditions exhibits extraordinarily sensitive vagal reflexes. Thus, (*a*) pressure on the uterus, (*b*) release of pressure from the uterus, (*c*) simple induction of maternal hypoxia, or (*d*) applica-

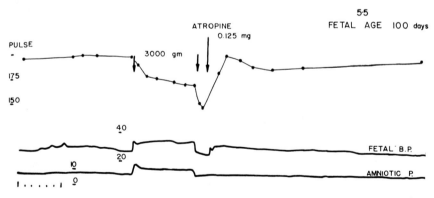

Fig. 3.   Evidence that vagal tone may be induced in fetal lambs by application of mechanical pressure (first arrow) on the uterus and again upon removal of pressure (second arrow). The slowing of the heart may be relieved by injection of atropine into the fetus (15).

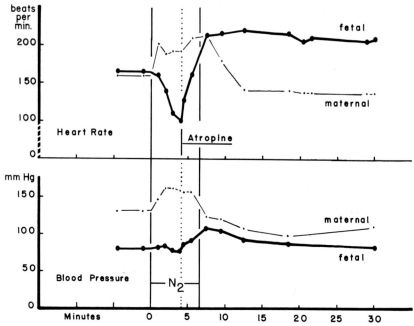

Fig. 4.   Slowing of the fetal heart rate by giving nitrogen to the ewe, and release from bradycardia during during the period of nitrogen administration by
injecting atropine into the fetus, showing that the slowing was vagal in origin (15).

tions of various types of maternal hemodynamic stress induce vagal
tone (Figs. 3–6), which may be long lasting, and which is abolished
by injection of atropine into the fetus. I am forced to conclude that
when the lamb fetus is lying undisturbed in its normal habitat its
heart is free of vagal tone even near term under conditions of rest but
that stressful stimuli of a mechanical, chemical, or hemodynamic nature readily induce slowing of the heart through a vagal mechanism.
I find no evidence that the carotid body or the accelerator nerves to
the heart have any effect (11, 12), but the vagus nerve alone in the fetal lamb may be brought into action and that at a very early stage of
development. Moreover, Dr. Dawes and his group (9) and I have
found independently that vagus section in the lamb results in vagal
slowing of the heart rate (Fig. 6), not vagal release resulting in cardiac acceleration, as in conventional laboratory experiments on dogs
and cats. It is necessary to conclude that in Barcroft's experiments

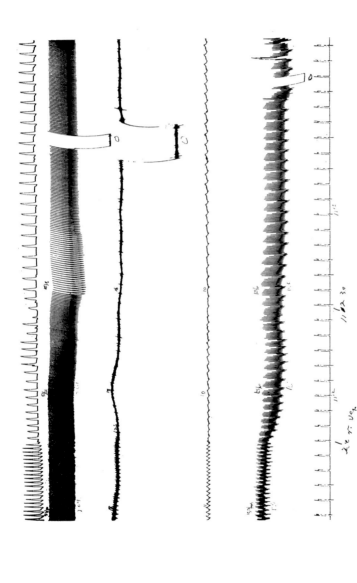

FIG. 5. Progressive fetal bradycardia resulting from tying of the left vagus nerve, with onset of sudden bradycardia to half the rate 45 seconds later. Top line, respiration in ewe; next line, fetal umbilical artery pressure; third, umbilical vein pressure, fourth, inferior vena cava pressure (ewe), and fifth, carotid artery pressure (ewe) (5). Time, 5-second intervals (from Reynolds and Bieniarz, unpublished).

CONTROL OF RESTING FETAL HEART RATE

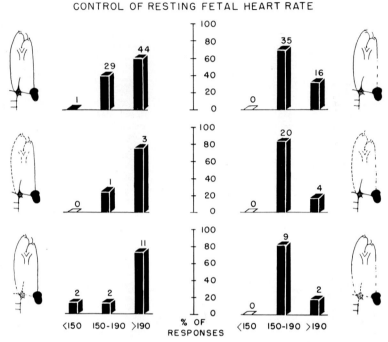

Fig. 6.   Graph showing primary role of the vagus in controlling resting fetal heart rate. Top left, vagus and sympathetic veins intact (60% of resting heart rates were over 190 or more beats per minute); second left, carotid bodies occluded; bottom left, stellate ganglion excluded; top right, both vagi cut; second, vagi cut and carotid bodies excluded; top right, both vagi cut; second, vagi cut and carotid bodies excluded; bottom, stellate ganglion removed. Note slower heart rate with vagi cut irrespective of the status of the carotid body and stellate ganglion (11).

the conditions were such that stressful conditions incident to the experiment actually induced homeostatic changes involving induction of vagal tone in the fetus. This, he regarded as "normal." Such a result may stem from the fact that Barcroft limited the acquisition of useful data to the first few minutes of an experiment immediately after operation at which time the manipulative effects of the operative procedures would still be apparent.

The blood pressure of the fetus requires brief consideration. A number of workers have shown that this increases as a fetus becomes larger. Carotid blood pressures are recorded in some experiments, umbilical artery and vein pressures, in others. In general, it appears

TABLE II. Fetal blood pressure near term (18)

Species	Artery, mm Hg	Vein, mm Hg
Rat	20	
Guinea pig		5–10
Rabbit	20	
Cat	30	7–13
Dog	40	
Sheep	76–84	18
Man	68–110	22–24

that the larger the fetus is, near term, the higher the pressure, a not entirely unsuspected observation (Table II). However, there is great variation, even under resting conditions, owing to the multiplicity of stimuli that affect the fetus (Fig. 7).

The interesting fact pertaining to blood pressure relates not to the changing levels of arterial blood pressure but rather to the umbilical vein pressure. Cohnstein and Zuntz (8) were the first to measure the latter in the lamb, and found the venous pressure to range between 16 and 34 mm Hg, a level not out of line with that observed by Haselhorst in the human (10). Barcroft is satisfied that umbilical vein pressures are higher than usual venous pressure, although he sets the level at between 5 and 18 mm Hg. Unlike arterial blood pressure, it does not increase as the fetus grows (Figs. 7, 8).

In our own work, we have found pressures covering all these ranges (Fig. 7). However, as far as we can determine, normal umbilical venous pressure is of the order of 15–25 mm Hg under what one might call resting conditions when the fetus is in good shape. Now, why it varies and for what purpose are not entirely clear. The reason for its being high is doubtless related to the observations of Barron (4) and Barclay, Franklin, and Prichard (2), who demonstrated a sphincter in the ductus venosus. This structure controls the exit of blood from the umbilical recess in the liver. The sphincter begins to form in the five-millimeter human embryo and is fully formed by the twentieth week of life (7). It is innervated by the vagus nerve (4, 7).

This resistance to venous outflow keeps the umbilical vein distended, as has been shown in the human when the cord is simultaneously clamped in two places while the blood is still flowing (13).

Measurements of diameters of the umbilical artery, the gradient of pressure loss along it and the volume flow of blood through it taken together show the importance for venous return of having a large diameter in the umbilical artery (14) (Fig. 9). If the same reasoning applies to the vein as it does to the artery, it is clear that this mechanism is one of vast importance to the fetus in assuring venous return from the placenta.

While I had the good fortune to be in Dr. Dawes laboratory in 1950–51, Dr. Ardran, Dr. Prichard, and I showed cineradiographically (unpublished) that modifying the venous return from the placenta

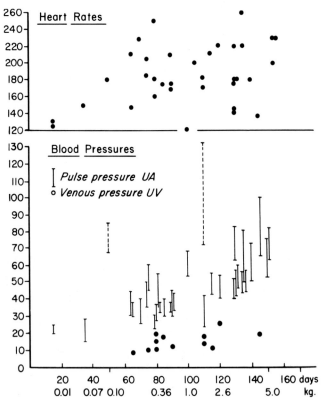

Fig. 7.   Graphs of fetal heart rate during pregnancy in sheep (top) and pulse pressure and venous pressure in umbilical vessels (bottom). See text for discussion.

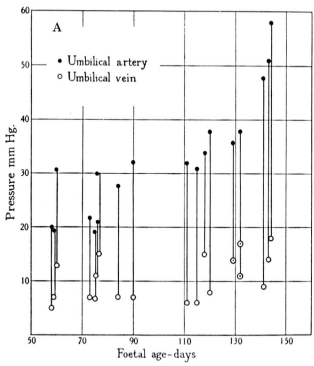

Fig. 8. Graph showing maintenance of umbilical vein pressure at a nearly constant high level during pregnancy as arterial blood pressure increases (3).

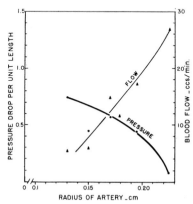

Fig. 9. Graph showing increased rate of blood flow and demonstrated loss of pressure by friction as diameter of an artery increases. Right ordinate, centimeters per second (14).

mechanically could cause the sphincter of the ductus venosus to open partially or wholly. The physiological mechanisms involved have not yet been explored, though in order to maintain the fetus alive, it is clear that this is a vital aspect of fetal circulatory physiology that deserves our attention. The sphincter, when closed, directs blood returning from the placenta into the liver and thence to the inferior vena cava. By so doing, it maintains a vis-a-tergo in the entire placental organ so that it is an erectile organ (13).

In the pages above, we have reviewed in a cursory manner certain aspects of the fetal cardiovascular characteristics as the fetus develops and under conditions of rest and stress. We have seen that mechanical pressure upon the uterus, or a uterine contraction, hypoxia, or hemodynamic stress in the ewe may induce fetal cardiovascular responses. So far as heart rate is concerned, there are several types of change to be discerned. There may be slow, progressive slowing of the heart; there can be sudden slowing within a matter of seconds, or there may be instant slowing, between beats. There can be a mixture of these several kinds of cardiac slowing in a single record (Fig. 5). There may be also fetal cardiac acceleration to normal and higher than normal rates. What circumstances result in these several types of responses? We may take them up, one by one.

The rapid onset of bradycardia is experimentally shown independently by Barcroft and Bauer by temporary occlusion of the umbilical cord. We have found that this is so, also, and that the effect is abolished by vagotomy, but not by exclusion of the carotid body or the stellate ganglion (11, 12). This slowing of the heart is associated with a rise in arterial blood pressure when the cord is occluded (Fig. 10). However, it also occurs when the umbilical veins only are occluded and there is a fall in blood pressure (12). Such a bradycardia requiring 1–2 seconds to appear is not, therefore, a depressor reflex mechanism, but as Barcroft (3) first implied, an acute hypoxic effect, probably acting on the medullary centers directly.

It should be noted that equally rapid onset of bradycardia may be demonstrated, as mentioned above, by applying pressure on the arteries or by interfering with maternal blood flow through the uterus.

A slow onset of bradycardia is demonstrable in other ways. If the ewe is made hypoxic by breathing nitrogen-diluted air, a period of 10–20 minutes is required for the onset of bradycardia (6, 16). The initial phase of this is vagal in origin since it can be blocked by atropine injected into the fetus (Fig. 4) (16). The slowing of the heart may be gradual, or it may be preceded or associated with atrioventricular block. These episodes, too, may be blocked by atropine. In either case, the initial disturbance is a vagal one, and has not been shown to be due to the action of chemoreceptors. Ultimately,

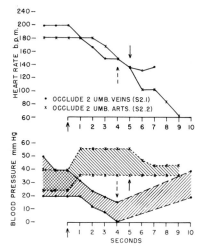

Fig. 10. Slowing of the fetal heart of lamb by occlusion of either the umbilical arteries (with a rise of fetal blood pressure) or the umbilical veins (with a fall in blood pressure) (11).

the cardiac slowing is related to direct depression of the myocardium, as may be shown when the heart is denervated (12) or by the failure of atropine to elicit cardiac acceleration at this time.

When oxygen is restored to the fetus either by way of the ewe or release of the umbilical cord, the heart beats very rapidly (Fig. 11). This is due to endogenous adrenalin being secreted from the fetal adrenal glands (Fig. 12) (11).

Now let us turn to the periodic or rhythmic fluctuations that occur. These are usually associated with fluctuations in fetal blood pressure as well as with maternal blood pressure changes (Fig. 13). It has not been shown that these are vagally controlled, but my experience would suggest that this is so.

What is the common denominator to these vagally induced changes in fetal heart rate? A recent study has been made of this by Bieniarz and myself (5). We recorded (*a*) in the ewe, maternal respiration, carotid, blood pressure, and inferior vena cava blood pressure, amniotic pressure and (*b*) in the fetus, amniotic pressure, umbilical artery and umbilical vein pressures, and fetal heart rate. While we do not have perfect correspondence in all our experiments, it is clear that any maternal change in hemodynamics that causes a disproportionate rise in caval blood pressure or in arterial blood pressure will cause sudden, vagally induced changes in fetal heart rate. These changes compare with the changes induced by occlusion of the um-

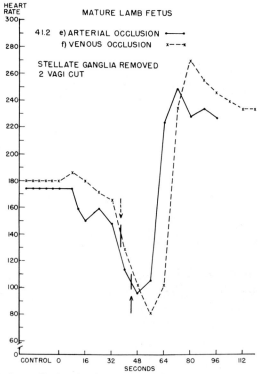

Fig. 11. Tachycardia in the fetus after release of cord occlusion (arteries *or* veins) with the heart completely denervated (11).

bilical arteries or the umbilical veins. It thus appears that a change in maternal hemodynamics which cause (*a*) passive congestion or (*b*) active congestion of the maternal placental circulation elicit transient, vagally induced changes in fetal heart rate. The changes compare, qualitatively, with the effect of occlusion of the umbilical arteries or the umbilical veins.

In view of the arrangement of the maternal and fetal circulations in the placenta of the sheep, as described by Barron (see reference 4) (Fig. 14), it is clear that such maternal hemodynamic changes can cause interference with venous drainage of fetal blood from a placental villus or of arterial inflow in the stem arteries of the villi. In either case, the effect on the fetal heart rate is the same, namely, vagal slowing of the heart. Occlusion of the umbilical arteries or veins produces a similar vagal reflex.

True fetal distress seems to differ from these typical fetal changes in the circulation. We have found that so long as the umbilical venous blood pressure remains high, the fetus will recover easily and well from a slow heart rate and even a low arterial blood pressure

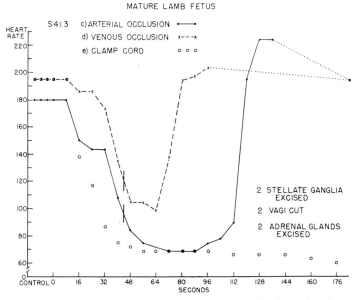

Fig. 12. Lack of tachycardia upon release of cord occlusion when heart is denervated and the fetal adrenals are clamped off. Demonstration with Fig. 11 of role of endogenous adrenaline in severe fetal distress (11).

S II a

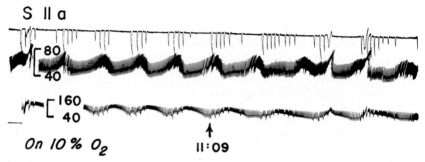

On 10% O₂   11:09

Fig. 13.   Effect of periodic breathing (top) in ewe, on arterial blood pressure (bottom), and fetal arterial blood pressure (middle). Fetus *in utero*. (See text) (16).

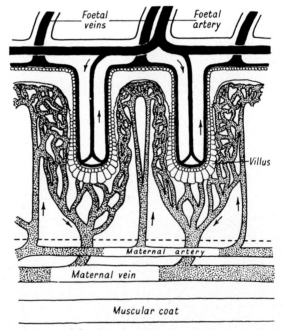

Fig. 14.   Arrangement of fetal and maternal vascular arrangement in sheep placenta. Venous engorgement in maternal circulation may occlude fetal venous outflow. Maternal arterial engorgement may lead to occlusion of the fetal villus stem artery. Either one causes fetal bradycardia (4).

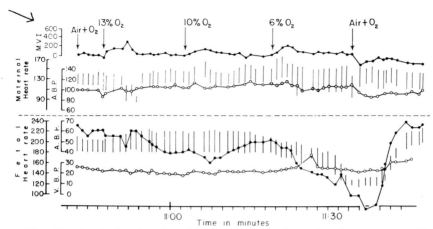

Fig. 15. Graph showing that the fetus recovers from slow heart rate (solid circles bottom) and low blood pressure (bottom vertical lines) if venous umbilical pressure remains high (bottom, open circles). Note, too, that there is no hemodynamic disturbance in the ewe (16).

(Fig. 15). However, in each case where venous pressure has fallen, the fetus lives lingeringly and ultimately dies. It has been pushed beyond its limit of homeostatic reserve. The factors that contribute to the fall and even to the regulation of umbilical vein pressure have not yet been investigated.

We may say, in conclusion, that it appears that the fetus *in utero* is not, physiologically, a small adult, as term approaches. It possesses the basic neural equipment for this, so far as its cardiovascular system is concerned, but it is only as gently stressful stimuli are brought to play upon the fetus *in utero* that it uses the parasympathetic mechanisms fleetingly. Thus it appears that uterine environmental stress rehearses, in a sense, the fetus for its neonatal life, and that the balance of homeostatic controlling mechanisms does not come into play until they are needed when the fetus encounters postnatal stresses. It is rehearsed in their use before it is born, but it does not depend upon them as a condition of maintaining an intrauterine existence.

REFERENCES

1. Bauer, J. J. *Physiol.* (*London*) **95**:187 (1939).
2. Barclay, A. E., Franklin, K. J., and Prichard, M. M. *The Foetal Circulation* Charles C Thomas, Springfield, Ill., 1945.

3. Barcroft, Sir Joseph. *Researches on Pre-Natal Life* Charles C Thomas, Springfield, Ill., 1947.
4. Barron, D. *Anat. Record* **82**:398 (1942).
5. Bieniarz, J., and Reynolds, S. R. M. *Am. J. Physiol.* **189**:128 (1960).
6. Born, G. V. R., Dawes, G. S., and Mott, J. C. *J. Physiol. (London)* **135**:1957
7. Chacko, A. W., and Reynolds, S. R. M. *Anat. Record* **115**:151 (1953).
8. Cohenstein, J., and Zuntz, N. *Pflüger's Anat. ges. Physiol.* **34**:173 (1884).
9. Dawes, G. S., Mott, J. C., and Rennick, B. R. *J. Physiol. (London)* **134**:139 (1956).
10. Haselhorst, G. *Z. Geburtshülfe u. Gynäkol.* **95**:400 (1929).
11. Reynolds, S. R. M. *Am. J. Physiol.* **176**:162 (1954).
12. Reynolds, S. R. M. *Am. J. Physiol.* **176**:169 (1954).
13. Reynolds, S. R. M. *Am. J. Obstet. Gynecol.* **70**:148 (1955).
14. Reynolds, S. R. M., Light, F. W., Ardran, G. M., and Prichard, M. M. *Bull. Johns Hopkins Hosp.* **91**:83 (1952).
15. Reynolds, S. R. M., and Paul W. M. *Bull. Johns Hopkins Hosp.* **97**:383 (1955).
16. Reynolds, S. R. M., and Paul, W. M. *Am. J. Physiol.* **193**:249 (1959).
17. Reynolds, S. R. M., Paul, W. M., and Huggett, A. St. G. *Bull. Johns Hopkins Hosp.* **95**:256 (1954).
18. Windle, W. F. *Physiology of the Fetus*, W. B. Saunders Company, Philadelphia, Pa., 1940.

Fetal and Neonatal Circulation in Relation to Congenital Heart Disease

G. S. DAWES

Nuffield Institute for Medical Research, University of Oxford, England

I propose to give a description of the principal features of the normal fetal circulation and of the changes which occur at birth. This description will be based very largely on experiments conducted on fetal and newborn lambs, the only species which as yet has been thoroughly investigated. This provides us with a model of what may be happening in a normal human infant, of the kind of physiological mechanisms which may be present in the fetus and at birth, and from which we may derive some insight as to the ability of the baby with congenital heart disease to survive, in spite of its deformity.

In the fetus the course of the circulation is quite different from that in the adult, because of the presence of the *foramen ovale* (which provides a large opening between the inferior vena cava and the left atrium) and of the *ductus arteriosus* (a very wide vessel joining the pulmonary trunk to the descending aorta). As a result of these arrangements the right and left sides of the heart work in parallel to pump blood from the great veins into the aorta. We may note at this point that since the two ventricles are in parallel, their output need not be equal; in the normal fetal lamb there is evidence that the output of the left ventricle is significantly greater than that of the right (7) (Fig. 1). The placenta, the lungs, and the other tissues of the fetus are also arranged in parallel between the arteries and the great veins. The volume of blood flow through the umbilical vessels (the fetal side of the placenta) has been measured directly by several methods, and is approximately 130 ml/kg/min in a mature fetal lamb (1). This constitutes more than half the combined output of both

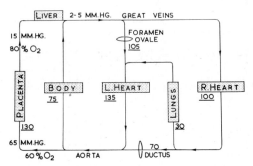

Fig. 1.   This is a simplified diagram of the fetal circulation, showing the pressure (in mm Hg), the O_2 per cent saturation, and the rate of flow (in ml/kg/min, underlined) in the great vessels.

ventricles. The distribution of blood flow through the other principal vessels of the fetus is shown in Fig. 1. It is important to note that 30–50% of the combined output of both ventricles passes through the foramen ovale and the ductus arteriosus. Pulmonary flow is comparatively small and amounts to only 30 ml/kg/min at the most.

The mean arterial pressure in a mature fetal lamb is about 65 mm Hg. Pulmonary arterial pressure is just above that in the descending aorta. The pressure in the umbilical vein is about 15 mm Hg and that in the great veins 2–5 mm Hg. There is, therefore, a pressure head of 50 mm Hg to drive blood through the placenta from the umbilical arteries to the umbilical vein, and of 10 mm Hg or more to drive blood through the liver from the umbilical vein to the inferior vena cava. There is good evidence that for some time before term the blood pressure is under the control of the autonomic nervous system (3). Thus a minor degree of anoxia or stimulation of the splanchnic nerves or of the stellate ganglion causes the heart beat to become more rapid and the blood pressure to rise. The presso- and chemoreceptor reflexes of the carotid bifurcations and the aortic arch are also present and functional both in lambs and in rabbits on the first day of life. Therefore, the mechanism of control of the circulation is unlikely to be very different from that of the adult, though there is no information as to how the blood volume is maintained.

The oxygen content of the blood and the oxygen partial pressure are very much less than those of the adult sheep. Blood returning from the placenta by the umbilical vein is about 80% saturated with oxygen. In the great veins and the heart it is mixed with venous blood returning from the fetal tissues, to a different extent in the right and left heart. Hence blood withdrawn from the carotid artery is 62% saturated, whereas blood returning to the placenta (and the lower half of the fetus) through the descending aorta is 58% saturated on the average, corresponding to a partial pressure of 25–30 mm Hg. This is much less than the arterial O_2 partial pressure of some 95 mm Hg in an adult, and drew from the late Sir Joseph Barcroft the analogy with the conditions at the summit of a high mountain, expressed in a very memorable phrase as "Mount Everest *in utero*." The point is well taken. Since his day it has proved possible to measure O_2 consumption directly in the fetal lamb (as the product of umbilical flow and arteriovenous oxygen difference), and it has been found that when the oxygen saturation of the arterial blood falls much below 50%, oxygen consumption is diminished (6). Therefore, the fetus really is in a potentially dangerous situation. On the other hand, it is well known that very young animals are well able to tolerate a period of total oxygen lack which would kill an adult of the same species. A fetal lamb, halfway through gestation, can survive for 40 minutes or more after its umbilical cord has been tied. During this time it derives energy by anaerobic glycolysis, particularly from the large stores of glycogen in its heart. When its cord is untied, its circulation rapidly returns to normal, and its respiratory center and power of neuromuscular coordination appear unimpaired by this astonishing period of total anoxia (Fig. 2). This ability to withstand acute anoxia is to some extent reduced as gestation proceeds, as is the quantity of glycogen stored in the fetal heart. This is one of the most fascinating phenomena of fetal physiology and is of crucial importance for surviving the gross asphyxia which is so frequent at birth.

The changes which occur in the circulation at birth result from four events: (*a*) the removal of the placenta, (*b*) the expansion of the lungs, (*c*) the rise in arterial O_2 partial pressure, and (*d*) the delivery of the fetus from a warm intrauterine environment into the cold external world. Let us see what happens.

When the lungs are expanded by the first few breaths, their resistance to blood flow drops to one-tenth or less of its former value.

Consequently pulmonary blood flow increases very greatly, and at the same time pulmonary arterial pressure falls toward (though it does not immediately reach) adult values, and left atrial pressure rises (9) (Fig. 3). Within two or three minutes of expansion of the lungs, therefore, great changes in the pressure relationships in the cardiovascular system have already taken place.

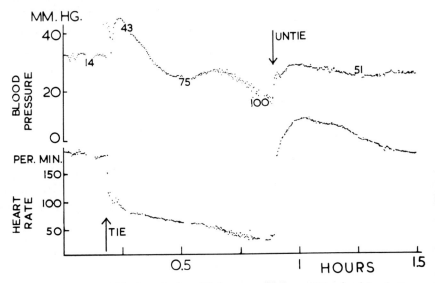

Fig. 2.   The umbilical cord of an 88-day gestation age, 350-g fetal lamb (term is 147 days) was tied. After 40 min complete oxygen lack, the cord was untied and the circulation was recovered. The blood lactate (indicated by the interpolated numerals in mg/100 ml) rose during anoxia and fell when the cord was untied.

The valve of the foramen ovale, which is on the atrial side of the orifice, is normally held open in fetal life during the greater part of the cardiac cycle. But when the lungs are ventilated, and pulmonary flow is thereby increased, left atrial pressure is raised. And since the placenta is removed, inferior vena caval flow is less and pressure reduced. Consequently, within a minute or two of the cord being tied and the lungs expanded, the valve of the foramen ovale becomes applied to the orifice during the whole of the cardiac cycle (8). The foramen ovale thus becomes functionally closed (Fig. 3).

Closure of the ductus arteriosus is more complicated. It is effected by contraction of the muscle fibers which constitute so large a part of the vessel wall, but it is not normally completed for many hours, or in some instances for some days after birth. Within a few minutes of birth in the normal lamb, calf, and foal, the ductus becomes partly constricted, and, because pulmonary arterial pressure has fallen below aortic, a loud murmur becomes audible owing to turbulent flow from aorta to the pulmonary trunk (Figs. 3 and 4). This initial constriction of the ductus is probably due to partial asphyxia at birth and, hence, liberation of sympathomimetic amines, in some lambs. However, there is also no doubt that a large rise

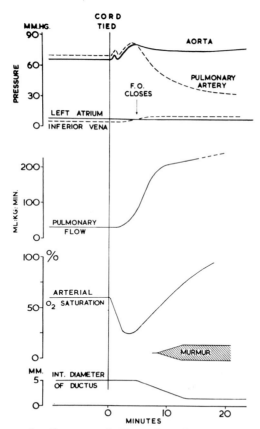

Fig 3. A composite diagram to indicate the principal changes in the circulation when the umbilical cord of a mature fetal lamb is tied, and breathing begins. A murmur becomes audible over the ductus arteriosus as it constricts.

a

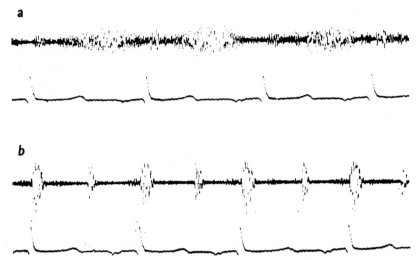

b

Fig. 4.   Records of the phonocardiogram (above) and electrocardiogram (below) from a 4-hour-old lamb, to show the murmur over the ductus arteriosus (*a*), as compared with the normal heart sounds from the apex beat (*b*) (8).

in the partial pressure of oxygen in the blood also causes the ductus to constrict, even in the absence of the central nervous system (Figs. 5 and 6), probably by a direct action on the muscle itself (4). This may be the most important single factor in the normal closure of the ductus arteriosus.

We may now pause for a moment to realize what a radical transformation of the circulation has been effected from the fetal to the neonatal condition (Fig. 7). It is a relatively new idea that there is a "neonatal circulation," an intermediate stage between the fetal and adult, which persists for several days after birth (5). This is characterized by the fact that the ductus arteriosus is still open, that blood flows through it (normally from left to right, from aorta to pulmonary trunk) in considerable quantities, and that the wall of the right ventricle is still almost as thick as that of the left. The continued patency of the ductus arteriosus for some while after birth has been observed, not only in animals but also subsequently in human infants after catheterization of the heart (2, 11). So long as this condition persists, the output of the left heart must be substantially greater than that of the right. It is not until the ductus arteriosus

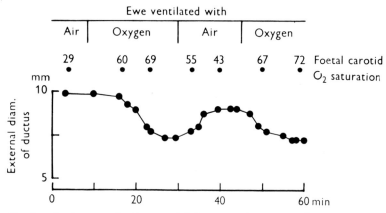

Fig. 5. An increase in the arterial O₂ saturation causes the ductus arteriosus to constrict in a fetal lamb (4).

is finally closed that the adult type of circulation is attained, in which the output of the left and right ventricles must be to all intents equal, since they now work in series to drive blood through the lungs and the systemic circulation.

I shall digress now to describe the change in O_2 consumption which takes place in the lamb at birth. Toward the end of gestation the rate of O_2 consumption of an anesthetized fetal lamb is, per unit body weight, about the same as that of its mother, 4–5 ml/kg/min. But at birth the lamb is removed from the intrauterine environment

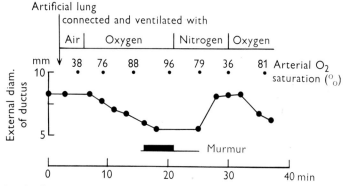

Fig. 6. An increase in the arterial O₂ saturation causes the ductus arteriosus to constrict in an isolated heart-ductus-artificial lung preparation (4).

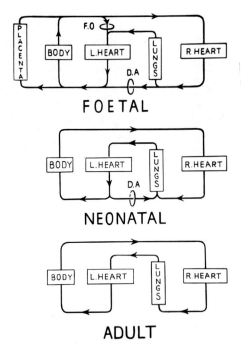

Fig 7.   A simple diagram of the principal changes in the circulation at birth to show the nature of the transitional neonatal circulation (5).

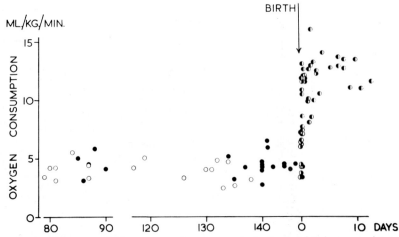

Fig. 8.   The rate of O_2 consumption, per unit body weight, is approximately constant during the latter half of gestation in the lamb, but is increases very considerably at birth.

TABLE I. Mean figures for blood flow in the fetal lamb and after birth

	Fetal	Newborn
	ml/kg, min	ml/kg, min
Pulmonary flow	30	325
Output of right ventricle	100	325
Systemic flow	75	325

of about 40°C, and thereafter lives at an environmental temperature of, say, 10–20°C. If it is to maintain its body temperature, it must increase its metabolic rate. In fact its rate of O_2 consumption increases threefold to about 12 ml/kg/min (6) (Fig. 8). This is probably related to the fact that whereas a lamb weighing 5 kg has a surface area of 0.33 m², a ewe weighing 50 kg has a surface area of only 1.0 m², i.e., the lamb has a threefold greater surface area per unit body weight.

We may now return to a consideration of the changes in cardiac output at birth. The only information available is in the lamb, where calculation suggests that ventricular output rises from about 100 ml/kg/min to 325 ml/kg/min, by a factor of threefold (Table I). It is interesting to note that these same calculations suggest that there may have been a fourfold increase in systemic blood flow, from 75 ml/kg/min up to 325 ml/kg/min. These are very striking changes, and it is most desirable that these calculations should be checked by measurements using different methods, and on other species. Nevertheless, the striking rise in O^2 consumption at birth does suggest a possible reason for the postulated increase in cardiac output and systemic blood flow. It is quite evident that any discussion of the changes in the circulation at birth should take account, not merely of the anatomical alterations in the course of the circulation associated with closure of the foramen ovale and ductus arteriosus, but also of the changes in the volume of blood flow through the heart and the systemic circulation. It is indeed curious that whereas the possibility of an increase in pulmonary blood flow at birth has been considered from Harvey's time (though not proved by direct experiment till within the last five years), the possibility of changes in cardiac output and in the systemic blood flow at birth has not been contemplated.

If we turn to congenital heart disease, there are several points which emerge from these experiments on the normal fetus and newborn animal. First, it is evident why so many gross congenital anomalies are compatible with survival until birth. The development of the heart is gradual, and the two ventricles work in parallel in the fetus. Thus, so long as one side of the heart is placed so that it can drive blood from the great veins to the aorta, survival should be possible. Indeed, as Jost (10) has shown in fetal rabbits, survival is possible even after removal of the head of the fetus. In this species not even the brain is required to regulate the circulation at the end of gestation. Secondly, it is clear that very radical changes take place at birth, which in the lamb affect not merely the course of the circulation but also lead to a large increase in O_2 consumption and probably in cardiac output. Also so long as the ductus arteriosus is open, the output of the left ventricle will be substantially greater than that of the right. Infants with some anomalies of the heart may be in peril at this time; in others, the persistence of the ductus arteriosus is necessary for survival. Thirdly, these experiments have thrown some light on the complex mechanisms which regulate normal constriction and closure of the ductus arteriosus. The ductus sometimes fails to close after birth, not only in human infants but also in animals such as the sheep or dog. Dr. Mott and I have come across one lamb during the last five years whose ductus arteriosus failed to constrict although it was well oxygenated. This anomaly also may be due to a developmental defect early in gestation rather than to cyanosis at birth. Finally it has been suggested that certain human cases of pulmonary hypertension might be due to persistence of the fetal condition, i.e., that the vascular resistance of the lungs remains high in the same way that it is high in the normal fetus. I do not think that this provocative suggestion will stand close examination. In the normal fetus expansion of the lungs causes a large fall of resistance and of pulmonary arterial pressure. If this fall does not take place when the lungs are well ventilated, then those lungs are not normal. I would plead that early investigation, soon after birth, of many types of congenital anomaly is required if we are to achieve a better understanding of their pathological physiology.

REFERENCES

1. Acheson, G. H., Dawes, G. S., and Mott, J. C. *J. Physiol. (London)* **135:**623 (1957).
2. Adams, F. H., and Lind, J. *Pediatrics* **19:**431 (1957).
3. Born, G. V. R., Dawes, G. S., and Mott, J. C. *J. Physiol. (London)* **134:**149 (1956).
4. Born, G. V. R., Dawes, G. S., Mott, J. C., and Rennick, B. R. *J. Physiol. (London)* **132:**304 (1956).
5. Born, G. V. R., Dawes, G. S., Mott, J. C., and Widdicombe, J. G. *Cold Spring Harbor Symposia Quant. Biol.* **19:**102 (1954).
6. Dawes, G. S., and Mott, J. C. *J. Physiol. (London)* in press.
7. Dawes, G. S., Mott, J. C., and Widdicombe, J. G. *J. Physiol (London)* **126:**563 (1954).
8. Dawes, G. S., Mott, J. C., and Widdicombe, J. G. *J. Physiol. (London)* **128:**344, 384 (1955).
9. Dawes, G. S., Mott, J. C., Widdicombe, J. G. and Wyatt, D. G. *J. Physiol. (London)* **121:**141 (1953).
10. Jost, A. *Cold Spring Harbor Symposia Quant. Biol.* **19:**167 (1954).
11. Rowe, R. D., and James, L. S. *J. Pediat.* **51:**1 (1957).

Fetal and Neonatal Circulation: Observations in Humans*

FORREST H. ADAMS and JOHN LIND

Departments of Pediatrics, University of California, Los Angeles, California, and the Karolinska Sjukhuset and the Wenner-Gren Cardiovascular Research Laboratory, Stockholm, Sweden

Barclay *et al.* (1) in their monograph on *The Foetal Circulation* have aptly stated, "however interesting and instructive work on lower animals may be, one's primary object . . . is to ascertain what happens in Man." They further state, "unfortunately, many of the investigations which have been carried out in the living lamb either cannot be repeated, or else have not been repeated in the human subject." The validity of these statements is self-evident; however, since publication of their monograph, much information even though fragmentary has been gained concerning the human fetal and neonatal circulation. Many of the techniques used to study this problem in humans are similar to those used by Barclay and his group and by his predecessors and by his followers. The purpose of this presentation is to bring up to date our present knowledge on the human fetal and neonatal circulation.

No attempt will be made to review those investigations performed on humans prior to the publication of Barclay's monograph since an excellent review of the literature on this subject is contained in it (1). Dr. Barry has already discussed the developmental anatomy in the human fetal circulation. How this is affected by or affects *the course of the blood flow in the human fetus* is not entirely clear at the present time, but there must be an interrelationship between the two.

* Supported by funds from the Los Angeles County Heart Association and The Association for Aid to Crippled Children.

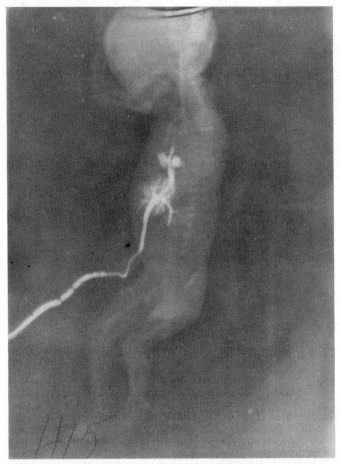

Fig. 1.   Roentgenogram showing course of radioopaque contrast media injected into umbilical vein of a living human fetus approximately 22 weeks of age. Note material filling both right and left atrium after passing through the liver.

Fetal Circulation

One of the first groups to apply to the human the methods developed by the Oxford group were Lind and Wegelius (2). These investigators performed angiocardiography in human fetuses from 18 to 22 weeks gestational age obtained at the time of legal abortion. The original equipment used in these studies permitted ten pictures per second. Although certain recent refinements in the technique have been made, they were able to demonstrate (in 1949 with pictures fairly high quality) both the venous and arterial fetal circulations. Figure 1 demonstrated the course of the radioopaque contrast media when injected into the umbilical vein. Figure 2 demonstrated the course of the contrast media when injected in a retrograde fashion through the umbilical artery. Later, Lind and Wegelius (3) performed similar studies in full term infants prior to and immediately

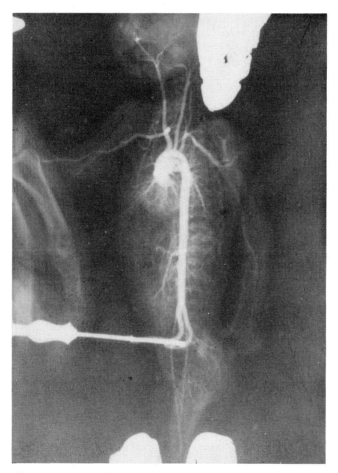

Fig. 2. Roentgenogram showing course of radioopaque material injected retrograde into the umbilical artery. All parts of the aorta and its branches are filled including the arch, the ductus arteriosus, and the pulmonary arteries.

after clamping of the umbilical cord. From these two investigations, they were able to conclude that the course of the human fetal and neonatal circulations were for all practical purposes similar to the fetal and newborn lamb.

Little additional information has been obtained since regarding the human fetal circulation. Crawford (4) has developed a technique for demonstrating the blood supply of the removed fetal placenta, but this work as yet has not demonstrated any new information.

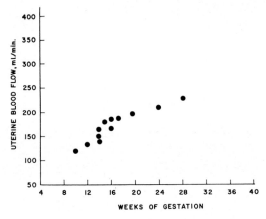

Fig. 3.   Uterine blood flow at various weeks of gestation as measured by the electromagnetic flow method. Note the progressive linear increase.

During 1957, Assali working with Lind *et al.* (5) made some very important observations on human uterine and fetal blood flow. Two different techniques were used by this group. The nitrous oxide technique was used for the uterine blood flow, and an electromagnetic flowmeter was used for both the uterine and fetal blood flows. The studies were performed on mothers and fetuses in Sweden and Finland undergoing legal abortion. Figure 3 shows the values of uterine blood flow obtained by the electromagnetic flowmeter method in various stages of early pregnancy. These ranged from 100 to 250 cc/min from 8 to 28 weeks gestation. Figure 4 shows the values obtained by the nitrous oxide method. With the electromagnetic flowmeter on the intact umbilical vein, fetal blood flows were also determined. The values ranged from 10 to 80 cc/min during the period from 8 to 28 weeks gestation (Fig. 5*a*). When the values were divided by the weight of the fetus, the blood flow remained almost constant over the period observed and compare favorably with the values obtained by Dawes in lambs as seen in Fig. 5*b*.

Neonatal Circulation

With the birth of the human infant, a number of important events take place which have a profound effect on the circulation. Probably

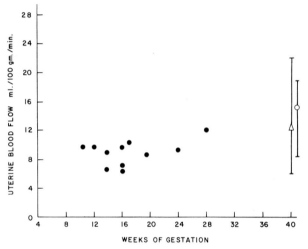

Fig. 4.   Uterine blood flow at various weeks of gestation as measured by the nitrous oxide method. The mean values with their ranges listed at 40 weeks are those obtained from previous studies and by others.

the most important of these events is the "first breath" with resultant inflation of the lungs and increased blood flow to the lungs. Prior to respiration, only a small portion of the blood flowing into the pulmonary artery reaches the lung parenchyma; the major portion bypasses the lungs via the ductus arteriosus. Based on Dawes' studies in the lamb (7) and simple logic, it would seem reasonable to assume that in the human infant prior to respiration, the pulmonary vascular resistance exceeds the systemic vascular resistance and that, with the first breath, there is a prompt drop in pulmonary resistance with a probable increase in systemic resistance, particularly if the umbilical cord is clamped simultaneously. Such a sudden shift in the balance

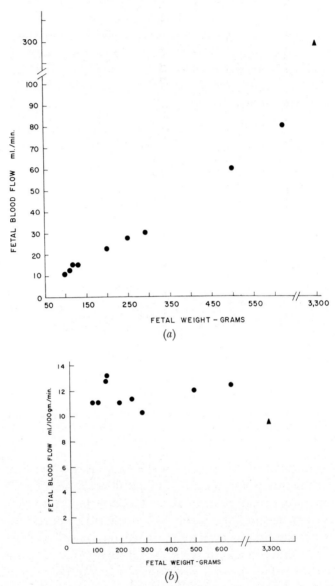

Fig. 5. (a) Fetal blood flow, measured with an electromagnetic flowmeter on the umbilical vein, correlated with fetal weight. Note the progressive and marked increase in flow with increasing weight. The value at 3300 g is from Dawes' data in sheep at term. (b) Fetal blood flow values from (a) expressed in terms of 100 g of fetal tissue. Note absence of marked changes with increasing weight.

of vascular resistance undoubtedly forces a large volume of blood into the pulmonary arterioles and capillaries.

Factors that initiate the "first breath" in the human infant are still not well documented. It is known, however, from studies by our group (9) that the major ingress of air into the newborn lung takes place very suddenly within 0.15 second. This is somewhat incompatible with the theory of "capillary erection" as a cause for lung expansion (10). Continued expansion of the newborn lung probably takes place over the next 24–96 hours (11). Figure 6 shows the physical arrangement used by us to study the newborn infant's "first breath." With this situation, rapid x-ray pictures at six films per second were taken in either the frontal (Fig. 7*a*) or lateral view (Fig. 7*b*).

The changes in intrathoracic pressure at birth likewise play a role in the filling of the lungs with blood as well as with air. As can be

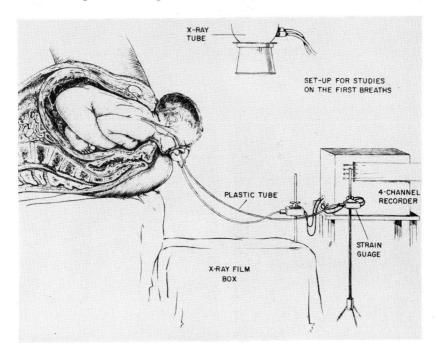

Fig. 6. Diagram illustrating physical arrangement for studying the "first breath."

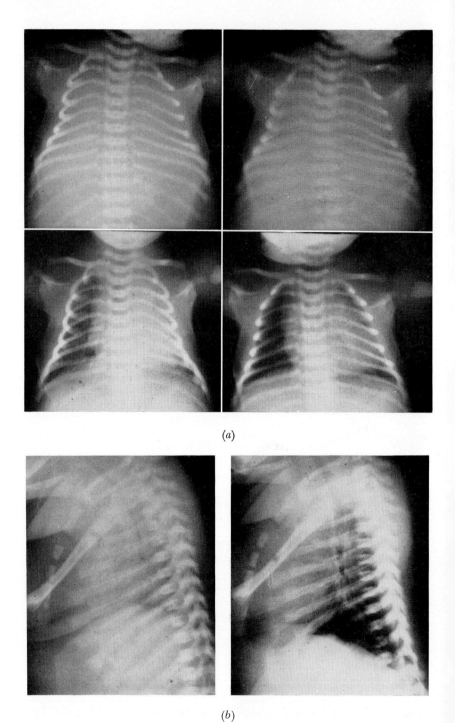

(a)

(b)

Fig. 7.   Roentgenograms taken at 6 frames per second in frontal view (a) and lateral view (b). The time interval between each film is approximately 0.15 second. Note rapid inflow of air particularly in the posterior parts of the lung.

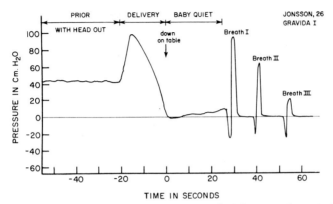

Fig. 8.   Diagrammatic representation of a typical intraesophogeal (intrathoracic?) pressure curve during delivery and the first breaths.

seen in Fig. 6, as the head emerged, a small plastic catheter was quickly inserted through the nose into the esophagus so that the tip was at the level of the carina. Pressure recordings were then made during the remainder of the delivery. A diagrammatic representation of a typical curve obtained under such circumstances is shown in Fig. 8. These studies showed that the process of normal vaginal delivery produces a moderate pressure effect on the infant's chest. In most instances, immediately following delivery the chest did not recoil producing a large negative pressure. Thus there appeared to be no "big squeeze" after effect. The first few breaths had a low pulmonary compliance, and the positive phase of respiration was very prominent. The range in pressures observed by us was from −70 to +100 cm of water.

With the increased pulmonary blood flow due to respiration, there occurs an increase in blood returning to the left atrium from the lungs. Under resting conditions this causes the flap on the foramen ovale to be closed and prevents the venoarterial shunt through it. Crying during the first several days of life may increase the pressure in the right atrium enough over that in the left atrium to reinstitute the venoarterial shunt through the foramen ovale and to produce systemic arterial desaturation (12).

In contrast to the rather prompt closure immediately after birth of the foramen ovale as a fetal channel, strong evidence now exists for the persistent patency of the ductus arteriosus for several days. As indirect evidence for patency of the ductus arteriosus are the observations of Eldridge *et al.* (13) and Prec and Cassels (14). The former found evidence of right to left shunting through the ductus arteriosus during the first several hours and days of life since the simultaneously determined arterial oxygen saturation in the foot was frequently lower than in the hand. Prec and Cassels (14), using dye dilution curves as a method for determining cardiac output, also found evidence of shunting which they reasoned probably was at the level of the ductus arteriosus. All the studies by Prec and Cassels were done in the quiet state and were indicative of a left-to-right shunt rather than a right-to-left shunt as found by Eldridge *et al.* (13). In order for a right-to-left shunt to occur, it was also reasoned that pulmonary hypertension must be present (13).

Direct observations by us and others using the right heart catheterization technique have confirmed the patency of the ductus arteriosus and the presence of pulmonary hypertension lasting up to several days of age (15, 16). In our studies, the left to right shunt through the ductus arteriosus was frequently quite large, but exact calculation of the amount was probably inaccurate due to poor mixing at the sampling site (15). A heart murmur could not be heard in any of the infants studied, and all had normal electrocardiograms and normal heart volume determinations for their age. The cardiac output, expressed as systemic blood flow, ranged from 298 ml/min to 846 ml/min (134 ml/min/kg to 187 ml/min/kg). The pulmonary hypertension observed by us (15) and Rowe and James (16) was frequently equal to the systemic pressure. The latter investigators found that short periods of hypoxia with 10% oxygen would increase the pulmonary artery pressure if the arterial oxygen saturation fell to fetal levels (17). Furthermore, Eldridge and Hultgren (18) showed that in those normal infants with a venoarterial shunt in room air, hypoxia would increase the veno-arterial shunt.

More recently we have been interested in evaluating the effect of drugs and gas mixtures on the neonatal cardiovascular system (19, 20). Comparable studies were performed in both animals and humans. The drugs were injected through an intracardiac catheter, and the

	LAMB		PIG		HUMAN	
	PRESSURE	PULSE	PRESSURE	PULSE	PRESSURE	PULSE
ACETYLCHOLINE 0.1 µg.	↓	↓	↓	O	O	O
ADRENALIN 0.5 µg.	↑	↑	↑	O^x	↑	↑^{x}
NORADRENALIN 0.5 µg.	↑	↑	↑	O	↑	↓
SEROTONIN 5.0 µg.	—	—	↓	H.B.	—	—
10% OXYGEN 5 min.	—	—	—	—	O	↑
100% OXYGEN 5 min.	—	—	—	—	O	↓

↓ = SIGNIFICANT DECREASE   H.B. = HEART BLOCK
↑ = SIGNIFICANT INCREASE   X = EXTRASYSTOLES
O = NO SIGNIFICANT CHANGE

Fig. 9. Chart showing the direction of response of the cardiovascular system in newborn infants and animals to various drugs and gas mixtures. Note the dissimilarities.

pressures and electrocardiogram were monitored. The direction of response of the cardiovascular system following the various procedures is summarized in Fig 9. From this it can be seen that relatively small amounts of acetylcholine, adrenaline, noradrenaline, and in a few instances serotonin were effective in eliciting a response in the animals. On the other hand, in the human neonates, acetylcholine even in large amounts produced no drop in pulmonary artery pressure or pulse rate. Likewise noradrenaline regularly caused a bradycardia in the humans whereas this was not observed in any of the animals studied. These studies would suggest that the human neonatal pulmonary vascular system is capable of *vasoconstriction*. As yet we have no evidence that it is capable of *vasorelaxation* as has been demonstrated in certain patients with left-to-right shunts where pulmonary hypertension exists (21, 22). Thus it is entirely possible that the pulmonary hypertension in the newborn infant is due to two factors: (*a*) increased resistance due to thick fetal pulmonary arteries, and (*b*) increased pulmonary blood flow due to the large left-to-right shunt through the ductus arteriosus.

As soon as the ductus arteriosus closes, the pulmonary hypertension disappears, so that probably the anatomical nature of the fetal pulmonary arteries is not the major factor in the production of the pulmonary hypertension.

It is obvious from what has been stated that there are many gaps in our knowledge of the normal fetal and neonatal circulation in humans. Continued animal and human research is necessary if we are to approach intelligently the problems of disease arising out of these periods.

REFERENCES

1. Barclay, A. E., Franklin, K. J., and Prichard, M. M. L. *The Foetal Circulation.* Charles C Thomas, Springfield, Ill., 1945.
2. Lind, J., and Wegelius, C. Angiocardiographic studies on the human foetal circulation. *Pediatrics* **4**:391–400 (1949).
3. Lind, J., and Wegelius, C. Human fetal circulation changes in the cardiovascular system at birth and disturbances in the postnatal closure of the foramen ovale and dictus arteriosus. *Cold Spring Harbor Symposia, Quant. Biol.* **19**:109 (1954).
4. Crawford, J. M. The foetal placental circulation. II. The gross anatomy. *J. Obstet. Gynaecol. Brit. Empire* **63**:87 (1956).
5. Assali, N., Lind, J., Rauramo, L., and Westin, B. Unpublished observations.
6. Dawes, G. S., Mott, J. C., Widdicombe, J. G., and Wyatt, D. G. Changes in the lungs of the newborn lamb. *J. Physiol. (London)* **121**:141 (1953).
7. Ardran, G. M., Dawes, G. S., Prichard, M. M. L., Reynolds, S. R. M., and Wyatt, D. G. The effect of ventilation of the fetal lungs upon the pulmonary circulation. *J. Physiol. (London)* **118**:12 (1952).
8. Adams, F. H., and Lind, J. Unpublished observations.
9. Adams, F. H., Karlberg, P., and Lind, J. Adaptations of the newborn infant's cardiovascular and pulmonary systems to extrauterine life. Presented before the American Pediatric Society, May 9, 1958, Atlantic City, N. J., *A.M.A. J. Diseases Children* **96**:603 (1958).
10. Jäykkä, S. Capillary erection and lung expansion. *Acta Paediatrica,* **Suppl. 109**, 1956.
11. Ahvenainen, E. K. Changes in dilatation and signs of aspiration in fetal and neonatal lungs: Experimental and histologic study. *Acta. Paediatrica* **35: Suppl. 3** (1948).
12. Prec. K. J., and Cassels, D. E. Oximeter studies in newborn infants during crying. *Pediatrics* **9**:756 (1952).
13. Eldridge, F. L., Hultgren, H. N., and Wigmore, M. E. Physiologic Closure of the ductus arteriosus in newborn infants. *Science* **119**:731 (1954)

14. Prec, K. J., and Cassels, D. E. Dye dilution curves and cardiac output in newborn infants. *Circulation* **11**:789 (1955).
15. Adams, F. H., and Lind, J. Physiologic studies on the cardiovascular status of normal newborn infants. *Pediatrics* **19**:431 (1957).
16. Rowe, R. D., and James, L. S. The normal pulmonary arterial pressures during the first year of life. *J. Pediat.* **51**:1 (1957).
17. James, L. S., and Rowe, R. D. The pattern of response of pulmonary and systemic arterial pressures in newborn and older infants to short periods of hypoxia. *J. Pediat.* **51**:5 (1957).
18. Eldridge, F. L., and Hultgren, H. N. The physiologic closure of the ductus arteriosus in the newborn infant. *J. Clin. Invest.* **34**:987 (1955).
19. Adams, F. H., Hirovenen, L., Lind, J., and Peltonen, T. Physiologic studies on the cardiovascular status of newborn pigs. *Études Neo-Natales* **7**:53 (1958).
20. Adams, F. H., Lind, J., and Rauramo, L. Physiologic studies on the cardiovascular status of normal newborn infants: Effect of adrenaline, noradrenaline, 10% oxygen and 100% oxygen. *Études Neo-Natales* **7**:62 (1958).
21. Harris, P. Influence of acetylcholine on pulmonary arterial pressure. *Brit. Heart J.* **19**:272 (1957).
22. Crittenden, I. H., and Adams, F. H. Effect of acetylcholine on pulmonary hypertension in left to right shunts. *A.M.A. J. Diseases Children* **96**:484 (1958).

Experimental Production of Congenital Cardiac Defects

JAMES G. WILSON

Department of Anatomy, College of Medicine, University of Florida, Gainesville, Florida

During the past eighteen years there has been a notable increase in interest in congenital malformations from both the clinical and experimental points of view. This is probably attributable to three sets of events. In 1940 Warkany and his collaborators (14) reported the first of a series of experiments in which developmental defects were produced in rats by means of maternal dietary deficiencies. Then in 1941 Gregg (7) found that an epidemic of German measles in Australia had resulted in congenital cataracts and other defects in human infants born to mothers who had been infected during early pregnancy. Throughout the 1940's and into the 1950's, such men as Blalock, Gross, Potts, and Crafoord made a series of bold surgical attacks on many types of congenital deformities previously regarded as inoperable, and showed that surgical repair is often feasible (2, 3, 8, 12). These events, by revealing that malformations may be determined by the environment and thereby preventable and that when not preventable may be subject to surgical correction, have done much to dispel the fatalistic attitudes that prevailed earlier.

Cardiovascular anomalies have figured prominently in this overall increase of interest in teratology. The spectacular breakthrough in the surgical repair of cardiovascular defects has focused attention particularly on this type of malformation. Subsequent experience in this field has raised many questions as to the etiology, development mechanics, and postnatal physiology of such anomalies. The need for an experimental method whereby cardiovascular defects could be produced at will in laboratory animals has frequently been expressed.

The first report of a method that produced significant numbers of anomalies comparable to those that occur in human infants came in 1949. Wilson and Warkany (18) found that maternal vitamin A deficiency during pregnancy in the rat caused embryonic maldevelopment of several organs, among them the heart and aortic arches (Figs. 1 and 2). The highest incidence of cardiovascular anomalies recorded was 33% of all abnormal animals, or about 26% of all offspring, but the true incidence at term was somewhat less, for these figures included a number of fetal stages. Since then several other methods have also become available (Table I). X-irradiation of developing rat embryos was found to be a very precise method for studying the effects of a teratogenic agent at a particular developmental stage (16) (Figs. 3–5). The incidence of cardiovascular defects, however, never exceeded 24% and was usually less. Pteroylglutamic acid deficiency in the pregnant rat was shown by Baird *et al.* (1) to produce a considerably higher incidence, and it had the further advantage that the time during which this agent acted upon the embryo could be restricted to a two-day period. Nelson *et al.* (11) found that maternal riboflavin deficiency, induced by feeding the antagonist galactoflavin, frequently caused defects in the interventricular septum of the offspring. In 1955 it was reported that the dye trypan blue when injected into pregnant rats caused cardiovascular anomalies in the offspring (15) (Figs. 1 and 2). Fox and Goss (4) refined this method by using more susceptible strains of rats and by performing microdissections of the hearts so that the yield of defects by this method was raised as high as 60%. Furthermore, the young born to mothers so treated were less severely malformed in other respects, which probably accounts for the fact that Richman, Thomas, and Konikov (13) were able to demonstrate that some of the young rats with cardiovascular anomalies were viable for at least thirty days. In 1958 Haring (9) reported that maintaining pregnant rats in an atmosphere containing an excess of CO_2 leads to cardiac maldevelopment in the offspring. It is probable that other known teratogenic agents also have caused cardiovascular defects which have not been detected because of the laborious technique required to study these anomalies.

Of the methods summarized in Table I, that involving the injection of trypan blue appears to be the most promising for in-

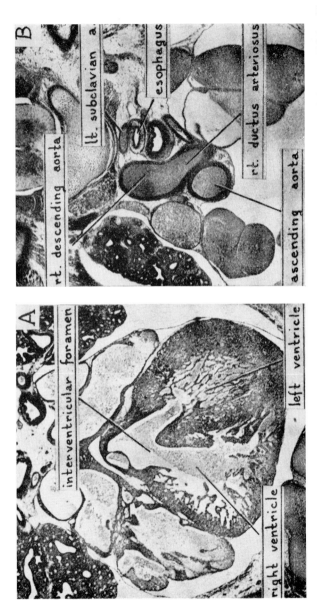

Fig. 1.   Hearts of newborn rats from vitamin A-deficient mothers. A. Interventricular septal defect. B. Right-sided arch of aorta and ductus arteriosus. Note that the left subclavian artery arises distally from the right-sided arch of aorta and passes dorsal to the esophagus to reach the left shoulder.

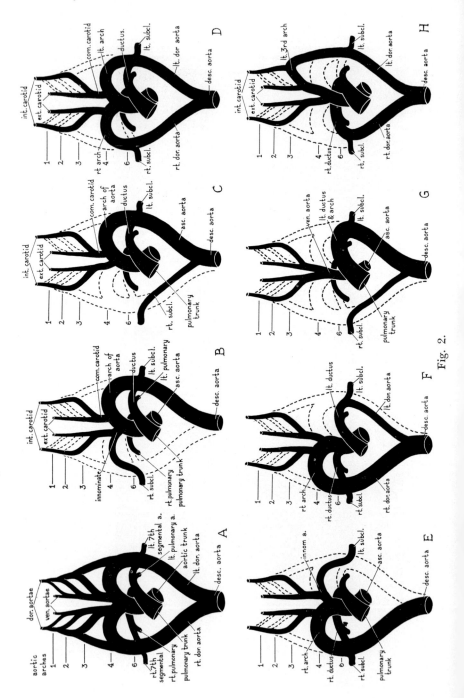

Fig. 2.

vestigations on such subjects as the developmental mechanics, the postnatal physiology, and the possibilities for surgical repair. In the first place this method is the easiest to apply and requires no special diets or apparatus. It yields a high incidence of cardiovascular anomalies, and frequently the offspring are viable and thus available for postnatal study. Furthermore, many of the defects are of the same types as occur in man. It only remains to be demonstrated that trypan blue is capable of causing these defects in larger animals, such as dogs and cats, which are more easily adapted to surgical and physiologic study. To date the dye has been shown to be teratogenic only in chicks, mice, hamsters, rats, and rabbits.

It is interesting to compare the patterns of malformations produced by three of the more productive agents (Table II). After maternal vitamin A deficiency, maternal pteroylglutamic acid deficiency, and trypan blue injection, interventricular septal defects occurred with considerable regularity in the three instances. Abnormal origin of the right subclavian artery from the distal part of the arch of the aorta was somewhat more common after pteroylglutamic acid deficiency than after either of the other agents. However, the occurrence of other types of aortic arch abnormalities was generally comparable for the three agents.

Fig. 2.   Schematic representations of some of the aortic arch anomalies found in the offspring of vitamin A-deficient rats. A. The embryonic aortic arch pattern showing all five pairs of arches cumulatively, as if all were present at one time. The dorsal aortae and the descending aorta are drawn on the same plane as the ventral aorta, but in reality the former lie dorsal to the trachea and esophagus and the latter ventral, the two being connected by the paired arches around either side of the trachea and esophagus. B. The definitive mammalian pattern of arteries derived from the embryonic system by retention of some parts and the deletion of others. C. Distally arising or retroesophageal right subclavian artery, resulting from absence of the right 4th arch and retention, instead, of the right dorsal aorta. D. Double arch of aorta, resulting from retention of both dorsal aortae as well as both 4th arches. E. Right-sided arch of aorta and ductus arteriosus, resulting from retention of right 4th and 6th arches and dorsal aorta instead of the left-sided members as normally occurs. F. Right arch-double ductus, resulting from retention of right (instead of left) 4th arch, both 6th arches and both dorsal aortae. G. Absence of aortic arch with the ductus arteriosus as the only connection between the heart and the descending aorta, resulting from absence of both 4th embryonic arches. H. Absence of aortic arch in which one 3rd and one 6th embryonic arches serve to connect the heart with the descending aorta, resulting from absence of both 4th embryonic arches.

TABLE I.   Experimental methods used to produce congenital cardio-vascular anomalies

Method	Time of Treatment (days of pregnancy)	Maximal Effect (% total young)	Reference
Vitamin A deficiency	Throughout pregnancy	26	Wilson and Warkany, 1949
X-irradiation, 100 r direct	9	24	Wilson, Jordan, and Brent, 1953
Pteroylglutamic acid deficiency	9 to 11	57	Baird, Nelson, Monie, and Evans, 1954
Riboflavin deficiency	7 to 11	24	Nelson, Baird, Wright, and Evans, 1956
Trypan blue, 3 injections, 1 cc of 1%	7, 8, 9	11	Wilson, 1955
Trypan blue, 1 injection, 1 cc of 1%	$8\frac{1}{2}$	60	Fox and Goss, 1956
CO_2 excess, 6% for 24 hr	8, 9, 10, or 11	11	Haring, 1958

Such similarity of incidence and types did not hold for defects involving the interatrial septum, the atrioventricular valves, the origins of the major arterial trunks, and the termination of the left superior vena cava (Table II). These anomalies occurred after trypan blue injection but not after maternal dietary deficiency of either vitamin A or pteroylglutamic acid. Although not represented in Table II, it is noteworthy that x-irradiation also caused these unusual types of cardiac defects and, in fact, the overall pattern of cardiovascular abnormalities were quite similar after treatment of the mothers with trypan blue and of the embryos with x-rays. It would appear, therefore, that we are dealing with two different patterns of abnormalities, the one produced by either of the dietary deficiencies and the other produced almost equally well by either trypan blue or x-rays.

The underlying reasons for these divergent patterns are obscure but they are, nevertheless, examples of what has been called *agent specificity* in teratology. In brief, this means that different teratogenic agents may, and frequently do, act upon the same developing systems

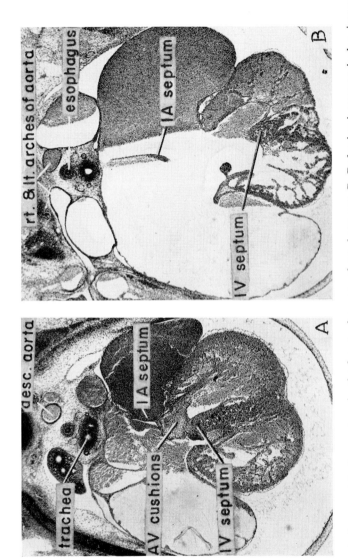

Fig. 3. A. Interventricular septum in the heart of a normal newborn rat. B. Defective interventricular, interatrial, and atrioventricular septa in the heart of a newborn rat irradiated with 100 r on the 9th day of gestation. Note the doubling of the aorta above the esophagus.

72   *J. G. Wilson*

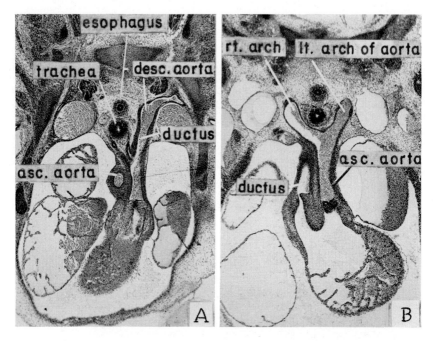

Fig. 4.   A. Ascending and descending aortae and ductus arteriosus in a normal newborn rat. B. Transposed ductus and aorta in a newborn rat irradiated with 100 r on the 9th day of gestation. Note the double arch of aorta, one going on either side of the trachea.

at the same times to produce different types of malformations. In other words, a particular set or syndrome of malformations may be associated with a specific teratogenic agent, although it is not necessarily limited to one agent. The implication is that an agent may act upon one aspect of the developmental process while another may act upon a different aspect to produce a different developmental outcome, or that two agents may act upon the same aspect to produce the same outcome. It would also appear that certain agents may act quite similarly in some respects and quite differently in others, as appears to be illustrated in Table II. Vitamin A deficiency and trypan blue act similarly on the interventricular septum but entirely differently on the positioning of the arterial trunks, for example.

The malformations resulting from maternal vitamin A deficiency, although not as promising for postnatal physiologic and surgical studies as those produced by trypan blue, have revealed some interesting facts regarding the developmental aspects of cardiovascular defects. In an experiment involving vitamin A deficiency, Wilson, Roth, and Warkany (17) demonstrated that the composition of the vitamin A deficiency syndrome could be changed by changing the time in pregnancy during which the agent was allowed to act (Table III). Unlike earlier experiments in which vitamin A deficiency was continued throughout pregnancy, in this experiment large doses of vitamin A were administered therapeutically on days 10, 11, 12, 13, 14, or 15, thus abruptly terminating the deficiency. In the first place, it

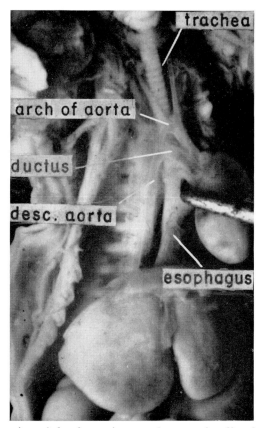

Fig. 5.   Dissection of the thorax in a newborn rat irradiated on the 9th day, showing arch of aorta and ductus arteriosus passing to the right of the trachea and esophagus.

TABLE II.   Comparison of the syndrome of cardiovascular anomalies produced by different methods in the rat

Type of Defect	Vitamin A Deficiency throughout Pregnancy[a]	Pteroylgluta-mic Acid Deficiency for 2-Day Period[b]	Trypan Blue Injection on Day 8½[c]
Interventricular septal defect	22%	33%	31%
Distal right subclavian artery	8	33	5
Double arch of aorta	4	4	2
Right-sided arch of aorta	6	9	4
Truncus arteriosus communis	2	6	1
Absence of functional ductus	6	4	1
Subclavian artery from pulmonary take	4	4	1
Absence of aortic (4th) arch	4	3	0
Transposition of arterial trunks	0	0	30
Interatrial septal defects	0	0	23
Abnormal termination left superior vena cava	0	0	11
Atrioventricular valvulis communis	0	0	6

[a] From reference 18.
[b] From reference 1.
[c] From reference 4.

TABLE III.   Cardiac malformations in the offspring of female rats maintained for varying periods during pregnancy on vitamin A deficiency[a]

	Percentage of Offspring Affected						
	After vitamin A therapy, days of pregnancy						Without therapy
	10th	11th	12th	13th	14th	15th	
Total defects	5	6	8	18	25	13	4
Interventricular septal defects	5	6	4	14	21	11	4
Truncoconal septal defects	0	0	0	6	11	7	4
Atrioventricular valvulis communis	0	3	4	0	0	0	0
Pulmonary stenosis	0	0	4	2	0	0	0

[a] Data taken from reference 17.

was found that to prevent all cardiac malformation therapy must be given earlier than the 10th day since that given at this time permits a low percentage of interventricular septal defects to occur. When therapy was delayed until the 12th day, interventricular defects again occurred, but this time in association with other abnormalities, namely, atrioventricular valvulis communis and stenosis of the pulmonary conus. Delaying therapy until the 14th or 15th day resulted in still further changes in the pattern: the incidence of interventricular defects increased, defects of the truncoconal septum began to appear, and valvulis communis was no longer observed. This suggests that vitamin A, or the lack of it, acts differently upon the embryonic heart at different stages in development.

It is noteworthy that animals given no therapy throughout pregnancy showed fewer malformations than those given therapy between the 10th and 15th days (Table III). The explanation is quite simple: many of the cardiovascular defects in the animals which received therapy were associated with other severe malformations. In the absence of therapy these more severely affected animals died *in utero,* but the giving of therapy salvaged many defective animals that otherwise would not have been seen at term. This exemplifies the manner in which so-called fetal wastage may be a blessing in that it tends to eliminate defective individuals before term.

A less striking change in the pattern of cardiovascular anomalies was noted by Baird *et al.* (1) when pteroylglutamic acid deficiency was applied for two-day periods at different times in pregnancy. The deficiency maintained from days 7 to 9, 9 to 11, or 10 to 12 caused changes in both the incidence and types of anomalies, with the greatest number and variety of defects following deficiency on days 9 to 11. An interesting difference was noted in the effects of time restriction of vitamin A deficiency and time restriction of pteroylglutamic acid deficiency. Variations in development of the vascular system were noted when the termination of vitamin A deficiency varied from the 10th through the 15th days of gestation, whereas no defects occurred when pteroylglutamic acid deficiency was started later than the 10th day. Although the two experiments differed in many respects, it nevertheless seems clear that these two vitamins do not influence cardiac de-

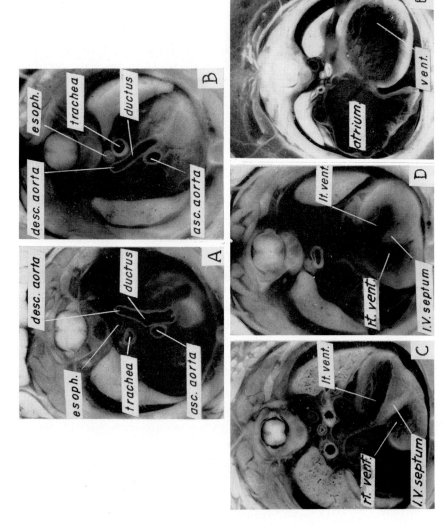

Fig. 6.

TABLE IV. Incidence of aortic arch anomalies and interventricular septaldefects in fetuses removed at progressively earlier ages from vitamin A-deficient mothers[a]

Gestational Age, days	Numbers of Fetuses Studied	Aortic Arch Anomalies, %	Interventricular Septal Defects, %
22	16	6	6
21	10	10	30
20	10	40	30
19	5	40	20
18	7	57	57
17	16	63	63

[a] Data from reference 18.

velopment in precisely the same way at the same time, despite similarities in the overall cardiovascular syndromes produced by each.

By their very nature, cardiovascular anomalies are expected to result in a certain level of mortality during the postnatal period. There is evidence from the animal experiments that this may also be true during the prenatal period (Table IV). When vitamin A-deficient mothers were killed at progressively earlier times in pregnancy and their offspring were removed and examined, it was found that the incidence of aortic arch and cardiac anomalies increased steadily. At term only 6% of surviving offspring were abnormal an this respect, whereas at 17 days of gestation 63% were abnormal. Obviously the intrauterine mortality is high among fetuses with cardiovascular defects during the last five days of gestation in the rat. The cardiovascular anomalies were not necessarily responsible for the increased mortality, but it is clear that they were at least associated with it. There are scattered data indicating that a similar situation exists in human abortuses as compared with stillborn and neonatal infants.

Fig. 6. Cardiac and aortic arch malformations in the offspring of female rats injected with trypan blue on the 7th, 8th, and 9th days of pregnancy. A. Razorblade section through the upper thorax showing the normal relations of the ascending and descending aortae and ductus arteriosus to the trachea and esophagus. B. Right-sided arch of aorta and ductus arteriosus, passing to the right of the trachea and esophagus, in a newborn from an injected female. C. Normal interventricular septum in a control newborn rat. D. Defective interventricular septum in a newborn rat from an injected female. E. Cor biloculare or two-chambered heart in which both the interatrial and interventricular septa failed to develop in a newborn from an injected female.

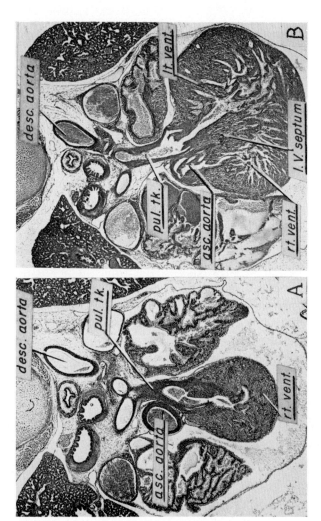

Fig. 7. Histologic sections through: A. Pulmonary trunk and ascending and descending aortae of a normal new-born rat. B. Similar section from a newborn rat whose mother was injected with trypan blue, showing the ascending aorta arising from the right ventricle and the pulmonary trunk arising from the left ventricle, constituting complete transposition of the arterial trunks.

TABLE V.   Variations in the aortic-arch pattern and in the condition of the interventricular septum among siblings from vitamin A deficient mothers. The aortic arch pattern is described in terms of the embryonic arches that persist and connect the heart with the descending aorta[a]

Litter	Sibling	Aortic Arch Pattern	Interventricular Foramen
I	a,b,c,d,	All normal	All closed
II	a	Normal	Closed
	b	Normal	Open, small
III	a	Normal	Closed
	b	rt. 4, lt. 6, rt. 6	Closed
IV	a	lt. 3, no 4, no 6	Open, moderate
	b	rt. 4, no 6	Open, moderate
V	a	rt. 4, rt. 6	Open, small
	b	rt. 6, no 4	Open, moderate
	c	lt. 3, no 4, rt. 6	Open, small
VI	a	Normal	Closed
	b	lt. 4, rt. 4, lt. 6, rt. 6	Closed
VII	a	lt. 3, rt. 3, no 4, no 6	Open, large
	b	lt. 3, rt, 3, no 4, no 6	Open, moderate
	c	Distal rt. subclavian artery	Open, large
VIII	a	rt. 4, no 6	Open, large
	b	rt. 4, lt, 6, rt. 6	Open, small
	c	Distal rt. subclavian artery	Open, moderate
	d	Normal	Open, small

[a] Data from reference 18.

Another principle of teratology is well illustrated by data that happened to involve cardiovascular malformations. In a vitamin A-deficiency experiment in which the mothers were allowed to continue to or nearly to term without receiving any therapy, the offspring were found to exhibit considerable variation as to the types of anomalies within members of the same litter (Table V). When the aortic arch pattern was abnormal in one member of a litter, it was not necessarily abnormal in all other members. When there was more than one individual with aortic arch abnormality, the abnormal individuals were rarely defective in the same way. Only once were identical abnormal aortic arch patterns found in two members of the same litter (sibs a and b, litter VII, Table V). In general, this sort of variation also existed with respect to interventricular septal defects. The siblings within a litter of rats, of course, correspond to diovular or multi-ovular twins. There are known instances of differing cardiovascular anomalies not only in human diovular twins but also in monovular or identical twins as well (10). These observations emphasize the need to consider intrauterine but nongenetic factors when thinking about the etiology of congenital heart disease. Relatively minor hemodynamic variations could conceivably alter the usual course of differentiation within the aortic arch system, and such things as variations in the position of the embryo *in utero* could certainly influence hemodynamic flow patterns in the aortic arch system.

Summary

Six experimental methods are known whereby cardiovascular malformations resembling those in human infants may be produced in laboratory animals. These include maternal vitamin A deficiency, x-irradiation of the embryos, maternal pteroylglutamic acid deficiency, maternal riboflavin deficiency, injection of trypan blue during pregnancy, and exposure of the maternal organism to excess CO_2.

The injection of trypan blue appears to be the most promising method for postnatal studies on congenital heart disease because of its higher yield of defective offspring and because the young are less abnormal otherwise and consequently are more likely to live beyond term.

The patterns of abnormalities produced by the different agents were similar in several respects but notably dissimilar in others, The defects caused by trypan blue and irradiation, included some not seen after vitamin A and pteroylglutamic acid deficiencies.

Analysis of available data seems to indicate that although the resulting anomalies are very much alike, vitamin A deficiency and pteroylglutamic acid deficiency do not exert their influence on the heart at the same period of development.

Cardiovascular anomalies were found to be frequently associated with intrauterine death although there is no proof that they are responsible for it in any large portion of cases.

The fact that the types and the degrees of abnormality varied considerably within the same litter of experimental animals, as within sets of human twins, was taken as an indication that nongenetic but intrauterine factors were operative in modifying if not initiating the maldevelopment.

REFERENCES

1. Baird, C. D. C., Nelson, M. M. Monie, I. W., and Evans, H. M. Congenital cardiovascular anomalies induced by pteroylglutamic acid deficiency during gestation in the rat. *Circulation Research* **2**: 544 (1954).
2. Blalock, A., and Taussig, H. B. The surgical treatment of malformations of the heart in which there is pulmonary stenosis or pulmonary atresia. *J. Am. Med. Assoc.* **128**: 189 (1945).
3. Crafoord, C., and Nylin, G. Congenital coarctation of the aorta and its surgical treatment. *J. Thoracic Surg.* **14**: 347 (1945).
4. Fox, M., and Goss, C. M. Experimental production of a syndrome of congenital cardiovascular defects in rats. *Anat. Record* **124**: 189 (1956).
5. Fox, M., and Goss, C. M. Experimentally produce malformation of the heart and great vessels in rat fetuses. Atrial and caval abnormalities. *Anat. Record* **129**: 309 (1957).
6. Fox, M., and Goss, C. M. Experimentally produced malformations of the heart and great vessels in rat fetuses. Transposition complexes and aortic arch abnormalities. *Am. J. Anat.* **102**: 65 (1958).
7. Gregg, N. McA. Congenital cataract following German measles in the mother. *Trans Ophthalmol. Soc. Australia* **3**: 35 (1941).
8. Gross, R. E. The patent ductus arteriosus. Observations on diagnosis and therapy in 525 surgically treated cases. *Am. J. Med.* **12**: 472 (1952).
9. Haring, O. Personal communication, 1958.
10. McClintock, K. Congenital malformations of the heart in one of identical twins. *Arch. Disease Childhood* **20**: 47 (1947).
11. Nelson, M. M., Baird, D. C., Wright, H. V., and Evans, H. M. Multiple congenital abnormalities in the rat, resulting from riboflavin deficiency induced by the antimetabolite galactoflavin. *J. Nutrition* **58**: 125 (1956).
12. Potts, W. J., Smith, S., and Gibson, S. Anastomosis of the aorta to a pulmonary artery. Certain types in congenital heart disease. *J. Am. Med. Assoc.* **132**: 627 (1946).
13. Richman, S. M., Thomas, W. A., and Konikov, N. Survival of rats with induced cardiovascular anomalies. *Arch. Pathol.* **63**: 43 (1957).
14. Warkany, J., and Nelson, R. C. Appearance of skeletal abnormalities in the offspring of rats reared on a deficient diet. *Science* **92**: 383 (1940).
15. Wilson, J. G. Teratogenic activity of several azo dyes chemically related to trypan blue. *Anat. Record* **123**: 313 (1955).
16. Wilson, J. G., Jordan, H. C., and Brent, R. L. Effects of irradiation on

embryonic development. II. X-rays on the ninth day of gestation in the rat. *Am. J. Anat.* **92:** 153 (1953).

17. Wilson, J. G., Roth, C. B., and Warkany, J. An analysis of the syndrome of malformations induced by maternal vitamin A deficiency. Effects of restoration of vitamin A at various times during gestation. *Am. J. Anat.* **92:** 189 (1953).

18. Wilson, J. G., and Warkany, J. Aortic arch and cardiac anomalies in the offspring of vitamin A deficient rats. *Am. J. Anat.* **85:** 113 (1949).

Etiologic Factors of Congenital Heart Disease

JOSEF WARKANY

College of Medicine, University of Cincinnati, Cincinnati, Ohio

Until twenty years ago fairly good agreement existed concerning the etiology of congenital heart disease (CHD). On anatomical grounds two types of cardiac anomalies were then distinguished. There were the malformations attributed to developmental errors and those thought to be due to fetal endocarditis. Fetal endocarditis in turn was ascribed to infectious or toxic agents which damaged the heart, particularly its valves, endocardium, or myocardium in the fetal period after normal development of the basic cardiac structures and after closure of the septa. Herxheimer (38), for instance, distinguished between the "vitia primae formationis" and cardiac anomalies due to congenital fetal inflammation. Maude Abbott (2) believed that the majority of cardiac defects was due to a primary arrest of development of unknown origin but that "in cases of stenosis of the pulmonary and tricuspid valves in which the interventricular septum is closed and the lesion is limited only to the thickened and fused valve leaflets, the cause is certainly a fetal endocarditis setting in in late embryonic life after the heart is fully formed. The cause of this fetal valvulitis might be any intercurrent infection including rheumatic fever, though the latter so rarely attacks the mother during her pregnancy that it must be regarded as an infrequent cause."

The concept of arrested development in cardiac defects can be traced to Meckel (57), who in 1802 compared such anomalies to the hearts of lower classes of animals, thus initiating the phylogenetic explanations which continued to flourish in our century. But Rokitansky (70), in 1875, at a time when the knowledge of human embryology afforded already a better understanding of ontogenetic processes, related most malformations to phases of arrested development of the human embryo. The concept of fetal endocarditis was apparently introduced by Kreysig (46), who early in the nineteenth century suggested that cases of pulmonary stenosis could be due to disease of the pulmonary artery and its valves, a concept subsequently accepted by many outstanding pathologists. Maternal rheumatic fever, bronchitis, and influenza thus were held responsible for certain forms of CHD (30, 38).

It must be stated, however, that not all investigators accepted the concept of fetal endocarditis. In 1941 Paul Gross (37) reviewed the literature on this subject and pointed out that the criteria for the diagnosis of fetal endocarditis were often very loose, entirely macroscopic, and based on a superficial resemblance of certain cardiac defects to postnatal rheumatic valvulitis. He pointed out that the acute form of this so-called inflammation had never been observed, that scar tissue is absent in the deformed valves, that the assumed etiologic pathogens in the reported cases have been either anamnestically absent or variable in identity, and he came to the conclusion that the occurrence of fetal endocarditis has not been established. Gross considered valvular and parietal endocardial changes previously attributed to fetal endocarditis as developmental defects since they showed no inflammatory residua.

By a strange coincidence it became known in the same year, 1941, that infection of the mother with the rubella virus can cause CHD in her child. This discovery of the opthalmologist Gregg (35) changed all the concepts of the relationship of infection to cardiac pathology. It showed that the results of this infection usually did not resemble anatomically those attributed to fetal endocarditis by the older pathologists and that the virus acting in the first months of gestation often led to cardiac malformations previously ascribed to arrested development. From the beginning Gregg (35) and Swan *et al.* (84) thought that patent ductus arteriosus was the leading malformation in the maternal rubella syndrome. When Rutstein *et al.* (72) reviewed the reported cases in which specific heart lesions were mentioned, they found that in 77 cases patent ductus arteriosus was diagnosed 42 times and septal defects 36 times. Rare diagnoses of tetralogy of Fallot, of coarctation of the aorta, and of patent foramen ovale had also been made. In the series of Gibson and Lewis (32), of 16 cases of CHD attributable to maternal rubella in early pregnancy, 14 had patent ductus, one a tetralogy of Fallot, and one an interatrial septal defect. Ten of the 14 cases of patent ductus were operated upon and 4 of them were found to be complicated by other lesions such as pulmonary stenosis, coarctation of the aorta, or interventricular septal defect. Jackson (39) reported 7 cases, all confirmed by operation or post mortem, showing patent ductus, one of them complicated by pulmonary stenosis and ventricular septal defect. Stuckey (81) observed patent ductus in 13 of his 27 patients. Four cases of patent ductus were complicated by ventricular septal defect or pulmonary valvular stenosis. In addition, there were in this series four patients with ventricular, and three with atrial septal defect, two with tetralogy of Fallot, and one each with aortic stenosis, coarctation of the aorta, pulmonary stenosis, and one with Eisenmenger syndrome. One instance of transposition of the great vessels in this series cannot be attributed to rubella since the maternal infection probably was too late to be accountable for the cardiac lesion. In the series of Lamy *et al.* (48), only 5 of 14 post-rubella cases were diagnosed as patent ductus. In an etiologic study of Campbell (12), there were no acyanotic cases with a history of rubella, all 4 patients with such a history showing signs of tetralogy of Fallot. In a prospective rubella study, Pitt (64) found one patient with patent ductus and one with tricuspid atresia, ventricular septal defect, and abnormal ductus. Thus, it was shown as time went on that the original impression of the Australian investigators, namely that acyanotic heart disease and patient ductus are the most common result of maternal rubella, was correct. However, it also became clear that many cases of patent ductus are complicated by other cardiovascular defects and that some cases of CHD without patent ductus, acyanotic or cyanotic, result from the prenatal infection. Thus, according to present evidence, maternal rubella may produce a wide variety of congenital heart defects in the child.

Quantitative estimates of the role played by rubella in CHD of children are difficult to obtain. Although some of the figures quoted in the literature are open to criticism, certain impressions can be gained from the material available. The risk of congenital malformations resulting from maternal rubella infection acquired during the first trimester of pregnancy has been variously estimated from 10 to 90% (47). In retrospective investigations, such as that of Swan *et al.* (84), "when a woman contracts rubella within the first two months of pregnancy, it would appear that the chances of her giving birth to a congenitally defective child are in the region of 100 per cent." Wesselhoeft (99) summarized many reports which included 656 congenitally deformed and 124 normal children of mothers who had had rubella during early pregnancy. Although he pointed out the fallacies of such retrospective studies, these reports were erroneously interpreted as suggesting an 80% risk of rubella during gestation. In prospective studies, the percentage of malformed children is found to be much lower. Greenberg *et al.* (34) summarized the results of prospective investigations and concluded that the available data indicate that after maternal rubella in the first trimester, about 12% of the children born are affected by congenital malformations. All the many reasons for these discrepancies cannot be discussed here, but it is clear that in retrospective studies cases of maternal rubella with normal outcome are likely to be overlooked.

Prospective studies in which nonepidemic cases are included are also fallible since many rashes diagnosed as rubella may actually have been caused by other etiologic agents. Many rashes can be mistaken for German measles. If such imitative diseases do not result in congenital malformations, it may appear that "German measles" of the mother does not affect her embryo.

Thus, rubella in a woman during the first four months of pregnancy represents a definite threat to her child, but reliable risk figures are not yet available. How many of the abnormal children are suffering from CHD is also not definitely established. Early estimates (35, 84) suggest that 40 to 50% of the children born with congenital malformations following maternal rubella are affected by CHD.

In large clinical retrospective surveys of children with all types of CHD, a history of maternal rubella in early pregnancy is obtained from the parents in about 1 to 2% of the cases (12, 20, 32, 39, 48, 81), but in large surveys of patients with patent ductus arteriosus, such a history of maternal rubella is obtained more often, namely in 2 to 6% of the cases (4, 53, 68, 72). This difference points out again the leading role of patent ductus among the cardiac lesions attributable to rubella during pregnancy.

Although maternal rubella accounts for only a small percentage of the cases of CHD, the discovery of this infection as an etiologic factor is of great theoretical importance. A possibility exists that other viral infections may play a similar role, but it is difficult to indict them. The experience with rubella has shown that the infection causes malformations in some children while others are spared. Sometimes women who are exposed to rubella without getting sick have children with the fully developed rubella syndrome (96). And in rare cases the syndrome is seen in children of mothers who are neither aware of exposure nor of illness during pregnancy (9, 84).

These lessons learned from rubella demonstrate how difficult it is to prove a causal connection between a prenatal virus infection and a congenital cardiac malformation without an experiment of nature like the Australian epidemic. One can suspect that other maternal viral or bacterial diseases during pregnancy are responsible for CHD in children (7, 20, 48), but convincing proof is lacking in most of the cases. Placental transmission of a number of viruses is well established (66) and may lead, in case of Coxsackie group B virus infection, to myocarditis in the late fetal or neonatal period (8, 40), but it has not been shown that this virus interferes with the development of the heart in its early formative periods.

Another point of interest is that rubella during the first trimester of gestation can lead to arrest of development immediately or as late as six or seven months later. In the case of septal defects, development is stopped during or soon after the infection. In the case of patent ductus arteriosus, arrest of development manifests itself many months after the infection. This example illustrates that one cannot assume generally that the time of causation of a defect coincides with the time at which arrest of development manifests itself as a malformation. The discovery showed that an infection may lead not only to forms of CHD such as valvular stenosis which had been attributed to fetal endocarditis in the past, but also to forms of arrested development such as septal defects or tetralogy of Fallot. The mechanism by which maternal rubella leads to arrest of development is not clear as yet. In embryos, fetuses, and children affected by cardiac anomalies of this type, only the end effects are known, but the initial pathologic processes have not been observed (82, 88). Nick (61), who examined four fetuses with septal defects, attributable to maternal rubella, found no microscopic changes, no abnormal tissue structure, and no infiltration in the cardiac tissues although microscopic changes were present in the lens, the inner ear, and the teeth of the abnormal fetuses. Therefore, it is not possible as yet to distinguish anatomically or histologically between cases of CHD caused by infection and those caused by other factors leading to developmental errors.

In the search for other environmental etiologic factors, hypoxia of differing origin has been repeatedly considered. Reports exist indicating that ductus arteriosus is more common in populations living in high altitudes than in those living near sea level. Alzamora *et al.* (3) reported from Lima, Peru, that in their clinical material of 42 cases of patent ductus, 26 or 62% were born at an altitude of over 3000 meters (9843 feet), although if equally distributed, only 15% of the patient population should have been born in these elevated areas. Dexter (18) stated that in Lima, Peru, only 0.8 per 100,000 population have patent ductus, whereas in Junin, an area of high altitude, 3 per 100,000, i.e., four times more, have patent ductus. However, this incidence of 3 per 100,000 is not impressive since in the United States, according to Anderson (4), 25 cases of patent ductus can be expected per 100,000 births. This suggests a very incomplete sampling in the Peru studies. That local factors other than altitude may influence the incidence of patent ductus is suggested by a report from Roscommon County, Ireland (42), which states that in this area, which does not rise over 417 meters (1377 feet), one in 616 school children, that is, 160 in 100,000, are affected by this anomaly.

To support the hypoxia theory one may cite that a few infants with CHD have been born of mothers with cyanotic CHD (76, 90). Before such observations are cited as proof of maternal hypoxia as a cause of CHD, a few other facts must be taken into consideration. A number of reports exist of normal though sometimes small children born to mothers with cyanotic CHD (10, 73, 77). Then there are also reports of mothers with noncyanotic CHD who transmitted CHD to their children (5, 17, 52). And there are observations of fathers with

CHD who had children with CHD (12, 24, 79, 85). These factors point to the possibility of involvement of genetic factors in the transmission of CHD from cyanotic or noncyanotic mothers to their children. It would appear that the role of hypoxia is difficult to prove by consideration of mothers with *congenital* heart disease. It would be much more convincing if *acquired* cyanotic heart disease would often result in cardiac or other congenital defects in the child. This, however, does not seem to be the case. There is no evidence that infants of women with acquired heart disease have children with an excess of congenital malformations (10). Thus, the evidence for hypoxia as an etiologic factor in CHD seems rather precarious at the present time.

If we turn now to the other side of the field of etiology of cardiac defects, we find some, though not overwhelming, evidence for genetic factors at work. They are disclosed in those rather rare instances of malformations of the heart or the great vessels which are transmitted through several generations. Such cases have been reported for patent ductus arteriosus (24, 60, 79). Walker and Ellis (95) mentioned a father with this defect who had eight children, four of them affected with the same anomaly. Taussig (85) reported patent ductus in three generations. Interventricular septal defect in parent and child has been seen repeatedly (17, 52, 75, 90). Apert and Cambessédès (5) observed an acyanotic mother with probable ventricular septal defects who had in each of two marriages a child with the same defect. Atrial septal defect was established by autopsy in a woman who had transmitted the same defect to her daughter and granddaughter (12). Another woman transmitted the anomaly to her son (98). Walker and Ellis (94, 95) reported the case of a father and son with coarctation of the aorta. Lewis *et al.* (50) reported a mother with pulmonary stenosis who had three children with similar malformations. A unique observation of a father and son with dextrocardia was made by Doolittle (21). Both father and son had normal twin sisters. Situs inversus transmitted through four generations was apparently observed by Lancisi (49).

In the cases mentioned so far the same anomaly was transmitted through two or more generations. Sometimes clinically differing anomalies occur in a pedigree. A mother with coarctation of the aorta had two children with patent ductus (80), or a mother with patent ductus, a daughter with aortic coarctation (12). More impressive pedigrees of this type were published in the older literature (31, 86), but the diagnosis was understandably doubtful in some of these early publications. Thus, the "morbus coeruleus" in four generations reported by Burwinkel (11) was probably not due to CHD but to hereditary noncardiac cyanosis as described by Thysell (87) more recently. These single case reports suggest that dominantly inherited CHD exists but it must be rare since in extensive surveys of cardiac patients no index cases have been found with parents affected by CHD (48), or the incidence in parents is not higher than that in the general population (54, 65).

The repeated occurrence of CHD in siblings is probably more frequent than transmission through several generations. However, such familial cases in the same generation are not convincing proof of genetic etiology since repetitive or persistent environmental or maternal factors could be responsible for cardiac defects in several children born to the same mother. To give some examples of cardiac defects in siblings, Joyce and O'Toole (42) reported three children with patent ductus and one with cyanotic CHD, and Kjaergaard (45) and Ekström (24) each observed three siblings with patent ductus. Two siblings with this anomaly have been seen in many families (24, 41, 54, 60, 79, 91). Ventricular septal defect has been reported in three (91) or in two siblings (25, 48, 54, 78, 91). Interatrial septal defect (19), interatrial septal defect with mitral stenosis (16), patent foramen ovale (48), congenital aortic stenosis (74), aortic coarctation (48), tetralogy of Fallot (48, 91), pulmonary valvular stenosis (14, 48), Eisenmenger complex (48), transposition of the great vessels (54), and endocardial fibroelastosis (22, 44, 71, 97) have been observed in siblings. Familial (fraternal) incidence of dextrocardia with situs inversus is a well-recognized phenomenon. There are reports of at least ten sibships with three affected and 29 with two affected by this anomaly (51).*

There are many observations of siblings affected by differing types

---

* Additional cases of familial occurrence of congenital heart disease can be found in R. A. Carleton, W. A. Abelmann, and E. W. Hancock. Familial occurrence of congenital heart disease. *New Engl. J. Med.* **259**: 1237 (1958).

of congenital cardiac anomalies (12, 15, 48, 54). Such isolated records of families with more than one affected member are paralleled by broader statistical studies on the familial incidence of congenital malformations of the heart. The data of McKeown *et al.* (54) suggest that the incidence of congenital cardiac malformation is raised in sibs but is not raised in parents and in cousins of affected individuals. Lamy *et al.* (48) also found an elevated familial incidence with a high rate of consanguineous marriages in their series of patients with CHD, suggesting that genetic factors are operative in the etiology of these disorders. In both studies it was found that the consanguinity rate varied in different clinical types. Because of a high familial incidence and a high incidence of parental consanguinity it has long been suspected that dextrocardia with situs inversus is in many instances genetically determined. Cockayne (15) believed that this anomaly is due to a single recessive autosomal gene, but other investigators assert that more complicated genetic mechanisms are at work (51, 89). On similar grounds Lamy *et al.* (48) suggest that in pulmonary stenosis genetic factors may be operative. This opinion is of special interest since, as pointed out before, pulmonary stenosis was considered by some as an example of a cardiac malformation produced by fetal endocarditis.

In rare instances genetic determination of cardiac anomalies can be proved because the changes of the heart are part of an established hereditary disorder or syndrome. It is very likely that atrial septal defects (63, 100), and it is certain that valvular changes and aortic or pulmonary aneurysms (33, 36, 55) occur as manifestations of the Marfan syndrome (arachnodactyly). Since arachnodactyly is due in most cases to a dominant pleiotropic gene, its cardiovascular components can be cited as rare, dominantly inherited cases of congenital heart disease. Although in many patients cardiovascular manifestations appear late, there can be no doubt that the basic anomaly is congenital. Ventricular and atrial septal defects occur in the Ellis van Creveld syndrome (26) associated with chondroectodermal dysplasia and polydactylism. For this syndrome, recessive inheritance seems well established (58, 59). The same mode of inheritance is considered for most cases of gargoylism, an inborn error of metabolism leading to endocardial, valvular, and coronary changes and often to heart failure. In other families gargoylism may be transmitted as a sex-linked recessive trait. Again it is worth pointing out that in some of these hereditary conditions valvular malformations occur which possibly have been attributed to fetal endocarditis by pathologists of the past. Genetic factors are now suspected also in the etiology of endocardial fibroelastosis (44, 71, 93), a disorder previously considered the prototype of fetal endocarditis (43). Cardiac rhabdomyoma may be a manifestation of tuberous sclerosis, a disorder attributable to a pleiotropic dominant gene. Although for some forms of CHD heredity can be held responsible, these cases are rare and only a few are found and recognized among the many patients of cardiac clinics and hospitals.

A number of observations indicate that the etiology of many cases and types of CHD cannot be explained as yet at the basis of our present day knowledge.

Studies of twins showing that discordance is more frequently observed than concordance (92) suggest that nongenetic factors play an important role in the determination of normality or abnormality of their hearts. Such twin studies afford interesting glimpses into the the etiology of CHD but interpretation of the observations is not always easy. The facts are that in pairs of identical twins (monozygotic twins) occasionally both members of the pair have congenital heart disease (concordance), but more often only one twin is affected (discordance). Nonidentical (dyzygotic) twins are usually discordant in regard to CHD. Monozygotic discordant twins, i.e., identical twins who differ in regard to cardiac defects, demonstrate that nongenetic factors play a role in the etiology of CHD. Since such monozygotic twins have identical genetic endowment, their difference must be attributed to nongenetic factors. Such twins also grow and develop in the same maternal environment. If their genetic endowment, their external or extrauterine maternal environment were at fault, both twins should be equally affected by adverse factors. Since this is not the case, it must be their intrauterine or their "microenvironments" that differ and decide that the heart of one twin develops normally and that of the other abnormally. About such microenvironmental factors we know little, if anything, at the present time.

Our ignorance of some etiologic factors is revealed by other observations. It is known, for instance, that mongolism is complicated by CHD in about 30% of clinical cases (91) and in about 60% of autopsied cases (27), and it can be concluded that whatever the causes of mongolism, they are also indirectly responsible for CHD in this syndrome. Unfortunately, nothing is known about the etiologic factors leading to mongolism except that a definite association exists between increasing maternal age and increasing risk to bearing a mongol child. The association is merely a statistical one and young mothers may also have mongoloid children. From whatever causes, mongolism occurs more often in older mothers than in younger. These causes have not been recognized. That they are already present either in the fertilized ovum or in the very young embryo is revealed by the fact that, in cases of identical twins, both twins are always mongoloid while in cases of nonidentical twins usually one twin only is affected. All one knows, therefore, about the etiology of CHD in mongols is that the acting factors are present more often in older mothers than in younger, and that they may be present already in the fertilized ovum, or that they operate in the earliest embryonic stages. This, of course, is not a satisfactory explanation of CHD in mongolism, but rather points out how much there is to be learned about the maternal age factor in embryologic pathology before this type of CHD will be understood.

Sex is another determinant disclosed by large-scale inquiries. CHD as a whole seems to be equally distributed in males and females (48). However, definite sex preponderance exists in certain anatomical and clinical entities. Of patients with patent ductus only about 30% are male and 70% female (1, 4, 68). Record and McKeown (68) point out that the proportion of affected males is related to the age of the patients at the time of observation as there is a higher early mortality of males with this anomaly. This differential mortality could to a certain extent account for the excess of female survivors. There seems to be general agreement also that atrial septal defects affect females and males in a proportion of 65 to 35% (6, 19, 43, 69).

The sex ratio is reversed in other cardiovascular anomalies. Of autopsy cases with aortic coarctation, 75% are males and 25% females (1, 38, 67). In clinical studies of this malformation, the differences of the sexes is not so marked, but there is still an incidence of over

60% males (48, 65). The prevalence of males in aortic stenosis seems also well established (13, 62). Transposition of the great vessels is another defect prevalent in males. In reported series of transposition, the patients were males in 59% (65), 72% (56), and 75% (23) of the cases. In the Children's Hospital of Cincinnati, of 83 patients with this diagnosis, 69 or 83% were males. More males than females seem to have tetralogy of Fallot (38, 48, 65), and congenital mitral stenosis (28, 29). These sex ratios must have some meaning, but their interpretation is not yet possible. While one could blame early male mortality for prevalence of females with ductus arteriosus in clinical populations, differential mortality does not account for excess of males with aortic defects or transposition of the great vessels. The true meaning of differing sex ratios may be concealed because of our ignorance of the relationship of chromosomal sex and cardiovascular malformations. It was known, for instance, that coarctation of the aorta and other congenital heart anomalies are not rare in girls with Turner's syndrome, but recently we have learned that most of these "girls" are chromatin-negative. Similar surprises may be in store for us in patients with other forms of CHD.

Thus it must be admitted that the etiology of most cases of CHD encountered in hospitals or clinics remains unexplained. However, a few important guideposts have been established in this vast field. These guideposts indicate only few etiologic factors and explain only few of the cases encountered, but they are important because they explain our ignorance and can guide us in the search for other etiologic factors in the future.

We have learned that maternal rubella is now a generally accepted cause of CHD, but that it explains only few of the cases. We have learned also that heredity plays a role in the etiology of certain cardiovascular malformations, but that it is proved for only few of the cases. If cardiac lesions are transmitted through several generations, dominant inheritance is made probable, but an increased incidence of CHD among siblings can be explained by environmental as well as genetic factors. To complicate matters, it is likely that sporadic cases of CHD are sometimes genetically determined. If some of the children with CHD who die in infancy or before reaching the reproductive period represent dominant lethal or semilethal mutations, these cannot be transmitted to subsequent generations. They would appear as sporadic cases in the pedigree and their genetic determination escape us. The conventional criteria for heredity or non-heredity (familial vs. sporadic occurrence) cannot be accepted in the search for etiologic factors.

The fact that in some instances heredity of a certain type of cardiac lesion has been proved does not permit the conclusion that this type is always of genetic origin. We have learned that identical or similar forms of CHD can be caused by genetic factors in some and by rubella in other cases.

We have learned that each known etiologic factor results in a spectrum of clinical forms of CHD. And from the overlapping of the spectra we have learned that for most types of CHD different causes can be responsible.

The association of CHD with syndromes such as mongolism or gonadal dysgenesis (Turner's syndrome) demonstrates that some cardiac defects are caused by processes which we cannot yet understand because the fundamental principles leading to these deviations of development are still obscure. Neither simple Mendelian inheritance nor obvious environmental factors account for these syndromes. The subtlety of nongenetic etiologic factors is also revealed by monozygotic twins who differ in regard to CHD.

After admission of our present ignorance, we need not feel too pessimistic about the future.* The guideposts described indicate the complexity of the problem and the need for further investigation of basic processes involved in normal and abnormal embryonic development. Phenomena apparently far removed from cardiology may be closely linked with the etiology of CHD. Unexpected contributions may come from distant fields. One of the basic discoveries in this subject was made in recent years by an ophthalmologist. In the future,

---

* This paper was presented on December 29, 1958. On January 26, 1959, J. Lejeune, M. Gautier, and R. Turpin [Les chromosomes humains en culture de tissus. *Compt. rend.* **248**: 602 (1959)] announced that they had found 47 chromosomes in three mongoloid boys, and several months later it was discovered that patients with Turner's syndrome also had chromosomal abnormalities [C. E. Ford, K. W. Jones, J. C. de Almeida, and J. H. Briggs. A sex-chromosome anomaly in a case of gonadal dysgenesis (Turner's syndrome). *Lancet* **1**: 711 (1959); J. H. Tjio, T. T. Puck, and A. Robinson. The somatic chromosomal constitution of some human subjects with genetic defects. *Proc. Natl. Acad. Sci.* **45**: 1008 (1959)].

progress in virology, genetics, embryology, experimental teratology and even in gerontology may bring about a better understanding in this area. Yet it should be pointed out that progress need not be left entirely to chance and that a better evaluation of patients with CHD, their mothers, and their families by cardiologists is also required. The present great interest in CHD is chiefly due to the possibility of repairing many defects and of restoring the health of the patients. The brilliant successes in cardiac diagnosis and surgery have been so rapid that few workers in this field have had time to extend their investigations beyond the patient's heart and to include etiologic studies in their activities. This is understandable but not desirable, and it is to be hoped that the cardiac teams active in so many medical centers at the present time will in the future include also persons with an interest in etiology of CHD.

REFERENCES

1. Abbott, M. E. *Atlas of Congenital Heart Disease*. American Heart Association, New York, 62 1936.
2. Abbott, M. E. (personal communication) cited by Gross, reference 37.
3. Alzamora, V., and others. On the possible influence of great altitudes on the determination of certain cardiovascular anomalies. *Pediatrics* 12:259 (1953).
4. Anderson, R. C. Causative factors underlying congenital heart malformations; patent ductus arteriosus. *Pediatrics* 14:143 (1954).
5. Apert, E., and Cambessédès. Malformations cardiaques (maladie de Roger) chez une mère et deux de ses enfants. *Bull. soc. Pédiat. Paris* 28:340 (1930).
6. Bailey, C. P., and others. Congenital interatrial communications: clinical and surgical considerations with description of new surgical technic: atrio-septopexy. *Ann. Internal Med.* 37: 888 (1952).
7. Bass, M. H. Diseases of pregnant woman affecting offspring. *Advances in Internal Med.* 5:15 (1952).
8. Benirschke, K., and Pendleton, M. E. Coxsackie virus infection. An important complication of pregnancy. *Obstet. Gynecol. Survey* 12: 305 (1958).
9. Beswick, R. C., Warner, R., and Warkany, J. Congenital anomalies following maternal rubella. *Am. J. Diseases Children* 78:334 (1949).
10. Burwell, C. S., and Metcalfe, J. *Heart Disease and Pregnancy: Physiology and Management*. Little, Brown, and Co., Boston, Mass., 1958.

11. Burwinkel, O. Morbus coeruleus bei vier Generationen. *Berlin. klin. Wochschr.* **47**:968 (1910).
12. Campbell, M. Genetic and environmental factors in congenital heart disease. *Quart. J. Med.* **18**:379 (1949).
13. Campbell, M., and Kauntze, R. Congenital aortic valvular stenosis. *Brit. Heart J.* **15**:179 (1953).
14. Coblentz, B., and Mathivat, A. Sténose pulmonaire congénitale chez deux soeurs. *Arch. maladies coeur et vaisseaux* **45**:490 (1952).
15. Cockayne, E. A. Genetics of transposition of viscera. *Quart J. Med.* **7**:479 (1938).
16. Courter, S. R., Felson, B., and McGuire, J. Familial interauricular septal defect with mitral stenosis (Lutembacher's syndrome). *Am. J. Med. Sci.* **216**:501 (1948).
17. Debré, R., Cordey, F., and Olivier. Une mère et son enfant atteints de maladie de Roger: hérédité similaire d'une cardiopathie congénitale. *Bull. mém. soc. méd. hôp. Paris,* **47**:1742 (1923).
18. Dexter, L. Congenital defects of heart in high altitudes. *New Engl. J. Med.* **247**:851 (1952).
19. Dexter, L. Atrial septal defects. (St. Cyres lecture, abridged). *Brit. Heart J.* **18**:209 (1956).
20. Dogramaci, I., and Green, H. Factors in etiology of congenital heart anomalies. *J. Pediat* **30**:295 (1947).
21. Doolittle, W. F. Congenital dexicardia. *Boston Med. Surg. J.* **157**:662 (1907).
22. Dordick, J. R. Diffuse endocardial fibrosis and cardiac hypertrophy in infancy; report of 2 cases in consecutive siblings. *Am. J. Clin. Pathol.* **21**:743 (1951).
23. Edwards, J. E. Congenital malformations of the heart and great vessels. *Pathology of the Heart,* S. E. Gould, Editor. Charles C Thomas, Springfield, Ill., 1953, pp. 266–503.
24. Ekström, G. The surgical treatment of patent ductus arteriosus; a clinical study of 290 cases. *Acta Chir. Scand.* **Suppl. 169,** 1952.
25. Ellis, R. W. B. Congenital morbus cordis in two sisters. *Brit. J. Children's Diseases* **33**:286 (1936).
26. Ellis, R. W. B., and van Creveld, S. Syndrome characterized by ectodermal dysplasia, polydactyly, chondrodysplasia and congenital morbus cordis; report of 3 cases. *Arch. Disease Childhood* **15**:65 (1940).
27. Engler, M. *Mongolism (Peristatic Amentia).* Wright, Bristol, England, 1949.
28. Ferencz, C., Johnson, A. L., and Wiglesworth, F. W. Congenital mitral stenosis. *Circulation* **9**:161 (1954).

29. Field, C. E. Congenital mitral stenosis. *Arch. Disease Childhood* 13:371 (1938).
30. Fischer, B. Ueber fötale Infektionskrankheiten und fötale Endokarditis, nebst Bemerkungen über Herzmuskelverkalkung. *Frankfurt. Z. Pathol.* 7:83 (1911).
31. Gänsslen, M., Lambrecht, K., and Werner, M. Die kongenitalen Missbildungen des Herzens. *Handbuch der Erbiologie des Menschen.* Springer, Berlin, 1940, Vol. 4, Pt. 2, pp. 198–217.
32. Gibson, S., and Lewis, K. C. Congenital heart disease following maternal rubella during pregnancy. *Am. J. Diseases Children* 83:317 (1952).
33. Goyette, E. M., and Palmer, P. W. Cardiovascular lesions in arachnodactyly. *Circulation* 7:373 (1953).
34. Greenberg, M., Pellitteri, O., and Barton, J. Frequency of defects in infants whose mothers had rubella during pregnancy. *J. Am. Med. Assoc.* 165:675 (1957).
35. Gregg, N. M. Congenital cataract following German measles in mother. *Trans. Ophthalmol. Soc. Australia* 3:35 (1942).
36. Griffin, J. F., and Koman, G. M. Severe aortic insufficiency in Marfan's syndrome. *Ann. Internal Med.* 48:174 (1958).
37. Gross, P. Concept of fetal endocarditis: a general review with report of an illustrative case. *Arch. Pathol.* 31:163 (1941).
38. Herxheimer, G. Missbildungen des Herzens und der grossen Gefässe, in E. Schwalbe, *Die Morphologie der Missbildungen des Menschen und der Tiere.* G. Fischer, Jena, 1909, Vol. 3, Pt. 3.
39. Jackson, A. V., in *Studies in Pathology*, E. S. J. King and others, Editors. Presented to Peter MacCallum. Melbourne University Press, Melbourne, Australia, 1950.
40. Javett, S. N., and others. Myocarditis in newborn infant; study of outbreak associated with Coxsackie group B virus infection in maternity home in Johannesburg. *J. Pediat.* 48:1 (1956).
41. Jewesbury, R. C. Two similar but somewhat unusual heart conditions in sisters. *Proc. Roy. Soc. Med.* 6:100 (1912–1913).
42. Joyce, J. C., and O'Toole, S. P. Congenital heart disease; report on unusually high incidence in one family. *Brit. Med. J.* 1:1241 (1954).
43. Keith, J. D., Rowe, R. D., and Vlad, P. *Heart Disease in Infancy and Childhood.* The Macmillan Company, New York, 1958.
44. Kelly, J., and Andersen, D. H. Congenital endocardial fibroelastosis. II. A clinical and pathologic investigation of those cases without associated cardiac malformations including report of two familial instances. *Pediatrics* 18: 539 (1956).
45. Kjaergaard, H. Patent ductus Botalli in 3 sisters. *Acta Med. Scand.* 125:339 (1946).

46. Kreysig, F. L. *Krankheiten des Herzens systematisch bearbeitet.* Berlin, 1814–1817, cited by Herxheimer.
47. Krugman, S., and Ward, R. Rubella problem; clinical aspects, risk of fetal abnormality, and methods of prevention. *J. Pediat* 44:489 (1954).
48. Lamy, M., De Grouchy, J., and Schweisguth, O. Genetic and nongenetic factors in the etiology of congenital heart disease: a study of 1188 cases. *Am. J. Human Genet.* 9:17 (1957).
49. Lancisi, cited by Gänsslen *et al.*, reference 31.
50. Lewis, S. M., Sonnenblick, B. P., Gilbert, L., and Biber, D. Familial pulmonary stenosis and deaf-mutism: clinical and genetic considerations. *Am. Heart J.* 55:458 (1958).
51. Lowe, C. R., and McKeown, T. Investigation of dextrocardia with and without transposition of abdominal viscera with report of case in one monozygotic twin. *Ann. Eugenics* 18:267 (1954).
52. Lund, C. J. Maternal congenital heart disease as obstetric problem. *Am. J. Obstet. Gynecol.* 55:244 (1948).
53. Lynxwiler, C. P., and Wells, C. R. E. Patent ductus arteriosus; report of 180 operations. *Southern Med. J.* 43:61 (1950).
54. McKeown, T., MacMahon, B., and Parsons, C. G. Familial incidence of congenital malformation of heart. *Brit. Heart J.* 15:273 (1953).
55. McKusick, V. A. Cardiovascular aspects of Marfan's syndrome: heritable disorder in connective tissue. *Circulation* 11:321 (1955).
56. MacMahon, B., McKeown, T., and Record, R. G. Incidence and life expectation of children with congenital heart disease. *Brit. Heart J.* 15:121 (1953).
57. Meckel, J. F. *De cordis conditionibus abnormibus.* Halae typ. Batheanis, 1802, cited by Herxheimer, reference 38.
58. Metrakos, J. D., and Fraser, F. C. Evidence for hereditary factor in chondroectodermal dysplasia (Ellis-van Creveld syndrome). *Am. J. Human Genet.* 6:260 (1954).
59. Mitchell, F. N., and Waddell, W. W., Jr. Ellis-van Creveld syndrome. Report of two cases in siblings. *Acta Paediat.* 47:142 (1958).
60. Nadas, A. S. *Pediatric Cardiology.* W. B. Saunders Company, Philadelphia, Pa., 1957.
61. Nick, J. Ueber die Untersuchungen von Herzen menschlicher Keimlinge mit den Zeichen einer Embryopathia rubeolica. *Schweiz. Z. Pathol. u. Bakteriol.* 16:653 (1953).
62. Ongley, P. A., Nadas, A. S., Paul, M. H., Rudolph, A. M., and Starkey, G. W. B. Aortic stenosis in infants and children. *Pediatrics* 21:207 (1958).
63. Piper, R. K., and Irvine-Jones, E. Arachnodactylia and its association with congenital heart disease, report of a case and review of literature. *Am. J. Diseases Children* 31:832 (1926).

64. Pitt, D. B. Congenital malformations and maternal rubella, *Med. J. Australia* 1:233 (1957).
65. Polani, P. E., and Campbell, M. Aetiological study of congenital heart disease. *Ann. Human Genet.* 19:209 (1955).
66. Potter, E. L. Placental transmission of viruses, with special reference to the intrauterine origin of cytomegalic inclusion body disease. *Am. J. Obstet. Gynecol.* 74:505 (1957).
67. Pritchard, J. A. Coarctation of the aorta and pregnancy. *Obstet. Gynecol. Survey* 8:775 (1953).
68. Record, R. G., and McKeown, T. Observations relating to aetiology of patent ductus arteriosus. *Brit. Heart J.* 15:376 (1953).
69. Roesler, H. Interatrial septal defect. *Arch. Internal Med.* 54:339 (1934).
70. von Rokitansky, C. *Die Defecte der Scheidewände des Herzens. Pathologisch-anatomische Abhandlung.* W. Braumüller, Wien, 1875.
71. Rosahn, P. D. Endocardial fibroelastosis: old and new concepts. *Bull. N. Y. Acad. Med.* 31:453 (1955).
72. Rutstein, D. D., Nickerson, R. J., and Herald, F. P. Seasonal incidence of patent ductus arteriosus and maternal rubella. *Am. J. Diseases Children* 84, Pt. 2: 199 (1952).
73. Scherlis, S., and Soloway, L. R. Pregnancy and labor in patient with cardiac anomaly, probable tetratology of Fallot. *Am. J. Obst. Gynecol.* 44:697 (1942).
74. Schöne, G. Ueber angeborene Herzfehler. Ein Beitrag zu ihrer Diagnostik, Zirkulationsgrösse und ihrem familiären Vorkommen. *Deut. Arch. klin. Med.* 184:129 (1939).
75. Seitz, R., and Baumann, H. Familiäres Vorkommen von angeborenen Herzfehlern. *Z. Kreislaufforsch.* 27:13 (1935).
76. Selzer, A., and Laqueur, G. L. Eisenmenger complex and its relation to uncomplicated defect of ventricular septum; review of 35 cases of Eisenmenger's complex including 2 new cases. *A. M. A. Arch. Internal Med.* 87:218 (1951).
77. Simon, D. L., and Lustberg, A. Case of truncus arteriosus communis compatible with full term pregnancy. *Am. Heart J.* 42: 617 (1951).
78. Snelling, D. B. Familial congenital heart disease: patent ductus arteriosus in sisters. *J. Am. Med. Assoc.* 108:1502 (1937).
79. Starer, F. Analysis of 50 cases of persistent ductus arteriosus. *Brit. Med. J.* 1:971 (1953).
80. Stein, I., and Barber, D. J. Congenital heart disease; case reports on 3 members of family. *Am. Heart J.* 30:118 (1945).
81. Stuckey, D. Congenital heart defects following maternal rubella during pregnancy. *Brit. Heart J.* 18:519 (1956).
82. Swan, C. A study of three infants dying from congenital defects follow-

ing maternal rubella in the early stages of pregnancy. *J. Pathol. Bacteriol.* **56**:289 (1944).

83. Swan, C., and Tostevin, A. L. Congenital malformations in infants following infectious diseases during pregnancy, with special reference to rubella. A third series of cases. *Med. J. Australia* **1**:645 (1946).

84. Swan, C., Tostevin, A. L., Moore, B., Mayo, H., and Black, G. H. B. Congenital defects in infants following infectious diseases during pregnancy, with special reference to relationship between German measles and cataract, deafmutism, heart disease, and microcephaly, and to period of pregnancy in which occurrence of rubella is followed by congenital abnormalities. *Med. J. Australia* **2**:201 (1943).

85. Taussig, H. B. *Congenital Malformations of the Heart.* Commonwealth Fund, New York, 1947.

86. Tedesco, P. A. Su due casi di cardiopatia congenita familiare. *Cuore e circolazione* **17**:76 (1933).

87. Thysell, T. Non-cardiac familiar cyanosis. *Acta paediat.* **30**:212 (1942–43).

88. Töndury, G. Les embryopathies causées par des viroses de la grossesse. *Études Néo-Natales* **2**:107 (1953).

89. Torgersen, J. Genic factors in visceral asymmetry and in development and pathologic changes of lungs, heart and abdominal organs. *Arch. Pathol.* **47**:566 (1949).

90. Tucker, A. W., Jr., and Kinney, T. D. Interventricular septal defect (Roger's disease) occurring in mother and her 6 month fetus. *Am. Heart J.* **30**:54 (1945).

91. Uchida, I. Familial occurrence of congenital heart disease, in J. D. Keith, R. D. Rowe, and P. Vlad, *Heart Disease in Infancy and Childhood.* The Macmillan Company, New York, 1958, pp. 129–132.

92. Uchida, I. A., and Rowe, R. D. Discordant heart anomalies in twins. *Am. J. Human Genet.* **9**:133 (1957).

93. Ullrich, O. Angeborene Herzhypertrophie mit Endokardfibrose bei zwei eineiigen Partnern von männlichen Drillingen. *Z. menschl. Verebungs-u. Konstitutionslehre* **21**:585 (1938).

94. Walker, W. G. Coarctation of the aorta in father and son. *New Engl. J. Med.* **211**:1192 (1934).

95. Walker, G. C., and Ellis, L. B. The familial occurrence of congenital cardiac anomalies. *Proc. New Engl. Heart Assoc.*, **1940–41**; 26.

96. Warkany, J. Etiology of congenital malformations. *Advances in Pediat.* **2**:1 (1947).

97. Weinberg, T., and Himmelfarb, A. J. Endocardial fibroelastosis (so-called fetal endocarditis); report of 2 cases occurring in siblings. *Bull. Johns Hopkins Hosp.* **72**:299 (1943).

98. Weinstein, A. Congenital heart disease in successive generations. In-

teratrial septal defect in a 63-year-old woman and her 31-year-old son. *J. Chronic Diseases* **8:**669 (1958).

99. Wesselhoeft, C. Medical Progress; rubella (German measles) and congenital deformities. *New Engl. J. Med.* **240:**258 (1949).

100. Wood, P., McDonald, L., and Emanuel, R. *The Clinical Picture Correlated with Physiological Observations in the Diagnosis of Congenital Heart Disease.* Pediatric Clinics of North America, W. B. Saunders Company, Philadelphia, Pa., 1958, p. 981.

II

PATHOLOGIC PHYSIOLOGY

Pathologic Anatomy of Congenital Intra- and Extracardiac Shunts Unassociated with Intracardiac Obstruction to Flow*

MAURICE LEV

Congenital Heart Disease Research and Training Center, Hektoen Institute, and the Department of Pathology, Northwestern University School of Medicine, Chicago, Illinois

Under the title of intracardiac shunts the following anomalies will be considered: (*a*) atrial septal defect, (*b*) ventricular septal defect, and (*c*) common atrioventricular orifice. The following extracardiac shunts will be discussed: (*a*) patent ductus arteriosus, (*b*) aorticopulmonary septal defect, and (*c*) anomalous pulmonary venous drainage. Conditions alluded to briefly will be (*a*) coronary arteriovenous (a-v) fistula, (*b*) ruptured aneurysm of an aortic sinus of Valsalva into the right side of the heart, and (*c*) pulmonary a-v fistula.

In the presentation of each anomaly the discussion will evolve about (*a*) the nature of the anomaly and (*b*) the nature of the cardiac pathologic complex associated with the anomaly. Such complexes include the reactions of the myocardium, endocardium, valves, orifices, and vessels to the anomaly. The reaction of the pulmonary vascular tree to the anomaly will not be discussed in this paper, and the reader is referred to the paper by Dr. Edwards.

In the present paper, the term *hypertrophy* of the myocardium of a chamber implies an increase in muscle mass of the chamber. The term *volume hypertrophy* signifies that the hypertrophy of the chamber is related to contraction on an increased volume. The term *pressure hypertrophy* implies that the hypertrophy of the chamber is related to contraction against increased peripheral resistance. This

---

* This investigation was supported by a Research Grant (H-3351) from the National Heart Institute of the National Institutes of Health, U.S. Public Health Service.

term includes pressure related to increased flow, with the pulmonary vascular resistance remaining normal, and pressure related to increased pulmonary vascular resistance. The term *dilatation* implies that the chamber is enlarged with respect to the size of the normal chamber at the respective age in the absence of failure. Thus, volume hypertrophy is associated with dilatation.

The term *endocardial hypertrophy* (fibroelastosis) signifies a process of focal or diffuse thickening of the endocardium (1–3). This is visible at the gross level as white streaks or plaques or a diffuse whitening or opacity. Histologically there is a proliferation of the smooth muscle, elastic and collagen fibers of the endocardium with or without a proliferation of the elements of the subendocardium. The term endocardial sclerosis signifies a process of degeneration occurring in endocardial hypertrophy. This consists of degenerative changes in the elastic, collagen, and muscle fibers in zones of hypertrophy. This process of hypertrophy and sclerosis occurs in aging and in heart disease. Both diffuse and focal endocardial hypertrophy and sclerosis are related to hemodynamic change. In aging, focal hypertrophy and sclerosis is apparently related to flow exacerbated by increased tension, whereas diffuse endocardial hypertrophy and sclerosis are apparently fundamentally related to increased tension. The term *hemodynamic changes* in a valve signifies changes which at the present time are considered to be due to altered hemodynamics in the valve region, the exact nature of which remains to be elucidated (4). In the atrioventricular valves they are characterized grossly by thickenings at the line of closure and whitening and thickening in the substance and sometimes at the base of the valve. In the semilunar valves, they are characterized grossly by thickening of the noduli, the line of closure, the base, and often the entire substance of the valve. Microscopically, they are characterized by endocardial hypertrophy and sclerosis of the proximalis and less the distalis, with elastosis and collagenosis of the spongiosa. These changes more or less resemble the "normal" aging changes of valves, but this problem needs further elucidation.

Atrial Septal Defect (5–16)

Atrial septal defects may be divided into (*a*) defects related to the fossa ovalis or "secundum" type defects; (*b*) persistent ostium primum,

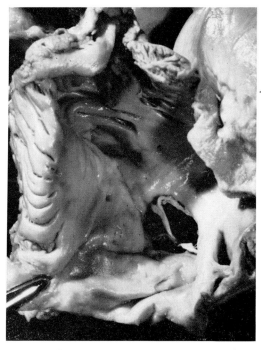

Fig. 1. Atrial septal defect of the secundum type. Right atrial view.

or "primum" type defects, and (*c*) defects related to the region proximal and cranial to the fossa ovalis.

A simple secundum type defect is restricted to the region of the fossa ovalis. It may be represented by a single or multiple perforations in the fossa (Fig. 1). However, secundum type defects, in addition to involving the fossa, may extend beyond the fossa, inferiorly so that it is almost in confluence with the mouth of the inferior vena cava (Fig. 2), superiorly so that its upper border is the roof of the atria (Fig. 3), or proximally and caudally so that there is no proximal atrial septum. The last anomaly may be associated with abnormal entry of the pulmonary veins or straddling inferior vena cava, entering both atria.

A primum type defect represents an opening in the atrial septum distal to and not involving the fossa ovalis. In the usual type, the lower margin of the defect is confluent with the central fibrous body and the adjacent portion of the mitral and tricuspid annuli (Fig. 4). Here, in almost all cases, there is a cleft anterior leaflet of the mitral

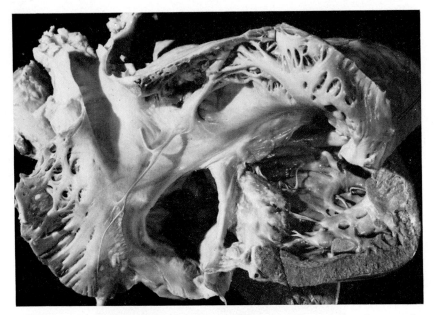

Fig. 2.   Atrial septal defect of the secundum type, with extension downward to mouth of inferior vena cava. Right atrial and right ventricular view.

valve (Fig. 5). In a few cases, in addition, the tricuspid valve is cleft (Fig. 6). In the unusual type, the defect does not extend to the central fibrous body, but a varying distance proximal to it, so that a small portion of atrial septum intervenes between the defect and the central fibrous body. Here the mitral and tricuspid valves are not cleft (Fig. 7).

The defect which is present proximal and cranial to the fossa ovalis is related to the orifice of the superior vena cava. Here the defect may be one or multiple, and may be associated with a superior vena cava which straddles the atrial septum or abnormal entry of the pulmonary veins. Some defects have both secundum and primum characteristics (Fig. 7). Various types of defects may be associated, and defects may be confluent resulting in almost or complete absence of the atrial septum.

The conduction system is usually not altered in secundum defects. In primum defects the a-v node and the beginning of the bundle are deviated posteriorly and hug the inferior and distal borders of the defect (17, 18).

Atrial septal defect of a primum or secundum type may be asso-

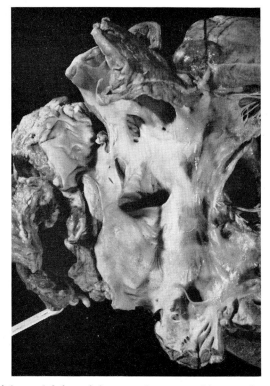

Fig. 3.   Atrial septal defect of the secundum type with extension upward to the roof of the right atrium. Right atrial view.

ciated with mitral stenosis (Lutembacher's). A secundum type defect is part of the complex of tricuspid atresia and stenosis, entry of the pulmonary veins into the right atrium, and hypoplasia of the aortic tract complexes. It is often associated with transposition complexes and with pulmonary stenosis with normal aortic root. These complexes are not discussed in this paper. An atrial septal defect may be complicated by subacute bacterial endocarditis and paradoxical embolism and brain abscess.

COMPLEX ASSOCIATED WITH ISOLATED ATRIAL SEPTAL DEFECT

In the metamorphosis of this complex, in the beginning the right atrium and ventricle present a volume hypertrophy owing to a left-to-right shunt at the atrial level. This may become associated with a

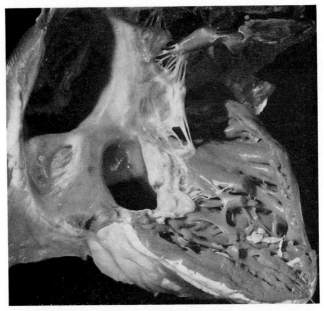

Fig. 4.   Atrial septal defect of the primum type. Right atrial and right ventricular view.

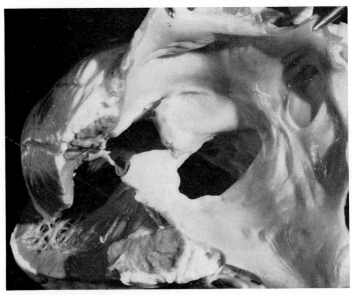

Fig. 5.   Atrial septal defect of the primum type. Left atrial and left ventricular view, showing cleft aortic leaflet of the mitral.

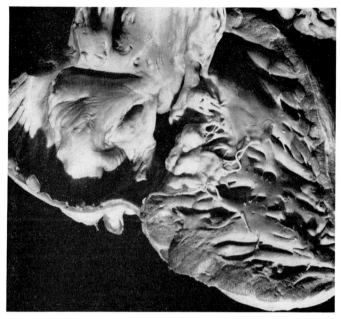

Fig. 6. Atrial septal defect of the primum type. Right atrial and right ventricular view showing cleft medial leaflet of the tricuspid.

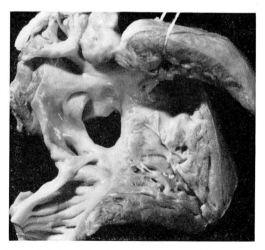

Fig. 7. Atrial septal defect. Mostly primum type, with an element of secundum type.

pressure hypertrophy related to flow, and eventually with a still further increment of pressure hypertrophy related to pulmonary arteriolar resistance. These chambers thus show considerable hypertrophy and marked dilatation (Fig. 2). The left atrium is normal in size, while the left ventricle is smaller than normal. Where there is increased pulmonary resistance and hence decreased left-sided flow, the left atrium and ventricle are both smaller than normal and presumably have a decreased muscle mass.

The tricuspid and pulmonic orifices are enlarged (often with pulmonary and tricuspid insufficiency), and the pulmonary artery is dilated. The mitral and aortic orifices are smaller than normal and there is hypoplasia of the aorta. The endocardium of the atria, especially the right, and the right ventricle, show increased focal endocardial hypertrophy and sclerosis. The right ventricle occasionally shows diffuse endocardial hypertrophy and sclerosis. The tricuspid and pulmonic valves likewise show hemodynamic change. Occasionally, the septal surface of the sinus of the right ventricle may present an altered muscular architecture, apparently related to altered hemodynamics in fetal life (Fig. 8).

The above described complex is typical of secundum defects. Primum defects show in addition the effects of changes in the central fibrous body and mitral and tricuspid valves. Here, in addition to

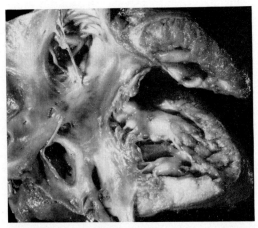

Fig. 8. Abnormal architecture of the trabecular pattern of the sinus of the right ventricle in atrial septal defect.

the effects of the defect, the left ventricle has a tendency to be hypertrophied, probably due to mitral regurgitation. This regurgitation also exacerbates the hypertrophy of the right side of the heart. There may also be tricuspid regurgitation with a further increment of volume hypertrophy on the right side. In addition, pressure hypertrophy is more common and more intense than in secundum defects. The a-v node and bundle may be congenitally interrupted or secondarily involved in fibrosis with varying degrees of heart block (18). The cause of death in atrial septal defect is related to right ventricular failure, pulmonary thrombosis, and pneumonitis.

Ventricular Septal Defects (12, 14, 19–31)

Ventricular septal defects are best divided according to size and position. According to size they are classified as small and large. The small defect presents little hemodynamic change in the myocardium, whereas the large presents important hemodynamic change in the myocardium.

With respect to position, for descriptive purposes, defects may be classified by their relationship to the anterior muscular, the posterior muscular septum and the pars membranacea (32). The anterior septum may be defined as that part anterior to the lower margin of the septal band of the crista. As seen from the left side, it is relatively brief, extending from the anterior part of the pars membranacea in an oblique manner a varying distance to the anterior wall. The posterior muscular septum is the remainder of the muscular septum. A defect may be present in the anterior part of the anterior septum, unrelated to the pars membranacea. As seen from the left side it lies beneath the left aortic cusp. As seen from the right, it lies just below the pulmonary artery, thus excavating the crista (Fig. 9). This is the high ventricular septal defect of Taussig. A defect may lie in the posterior part of the anterior septum with or without the involvement of the adjacent pars membranacea (Fig. 10). As seen from the left side it lies below the right aortic cusp and to a varying extent the posterior aortic cusp. As seen from the right side it lies in the posterior part of the conus just below the crista and in some cases the anterior part of the sinus, adjacent to the medial leaflet of the tricuspid. The crista is either excavated or deviated anteriorly. If this defect is con-

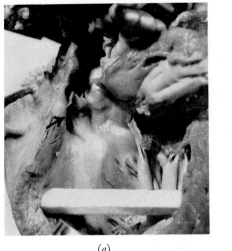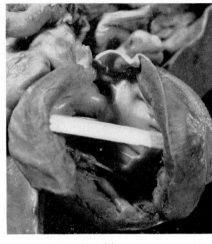

(a)   (b)

Fig. 9.   High ventricular septal defect of Taussig: (*a*) Left ventricular view. (*b*) Right ventricular view. Arrow points to the defect.

fluent with the mouth of the aorta, then the aorta overrides, and the architecture of the crista is disturbed. If the defect is not confluent with the mouth of the aorta, then the aorta may not override, and the crista is not deviated, but it may be excavated. A defect may lie in the posterior part of the anterior septum, unrelated to the pars membranacea, or in the general boundary between the two muscular septa. As seen from the left side the defect is at the base of the septum but away from the aorta, between the anterior wall of the left ventricle and the anterior leaflet of the mitral valve. As seen from the right side, it lies in the upper part of the sinus of the right ventricle, below the crista, and distal to the base of the tricuspid valve. A defect may lie in the pars membranacea, partially or completely replacing it (Fig. 11). As seen from the left side it lies below the junction of the right and posterior aortic cusps. As seen from the right side, it opens below the crista and into the anterior part of the medial leaflet of the tricuspid. A defect may be present in the posterior septum at the base (Fig. 12). As seen from the left side, it lies adjacent or distal to the annulus of the aortic leaflet of the mitral valve, unrelated to the pars membranacea. As seen from the right side it opens into the sinus of the right ventricle at the base adjacent to the tricuspid valve or distal

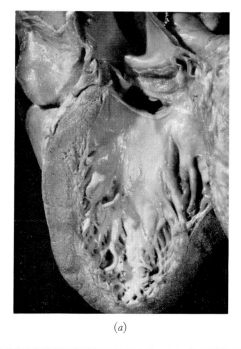

(*a*)

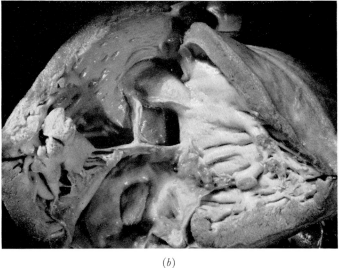

(*b*)

Fig. 10.   Ventricular septal defect in posterior part of the anterior muscular septum, involving part of the pars membranacea. The defect is confluent with the mouth of the aorta. (*a*) Left ventricular view. (*b*) Right ventricular view.

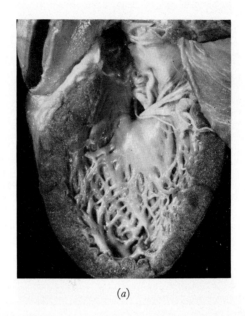

(a)

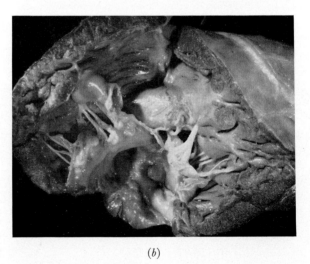

(b)

Fig. 11. Ventricular septal defect involving the pars membranacea. (a) Left
ventricular view. (b) Right ventricular view.

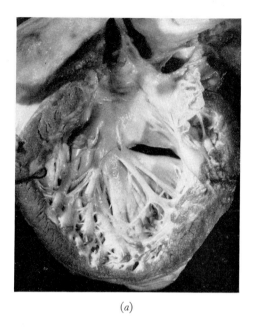

(a)

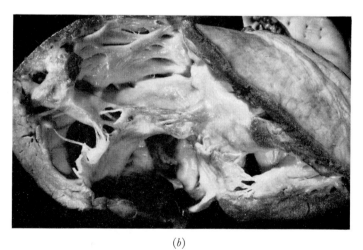

(b)

Fig. 12. Ventricular septal defect involving the basal part of the posterior ventricular septum. (a) Left ventricular view. (b) Right ventricular view.

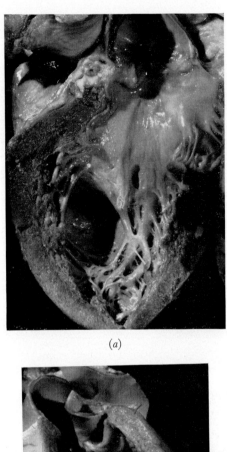

(a)

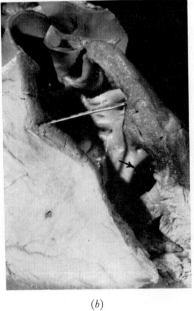

(b)

Fig. 13. Ventricular septal defect involving the near apical region of the posterior ventricular septum. (a) Left ventricular view. (b) Left lateral right ventricular view. Arrow points to the defect in (b).

118

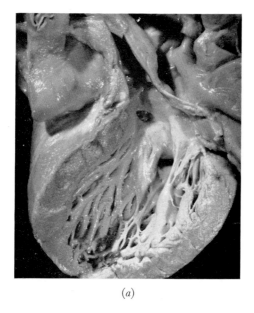

(a)

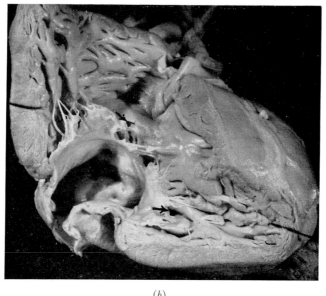

(b)

Fig. 14. Two ventricular septal defects, one involving the posterior part of the anterior ventricular septum and one involving the basal part of the posterior ventricular septum. (a) Left ventricular view. (b) Right ventricular view. Arrows point to the defects in (b).

to it. A defect may be present in the posterior septum at the apical portion (Fig. 13). Here it lies in the apical portion of the right and left ventricles unrelated to the valves. Multiple defects are not rare (Fig. 14). In subaortic defects the a-v bundle courses along the posterior and distal walls of the defect (17, 18, 33–35) (Fig. 15).

A ventricular septal defect may be part of many complexes, such as transposition complexes, tricuspid atresia and stenosis complexes, and pulmonary stenosis with normal aortic root. It may form an associated complex with coarctation of the aorta, patent ductus arteriosus, and atrial septal defect. These complexes are not the subject of the present discussion. Where the aorta overrides or comes out

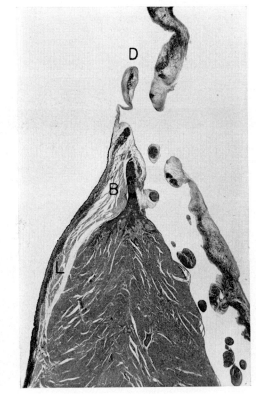

Fig. 15.   Photomicrograph of the bundle of His in ventricular septal defect. Weigert-van Gieson stain X12. B. Bundle of His. L. Left bundle branch. D. Defect of the ventricular septum.

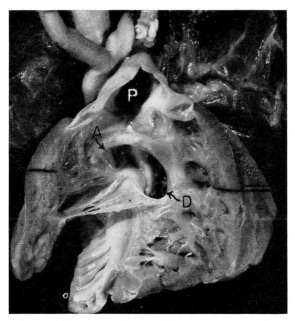

Fig. 16. Double outlet right ventricle (partial transposition) with large pulmonary tract. Right ventricular view. A. Aortic ostium. D. Ventricular septal defect. P. Pulmonary artery.

completely from the right ventricle, the anatomy of the outflow tract of the right ventricle is markedly disturbed, yet the physiology may be that of isolated ventricular septal defect (Fig. 16). This may be called overriding aorta with ventricular septal defect (anatomic Eisenmenger complex), or partial transposition with large pulmonary tract, dependent upon the position of the aorta. This is not the same as the Eisenmenger syndrome of the clinicians. Ventricular septal defects may be associated with right aortic arch, vascular rings, bicuspid aortic and pulmonic valve, and left superior vena cava.

COMPLEX ASSOCIATED WITH ISOLATED VENTRICULAR SEPTAL DEFECT

Where the defect is small, there is probably always a small amount of volume hypertrophy of the right ventricle. This, however, is probably insufficient to reach the clinical level. In the metamorphosis of the complex associated with large defects, the right ventricle in the

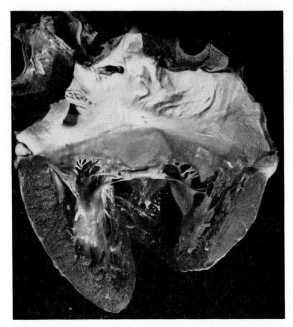

Fig. 17.   Ventricular septal defect complex. Left atrial and ventricular view. Note the hypertrophy and dilatation of both chambers, and hemodynamic changes on the aortic leaflet of the mitral valve.

beginning may present only a volume hypertrophy, which early or later may have an increment of pressure hypertrophy due to flow. The left atrium also shows a volume hypertrophy. Thus, the right ventricle and left atrium are hypertrophied and dilated (Figs. 17, 18). The left ventricle is dilated, and in many cases it is hypertrophied (Fig. 17), but apparently not in all. This is related to the opposing tendencies of increased volume and decreased peripheral resistance. In the later stages, the right ventricle shows an increment of pressure hypertrophy due to increased pulmonary vascular resistance with a lesser hypertrophy and dilatation of the left atrium. In still later stages, the right ventricle is tremendously hypertrophied due to pressure, while the left atrium and ventricle are normal in size and thickness or atrophied.

The tricuspid orifice is normal while the pulmonary orifice is dilated (in some cases with pulmonary insufficiency). The mitral orifice is dilated in the early stages (Fig. 17), while the aortic orifice is smaller

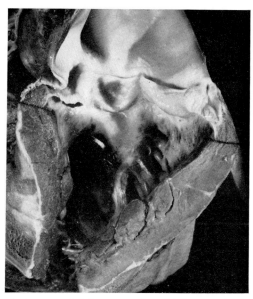

Fig. 18.   Ventricular septal defect complex. Right ventricular view. Note the marked hypertrophy of the right ventricle and hemodynamic changes of the pulmonic valve.

than normal at all times. With increase in pulmonary resistance, the mitral orifice becomes normal again. The endocardium of the right ventricle shows increased focal endocardial hypertrophy, while the left atrium and ventricle show a more generalized endocardial hypertrophy. The endocardial hypertrophy is in general more marked in the region of the defect. The tricuspid and pulmonic valves show hemodynamic changes (Figs. 18, 19). This may be present in the mitral valve (Fig. 17), and if the defect is confluent or close to the aorta, parts of the aortic valve may likewise show such changes.

Ventricular septal defect may show, in addition, hemodynamic effects which may have occurred in fetal life. Thus the trabecular architecture of the left and right ventricles may be altered (Fig. 20), and the mitral valve itself may have a second opening. In a remarkable case of aortic stenosis with ventricular septal defect, both the mitral and tricuspid orifices showed secondary openings which I assume to be related to altered hemodynamics created by the defect (Fig. 21).

Ventricular septal defect is more often complicated by subacute bac-

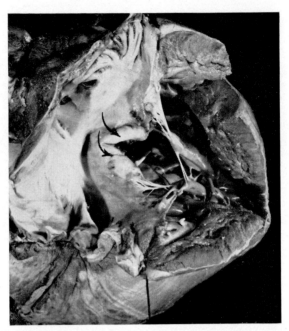

Fig. 19. Ventricular septal defect complex. Right atrial and right ventricular view. Note the hemodynamic changes of the adjacent portions of the anterior and medial leaflets of the tricuspid valve. Arrows point to the lesion.

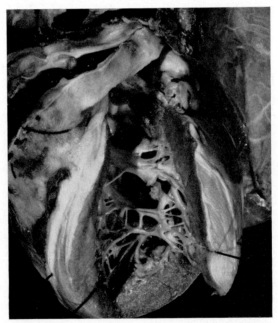

Fig. 20. Ventricular septal defect complex. Left ventricular view. Note the abnormal trabeculation of this chamber.

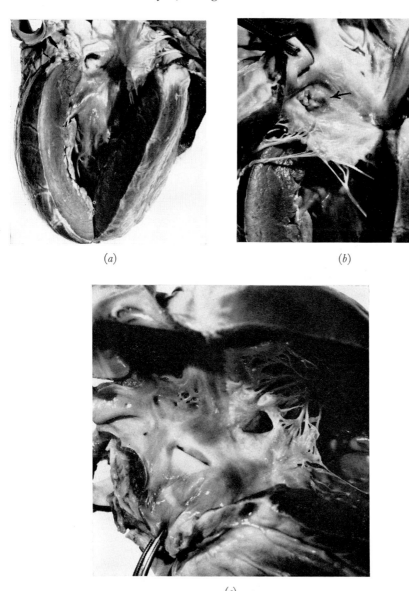

(a)

(b)

(c)

Fig. 21. Aortic stenosis with ventricular septal defect associated with accessory mitral and tricuspid orifices. (a) Left ventricular view, showing the defect. (b) Left atrial and left ventricular view showing accessory orifice in the anterior leaflet of the mitral valve. (c) Right atrial and right ventricular view showing accessory orifice in the tricuspid valve. Arrow in (b) points to the accessory orifice in the mitral valve.

terial endocarditis than is atrial septal defect. In addition, the defect
may pull down, herniate, or deform the aortic valve to produce aortic
insufficiency. It may become adherent to the tricuspid valve to produce
tricuspid insufficiency. And it may result in secondary fibrotic changes
in the region of the bundle of His to produce congenital heart block
or acquired heart block in congenital heart disease. The cause of death
in isolated ventricular septal defect complex is related to left ventricular failure in children, right ventricular failure in both children
and adults, pneumonitis, and subacute bacterial endocarditis.

Common Atrioventricular Orifice (canal) (12, 14, 36–40)

In this anomaly the mitral and tricuspid orifices are represented
by a common orifice (Fig. 22). This orifice is guarded by a varying
arrangement of valves. There are always two small lateral or inferior
leaflets, one on the right and one on the left side. These represent
the corresponding normal right and left inferior or posterior leaflets.
There is almost always a large posterior leaflet representing a fusion
of the entire or part of the normal medial leaflet of the tricuspid with
the inferior portion of the normal aortic leaflet of the mitral. There is
a varying architecture in the remainder of the valve. Often there is a
large anterior leaflet representing the fusion of the anterior portion
of the normal aortic leaflet of the mitral with either part of the normal medial leaflet of the tricuspid or with the anterolateral leaflet of
the tricuspid. Or there may be a separate left anterior leaflet representing the anterior part of the normal anterior leaflet of the mitral,
accompanied by a separate right anterior leaflet representing the normal anterolateral leaflet of the tricuspid. The attachments of the
valve structures representing the right anterior and inferior leaflets
of the tricuspid and the cleft or uncleft medial leaflet of the tricuspid
are normal. In the left ventricle, however, it is common to have
either a small posterior papillary muscle, a ridgelike structure remi-
niscent of the posterior papillary muscle, or no papillary muscle at
all. The anterior papillary muscle is usually normal. Accordingly, the
valve structure representing the anterior portion of the aortic leaflet
of the mitral valve is attached to the anterior papillary muscle and by
chordae to the septum. That representing the posterior portion of
the aortic leaflet of the mitral is attached to the inferior papillary

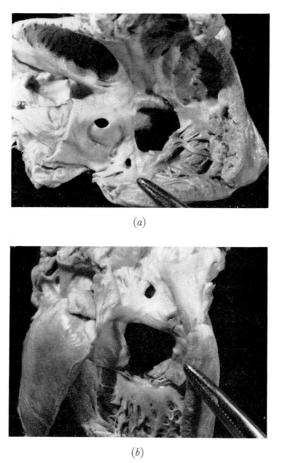

(*a*)

(*b*)

Fig. 22.   Common a-v orifice. (*a*) Right atrial and right ventricular view. (*b*) Left atrial and left ventricular view.

muscle when present, and by chordae to the septum. That representing the inferior leaflet on the left side is either attached to both papillary muscles and where the posterior papillary muscle is absent, to only the anterior papillary muscle and by chordae to the septum.

Associated with a common a-v orifice there is always a combined defect consisting of a patent foramen primum and a ventricular septal defect, both of varying size. In many instances there is also a patent foramen ovale, and in some cases the atrial septal defect begins at the proximal border of the limbus, so that the atrial portion of the defect is a combined foramen ovale and foramen primum (cor triloculare biventriculosum). The ventricular septal component of the defect consists of an absence of the pars membranacea and the adjacent portion of the posterior septum. In a few instances the posterior ventricular septum may be markedly defective. Sometimes the adjacent portion of the anterior ventricular septum is also involved. The a-v node is displaced posteriorly, and the a-v bundle courses on the posterior and distal rim of the combined defect (17) (Fig. 23). The tricuspid portion of the orifice is usually larger than the mitral, the two may be equal in size, or uncommonly the left may be larger. In some cases the atrial septum is shifted to the left beyond the plane of the ventricular septum so that the tricuspid portion of the orifice points in part toward the left ventricle. A common a-v orifice may be associated rarely with overriding aorta or partial transposition, or more commonly with complete transposition of the arterial trunks. This paper does not deal with these complexes.

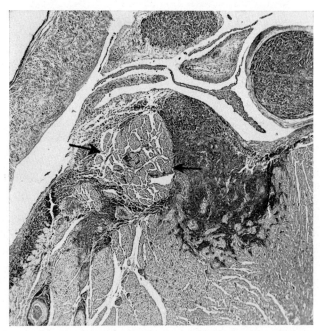

Fig. 23.   Photomicrograph of the bundle of His in common a-v orifice. Weigert-van Gieson stain ×45. Arrows point to the bundle lying on the lower margin of the defect.

There is a tendency to group common a-v orifice and patent foramen primum together. It is best to distinguish between these anomalies even though there are intermediate forms where the distinction is difficult to make. This distinction is valuable to the clinician and surgeon because of the difference in outlook in the two conditions and in the surgical approach and result.

COMPLEX ASSOCIATED WITH ISOLATED COMMON A-V ORIFICE

The effects of the anomaly are related to the atrial and ventricular septal defects, possibly complicated by the insufficiency of the common valve. The right atrium and ventricle present a volume and pressure hypertrophy early. With the increase in pulmonary resistance there is a further increment of pressure hypertrophy. Thus these chambers show hypertrophy and dilatation. The effect of the possible insufficiency of the common valve cannot be gaged. The left atrium is usually small in size and thin, while the left ventricle varies in size and thickness, related to the size of the ventricular septal defect, the position of the atrial septum, the amount of pulmonary resistance, and the amount of insufficiency of the mitral portion of the a-v valve. In some cases this chamber appears to present a volume hypertrophy, but in others the chamber is normal in size or small, and normal in thickness or atrophied.

The tricuspid and pulmonic orifices are enlarged on account of increased flow. The aortic orifice is small on account of decreased flow. The endocardium of the atria and ventricles shows increased focal endocardial hypertrophy and sclerosis. The common a-v valve and the pulmonic valve show increased hemodynamic change. The cause of death in this complex is usually right ventricular failure.

Patent Ductus Arteriosus (12, 14, 41–49)

A ductus which is patent after three months of age is abnormal. However, a ductus whose diameter equals that of the main pulmonary artery is abnormal at any time after birth. The patent ductus varies in size and diameter. It may be more than a centimeter long, or so brief as to constitute a window joining the aorta and left pulmonary artery at the normal site of the ductus. Its diameter may equal as much as 2 cm. It enters the aorta distal to the isthmus, and the left pulmonary artery close to the bifurcation into right and left pulmonary arteries. Its aortic orifice may be wider than that at the pulmonary orifice and funnel-shaped.

A ductus arteriosus may be part of a hypoplasia of the aortic tract complex, fetal coarctation complex, and may be associated with transposition complexes, adult coarctation and almost any other complex. It may also be associated with bicuspid aortic valve, subaortic stenosis, ventricular septal defect, and pulmonary stenosis. These complexes are not the subject of the present discussion.

COMPLEX ASSOCIATED WITH ISOLATED PATENT DUCTUS ARTERIOSUS

In the earlier phase of the complex, with a left-to-right shunt and normal pulmonary resistance, the left atrium and ventricle are the seat of a volume hypertrophy (Fig. 24). They are thus dilated as well as hypertrophied. The right atrium and ventricle are normal in size and thickness. The pulmonary artery is dilated, and the base of the aorta is enlarged. There may be diffuse endocardial hypertrophy of the left atrium and ventricle. The mitral, aortic, and pulmonic valves may show increased hemodynamic change. The pulmonary artery may show sclerotic change. If the left-to-right shunt is great, there may be a pressure hypertrophy of the right ventricle due to flow and, perhaps, back pressure.

Where the pulmonary resistance becomes increased, the right ventricle shows a further increment of pressure hypertrophy, while the left atrium and ventricle are still hypertrophied and dilated. The right ventricle may now show increased focal endocardial hypertrophy and the pulmonic valve increased hemodynamic change. Where pulmonary resistance becomes markedly increased with decreased pulmonary flow, the left atrium and ventricle are normal or small in size, and normal or atrophied in thickness.

In the unusual ductus (Fig. 25) with marked increase in pulmonary resistance early (or perhaps from birth) the massive hypertrophy of the right ventricle is in marked contrast with the normal or small left ventricle. In still another poorly understood type (Fig. 26), there is a marked hypoplasia of the ascending aorta associated with biventricular hypertrophy. This may be a conversion from a hypoplasia of

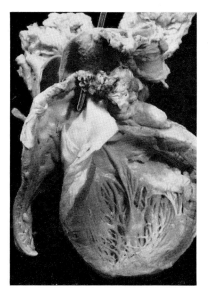

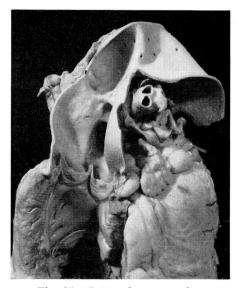

Fig. 24. Patent ductus arteriosus complex. Probe is in the ductus. Note the marked hypertrophy and dilatation of the left ventricle.

Fig. 25. Patent ductus arteriosus complex with early development of pulmonary hypertension. Right ventricular view showing the widely patent window type ductus, and the marked right ventricular hypertrophy.

the aortic tract complex. The cause of death in patent ductus arteriosus is usually left or right ventricular failure, subacute bacterial endocarditis, or pulmonary embolus.

Aorticopulmonary Septal Defect (12, 14, 50–53)

In this anomaly there is a round or oval smooth-edged opening 2–16 mm in diameter between the aorta and the pulmonary artery (Fig. 27). It is usually situated in the first few centimeters above the aortic valve, but it may be present midway between the valve and the innominate artery. This anomaly may be associated with a perforation of the pulmonary valve, bicuspid aortic valve, a ventricular septal defect, patent ductus arteriosus, patent foramen ovale, infantile coarctation, or origin of the right pulmonary artery from the aorta.

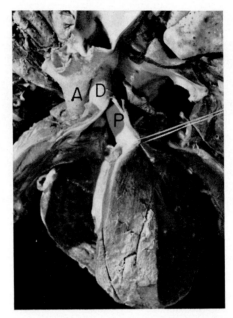

Fig. 26. Patent ductus arteriosus complex with hypoplasia of the aorta. Note the right and left ventricular hypertrophy. A. Aorta. D. Ductus arteriosus. P. Pulmonary artery.

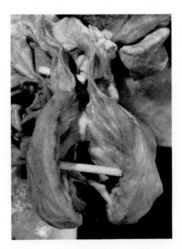

Fig. 27. Aorticopulmonary septal defect complex. Right ventricular view. Upper wooden rod passes through the defect.

COMPLEX ASSOCIATED WITH AORTICOPULMONARY SEPTAL DEFECT

This resembles that of patent ductus arteriosus with a greater tendency toward pulmonary hypertension of flow and vascular resistance type and hence more right ventricular hypertrophy. The left atrium and ventricle exhibit a volume hypertrophy where there is increased pulmonary flow. Hemodynamic changes in endocardium and valves resemble those in patent ductus.

Anomalous Pulmonary Venous Drainage into the Systemic Venous Circuit (12, 14, 54–65)

In this anomaly, one, two, or all four pulmonary veins enter directly or indirectly into the right atrium. In total anomalous pulmonary venous drainage, all pulmonary veins usually enter a persistent left superior vena cava, the left innominate (Fig. 28), the coronary sinus or the right atrium. Less frequently they enter into the right superior vena cava, the inferior vena cava, the portal vein, the ductus venosus, or the pancreatic vein. Where only one or two veins enter abnormally, on the right side they usually enter the right superior vena cava, or the right atrium, and on the left side the innominate, the left superior vena cava, or the coronary sinus. One or two pulmonary veins may also enter the azygos, inferior vena cava, or left subclavian. Where there is complete aberrant drainage of the pulmonary veins, they usually form a single channel prior to joining the systemic veins, except where they join the right atrium directly. In the latter group, they may join by multiple channels, or they may enter into an antechamber located in the postero-superior wall of the right atrium, to the left of the superior and inferior venae cavae and superior to the coronary sinus. There is always an associated atrial septal defect in total anomalous pulmonary venous drainage, and often in partial. Occasionally there is mild pulmonary and mitral stenosis.

COMPLEX ASSOCIATED WITH TOTAL ANOMALOUS PULMONARY VENOUS
   DRAINAGE

There are two types of complexes: (*a*) the supradiaphragmatic and (*b*) the infradiaphragmatic.

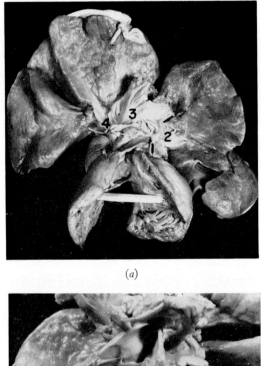

(a)

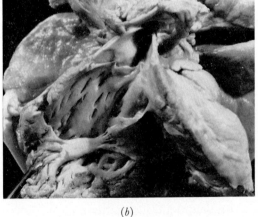

(b)

Fig. 28.   Complex associated with entry of the pulmonary veins into the left innominate vein. (a) View of the heart and lungs, and thoracic veins: 1, confluence of the pulmonary veins; 2, left pulmonary veins; 3, left innominate vein; 4, beginning of right superior vena cava. (b) Right ventricular view.

Supradiaphragmatic. The right atrium and ventricle show a marked volume hypertrophy (Fig. 28). Thus they are also dilated. In some cases early there is also a pressure hypertrophy with or without increase in pulmonary vascular resistance. The left atrial and ventricular chambers are much smaller than normal and they are atrophied. The pulmonary artery is dilated and the aorta is small. The endocardium of the right atrium and ventricle shows increased focal endocardial hypertrophy. Occasionally the right ventricle may show diffuse endocardial hypertrophy (Fig. 29). The tricuspid and pulmonic valves show hemodynamic change.

Infradiaphragmatic. When the pulmonary veins enter the portal vein, the complex is modified by pulmonary venous obstruction. The entire heart is said not to be enlarged, even though the hypertrophy of the various chambers is as in the usual complex. In addition to the changes in the lungs, not discussed here, there is an increment of pressure hypertrophy of the right ventricle.

COMPLEX ASSOCIATED WITH PARTIAL ANOMALOUS PULMONARY VENOUS
   DRAINAGE

Here the effects on the right atrium and ventricle and the opposite effects on the left atrium and ventricle are much less.

Cornary a-v Fistula (66–68) and Ruptured Aneurysm of a Sinus of Valsalva into Right Side of Heart

The right coronary artery may communicate with the coronary sinus, a coronary vein, the right atrium, and the right ventricle or pulmonary artery. Less commonly a coronary artery may communicate with the left atrium or left ventricle. These communications usually appear as circoid aneurysms. Dependent upon the chamber or vessel they enter, they may produce a volume hypertrophy, and the patient may die in cardiac failure. Similarly, there may be a fistulous communication between the aorta and the right atrium or right ventricle, or a rupture of an aneurysm of the sinus of Valsalva into the right atrium or right ventricle.

Pulmonary a-v Fistula (69, 70)

They usually consist of a distended afferent artery, a distended efferent vein, and an intervening loculated vascular sac or labyrinth of distended vessels. There is usually no association with the bronchial arterial tree or other vessel coming from the aorta. Such fistulae are

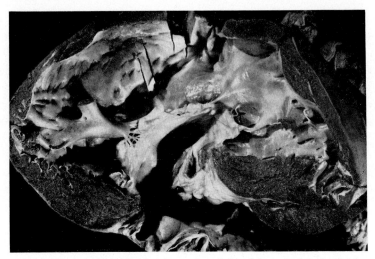

Fig. 29.   Diffuse endocardial hypertrophy of the right ventricle in total anomalous pulmonary venous drainage.

often multiple. In most cases the increase in cardiac work is insufficient to produce hypertrophy of the heart. Where there is a communication with the bronchial arterial tree, the left ventricle may be hypertrophied.

ACKNOWLEDGMENT

Figures 9, 22, 24, 25, 27, and 28 are reproduced by permission from M. Lev, *Autopsy Diagnosis of Congenitally Malformed Hearts.* Copyright 1953, Charles C Thomas, Springfield, Ill.

REFERENCES

1. Lev, M. The histology of the heart and its changes with age. *Military Med.* **120:**257 (1957).
2. McMillan, J. B., and Lev, M. The aging heart. I. Endocardium. *J. Gerontol.* **14:**268 (1959).
3. Lev, M., and McMillan, J. B. Aging changes in the heart. *Bourne's Cellular Changes in Ageing.* In press.
4. McMillan, J. B., and Lev, M. The aging heart. II. The valves. To be published.
5. Keith, J. D., and Forsyth, C. C. Auricular septal defects in children. *J. Pediat.* **38:**172 (1951).

6. Braudo, J. L., Nadas, A. S., Rudolph, A. M., and Neuhauser, E. B. D. Atrial septal defects in children: A clinical study with special emphasis on indications for operative repair. *Pediatrics* **14**:618 (1954).
7. Disenhouse, R. B., Anderson, R. C., Adams, P., Jr., Novick, R., Jorgens, J., and Levin, B. Atrial septal defect in infants and children. *J. Pediat.* **44**:269 (1954).
8. Swan, H., Blount, S. G., Jr., and Virtue, R. W. Direct vision suture of interatrial septal defect during hypothermia. *Surgery* **38**:858 (1955).
9. Lewis, F. J., Taufic, M., Varco, R. L., and Niazi, S. The surgical anatomy of atrial septal defects: experiences with repair under direct vision. *Ann. Surg.* **142**:401 (1955).
10. Kirklin, J. W., and Ellis, F. H., Jr. Atrial septal defect. *Surg. Clin. North Am.* **35**:989 (1955).
11. Blount, S. G., Jr., Balchum, O. J., and Gensini, G. The persistent ostium primum. *Circulation* **13**:499 (1956).
12. Lev, M. *Congenital Heart Disease in Systemic Pathology*, Vol. I, O. Saphir, Editor. Grune and Stratton, New York, 1958.
13. Lev, M. The pathology of congenital heart disease, in *Cardiology*, A. Luisada, Editor. Blakiston Publishing Division, McGraw-Hill Book Co., New York, 1959.
14. Edwards, J. E. Congenital malformations of the heart and great vessels, in *Pathology of the Heart*, S. E. Gould, Editor. Charles C Thomas, Springfield, Ill., 1953, p. 266.
15. Dexter, L. Atrial septal defect. *Brit. Heart J.* **18**:209 (1956).
16. Campbell, M., Neill, C., and Suzman, S. The prognosis of atrial septal defect. *Brit. Med. J.* **1**:1375 (1957).
17. Lev, M. The architecture of the conduction system in congenital heart disease. I. Common atrioventricular orifice. *A.M.A. Arch. Pathol.* **65**:174 (1958).
18. Lev, M. The conduction system, in *Pathology of the Heart*, 2nd ed., S. E. Gould, Editor. Charles C Thomas, Springfield, Ill., 1959.
19. Selzer, A. Defect of the ventricular septum: summary of twelve cases and review of the literature. *Arch. Internal Med.* **84**:798 (1949).
20. Engle, M. A. Ventricular septal defect in infancy. *Pediatrics* **14**:16 (1954).
21. Wood, P., Magidson, O., and Wilson, P. A. O. Ventricular septal defect with a note on acyanotic Fallot's tetralogy. *Brit. Med. J.* **16**:387 (1954).
22. Blount, S. G., Jr., Mueller, H., and McCord, M. C. Ventricular septal defect. *Am. J. Med.* **18**:871 (1955).
23. Harned, H. S., Jr., Crothers, C. N., and Whittemore, R. Diagnosis of atrial and ventricular septal defects. *Am. J. Diseases Children* **90**:211 (1955).
24. Becu, L. M., Fontana, R. S., DuShane, J. W., Kirklin, J. W., Burchell,

H. B., and Edwards, J. E. Anatomic and pathologic studies in ventricular septal defect. *Circulation* 14:349 (1956).

25. Heath, O., Brown, J. W., and Whitaker, W. Muscular defects in the ventricular septum. *Brit. Heart J.* 18:1 (1956).

26. Brostoff, P., and Rodbard, S. Hydrodynamics in ventricular septal defects. *Am. Heart J.* 51:325 (1956).

27. Warden, H. E., DeWall, R. A., Cohen, M., Varco, R. L., and Lillehei, C. W. A surgical-pathologic classification for isolated ventricular septal defects and for those in Fallot's tetralogy based on observations made on 120 patients during repair under direct vision. *J. Thoracic Surg.* 33:21 (1957).

28. Gasul, B. M., Dillon, R. F., Vrla, V., and Hait, G. Ventricular septal defects. Their natural transformation into those with infundibular stenosis or into the cyanotic or non-cyanotic type of tetralogy of Fallot. *J. Am. Med. Assoc.* 164:847 (1957).

29. Zacharioudakis, S. C., Terplan, K., and Lambert, E. C. Ventricular septal defects in the infant age group. *Circulation* 16:374 (1957).

30. Manheimer, E., Ikkos, D., and Jonsson, B. Prognosis of isolated ventricular septal defects. *Brit. Heart J.* 19:333 (1957).

31. Brotmacher, L., and Campbell, M. The natural history of ventricular septal defect. *Brit. Heart J.* 20:97 (1958).

32. Lev, M. The pathologic anatomy of ventricular septal defect. *Diseases of Chest* 35:533 (1959).

33. Truex, R. C., and Bishof, J. K. Conduction system in human hearts with interventricular septal defects. *J. Thoracic Surg.* 35:421 (1958).

34. Reemtsma, K., and Copenhaver, W. M. Anatomic studies of the cardiac conduction system in congenital malformations of the heart. *Circulation* 17:271 (1958.

35. Lev, M. The architecture of the conduction system in congenital heart disease. III. Ventricular septal defect. *A.M.A. Arch. Pathol.* In press.

36. Rogers, H. M., and Edwards, J. E. Incomplete division of the atrioventricular canal with patent interatrial foramen primum (persistent common a-v ostium). *Am. Heart J.* 36:28 (1948).

37. Wakai, C. S., and Edwards, J. E. Developmental and pathologic considerations in persistent common atrioventricular canal. *Proc. Staff Meetings Mayo Clinic* 31:487 (1956).

38. Giraud, G., Latour, H., Puech, P., and Roujon, J. Les formes anatomiques et les bases du diagnostic de la persistance du canal auriculoventriculaire commun. *Arch. maladies coeur et vaisseaux.* 50:909 (1957).

39. Campbell, M., and Missen, G. A. K. Endocardial cushion defects; common atrioventricular canal and ostium primum. *Brit. Heart J.* 19:403 (1957).

D., Rowe, R. D., Vlad, P., and O'Hanley, J. H. Complete
ıs pulmonary venous drainage. *Am. J. Med.* **16**:23 (1954).

R. P. Anomalous pulmonary veins; report of nine cases.
ernal Med. **42**:11 (1955).

da, G., Lukas, D. S., and Steinberg, I. Anomalous drainage of
ary veins. Clinical, physiologic and angiocardiographic fea-
m. J. Med. **18**:883 (1955).

. H., Jr., and Kirklin, J. W. Anomalous pulmonary venous con-
ns. *Surg. Clin. North Am.* **35**:997 (1955).

V. L., Lester, R. G., Lillehei, C. W., and Varco, R. L. Total
alous pulmonary return. An analysis of thirty cases. *Circulation*
3 (1956).

enfeld, I., Silverblatt, M. L., and Strauss, L. Total anomalous
monary venous drainage into the portal vein. *Am. Heart J.* **53**:616
57).

hnson, A. L., Wiglesworth, F. W., Dunbar, J. S., Siddoo, S., and
rajo, M. Infradiaphragmatic total anomalous pulmonary venous
onnection. *Circulation* **17**:340 (1958).

wan, H. J. C., Kirklin, J. W., Becu, L. M., and Wood, E. H. Anomalous
onnection of right pulmonary veins to superior vena cava with interatrial communications. Hemodynamic data in eight cases. *Circulation*
16:54 (1957).

Guntheroth, W. G., Nadas, A. S., and Gross, R. E. Transposition of
the pulmonary veins. *Circulation* **18**:117 (1958).

. Knoblich, R., and Rawson, A. J. Arteriovenous fistula of the heart.
Am. Heart J. **52**:474 (1956).

7. Steinberg, I., Baldwin, J. S., and Dotter, C. T. Coronary arteriovenous
fistula. *Circulation* **17**:372 (1958).

68. Edwards, J. E., Gladding, T. C., and Weir, A. B., Jr. Congenital communication between the right coronary artery and the right atrium.
J. Thoracic Surg. **35**:662 (1958).

69. Yater, W. M., Finnegan, J., and Griffin, H. M. Pulmonary arteriovenous fistula (Varix). Review of the literature and report of two cases.
J. Am. Med. Assoc. **141**:581 (1949).

70. Claiborne, T. S., and Hopkins, W. A. Aorta-pulmonary artery communication through the lungs. *Circulation* **14**:1090 (1956).

40. Paul, M. H. Endocardial cu...
    ventricular canal and persister...
    Am. Nov. 1958.
41. Gross, R. E., and Longino, L. A...
    tions from 412 surgically treated...
42. Gross, R. E. The patent ductus a...
    and therapy in 525 surgically treat...
43. Yu, P. N., Lovejoy, F. W., Joos, H...
    Studies of pulmonary hypertension. \...
    arteriosus with marked pulmonary hy...
    (1954).
44. Lyon, R. A., and Kaplan, S. Patent duc...
    atrics **13**:357 (1954).
45. Gordon, A. J., Donoso, E., Kuhn, L. A., R...
    stein, A. Patent ductus arteriosus with rev...
    Med. **251**:923 (1954).
46. Whitaker, W., Heath, D., and Brown, J. W...
    with pulmonary hypertension. *Brit. Heart J.*...
47. Harris, P. Patent ductus arteriosus with pu...
    Brit. Heart J. **17**:85 (1955).
48. Cosh, J. A. Patent ductus arteriosus, a follow-...
    Brit. Heart J. **19**:13 (1957).
49. Heiner, D. C., and Nadas, A. S. Patent ductus arter...
    with pulmonic stenosis; a report of six cases with add...
    congenital anomalies. *Circulation* **17**:232 (1958).
50. Spencer, H., and Dworken, H. J. Congenital aortic s...
    communication between aorta and pulmonary artery...
    880 (1950).
51. Downing, D. F. Congenital aortic septal defect. *Am. H...*
    (1950).
52. Sprengel, R. A., and Brown, A. F. Aortic septal defect. *A...*
    48:796 (1954).
53. Kirklin, J. W., Ellis, F. H., Jr., and Clagett, O. T. Aortico-p...
    septal defect. *Surg. Clin. North Am.* **35**:975 (1955).
54. Brody, H. Drainage of the pulmonary veins into the right sid...
    heart. *Arch. Pathol.* **33**:221 (1942).
55. Edwards, J. E., and DuShane, J. W. Thoracic venous anomalies. ...
    cular drainage of the left atrium and the left innominate vein (...
    atria-cardinal vein) associated with mitral atresia and prema...
    closure of the foramen ovale (case 1). II. Pulmonary veins drain...
    wholly into the ductus venosus (case 2). *Arch. Pathol.* **49**:517 (1950).
56. Healey, J. E. An anatomic survey of anomalous pulmonary veins: thei...
    clinical significance. *J. Thoracic Surg.* **23**:433 (1952).

57. Keith, J...
    anomalo...
58. Johnson...
    Ann. In...
59. Sepulve...
    pulmor...
    tures. ...
60. Ellis, ...
    nectic...
61. Gott...
    anor...
    13:5...
62. Ros...
    pu...
    (1...
63. Jo...
    G...
    c...
64. S...
    ...
65...

66...

6...

Hemodynamic Alterations Associated with Ventricular Septal Defects*

MARC SAVARD, H. J. C. SWAN, JOHN W. KIRKLIN, EARL H. WOOD

Mayo Clinic and Mayo Foundation,† Rochester, Minnesota

This discussion of the hemodynamic alterations associated with ventricular septal defect will be restricted to general considerations concerning the physical factors that determine the direction and magnitude of blood flow across such defects. The concepts to be presented are not new since they have been discussed previously by such authors as Selzer (1), Wood and co-workers (2), Blount and associates (3), Brotmacher and Campbell (4), and Grosse-Brockhoff (5). However, heretofore such discussions have been largely theoretical in nature since data relating the actual size, that is, the area of the defect, to the hemodynamic alterations associated with such a defect *in vivo* have been scarce or completely lacking.

With the advent of surgical correction of ventricular septal defects under direct vision, it became possible to measure the dimension of these defects in living patients and relate these measurements to the associated hemodynamic alterations as determined at preoperative cardiac catheterization (6) or during operation just prior to the cardiotomy (7). It is the object of this discussion to present data which demonstrate that the hemodynamic alterations associated with a ventricular septal defect are determined chiefly by two factors: (*a*) the area of the defect and (*b*) the reactions of the pulmonary vasculature, that is, changes in resistance to pulmonary blood flow, associated with the defect.

* This study was supported in part by research grant no. H-3532 from the National Institutes of Health, Public Health Service.

† The Mayo Foundation, Rochester, Minnesota, is a part of the Graduate School of the University of Minnesota.

141

For purposes of simplifying this discussion, ventricular septal defects will be separated into the two categories, large and small, on the basis of the cross-sectional area of the defect. Figure 1 shows a diagram of the central circulation in the presence of a small and of a large ventricular septal defect. It is recognized that there are many defects whose size is intermediate between these two categories.

A small ventricular septal defect is defined as one the size of which provides a significant resistance to blood flow between the left and the right ventricle. On the basis of the data to be presented subsequently, it is believed that the area of such a defect is less than 1 square centimeter per square meter of body surface (cm^2/m^2). Since such a defect provides a considerable resistance to blood flow across the defect, the ventricular septum still constitutes an effective, albeit incomplete, barrier between the left ventricle and the right ventricle.

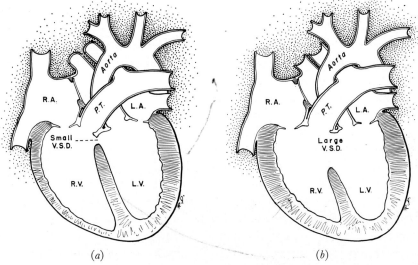

(a)   (b)

Fig. 1. Diagram of the heart and great vessels in the presence of (*a*) a small ventricular septal defect (V.S.D.) and (*b*) a large V.S.D. R.A. and L.A. indicate the right and left atria, R.V. and L.V. the ventricles, and P.T. the pulmonary artery. The small V.S.D. (area less than 1 cm^2/m^2) offers a high resistance to blood flow across it so that the relationship of left-to-right ventricular pressures is maintained essentially normal. The large V.S.D. (area more than 1 cm^2/m^2) has such a low resistance to blood flow that the ventricular septum is ineffectual. Consequently, right ventricular pressure is elevated toward or equal to left ventricular pressure.

It would be expected, therefore, that the pressure in the right ventricle would be significantly lower than that in the left ventricle and would approach the situation that prevails in the normal circulation. Under such circumstances the magnitude of a left-to-right shunt is determined chiefly by the size of the defect, that is, the resistance of blood flow across it.

A large ventricular septal defect is defined as one whose size is such that the resistance to blood flow through the defect is very small, and therefore the function of the ventricular septum as a barrier between the left and right ventricles is ineffectual. In this situation the pressure in the right ventricle and that in the left ventricle are maintained essentially equal since the large septal defect acts as a pressure equalizer between the two ventricles. The magnitude and the direction of the blood flow through such a defect is not determined primarily by the size of the defect but rather by the relative resistances to the outflow of blood from these two common-pressure chambers via the aorta on the left and the pulmonary artery on the right side of the incomplete septum. The resistances to blood flow out through the aorta and the pulmonary artery are determined in turn by the magnitude of the systemic vascular resistance on the one hand and the pulmonary vascular resistance on the other. If pulmonary vascular resistance is low in relation to systemic vascular resistance, a large left-to-right shunt will be present and vice versa.

The two most important factors in determining the hemodynamics associated with a ventricular septal defect are therefore (*a*) the resistance to blood flow across the defect, that is, the size of the defect, and (*b*) the relation of the pulmonary to the systemic vascular resistance. Since systemic vascular resistance has been demonstrated to remain essentially normal in patients with ventricular septal defects, the alterations in pulmonary vascular resistance that are frequently associated with this disease are of great importance in determining the hemodynamic effects associated with the defect.

Material and Methods

Direct measurements of the maximal and minimal dimensions of ventricular septal defects visualized during open cardiotomy under conditions of total body perfusion have been made in a series of 43 patients. The defects were assumed to be elliptical, and their areas were calculated by means of the equation relating the area of an ellipse to the magnitude of the major and minor axes. Each of these patients was studied by cardiac catheterization prior to operation. These studies included determination of the pulmonary and systemic blood flows and the simultaneous recording of pulmonary-artery and systemic arterial pressure and of right ventricular and systemic arterial pressure (6). In the large majority of these patients the determinations were carried out both when the patient was breathing air and when breathing oxygen.

The resistance to blood flow across the ventricular septal defects was assumed to be related to a pressure/flow ratio which was calculated as follows. The pressure gradient across the ventricular septal defect was assumed to be directly related to the difference between the systolic arterial pressure recorded at the radial artery and the systolic pressure recorded simultaneously from the right ventricle, expressed in millimeters of mercury. A figure related to the pressure/flow ratio across the defect was then calculated by dividing this difference in systolic pressure by the estimated magnitude of the left-to-right shunt expressed in liters per minute.

Results

A significant relationship between the areas of the ventricular septal defects measured in this series of patients and the calculated resistances to blood flow across these defects as determined at cardiac catheterization is demonstrable as shown in Fig. 2. The pressure/flow indexes obtained both while the patients were breathing air and while they were breathing oxygen are included. The fact that these two determinations of the resistance to blood flow across the defect made in the same patients were in general closely similar suggests that the value for the resistance to blood flow obtained in this manner is reasonably reproducible and presumably, therefore, of some validity. Similarly, the presence of a demonstrable relationship between these resistance values and the estimated areas of the defects suggests that the measurements of the dimensions of these defects made during ventriculotomy are related to the actual size assumed by these defects when the circulation was intact.

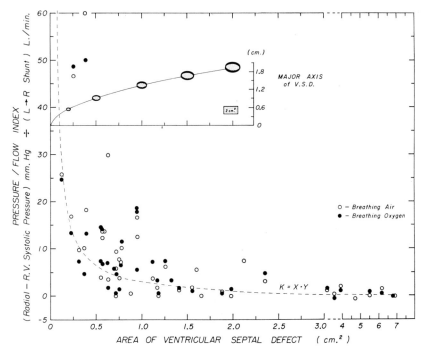

Fig. 2. Relationship between the size (area) of the defect and the "resistance" to blood flow across ventricular septal defects. Inset shows the relationship between the area of an ellipse in square centimeters and the magnitude of the major axis, which is 125% of the minor axis. In the series of patients studied the maximal dimension of the ventricular septal defect averaged 125% of the minimal dimension. The broken line indicates the rectangular hyperbola, $K = X \cdot Y$, in which K equals the average product of ordinate (Y) values for the pressure/flow indexes and the abscissa (X) values for the areas of the defects. See text for discussion.

The data shown in Fig. 2 indicate that for defects of an area of less than 1 cm² the resistance to blood flow across the defect increases rapidly with a decrease in the size of the defect. In accord with the previously stated definitions and discussion, defects of this size have therefore been classified as small defects.

The resistance to blood flow across defects with an area of more than 1 cm² falls to practically zero. Therefore, since defects of this size offer little resistance to blood flow across them, they have been classified as large defects.

The inset in Fig. 2 has been prepared in an attempt to provide a better visual impression as to the size of these defects. The diagram-

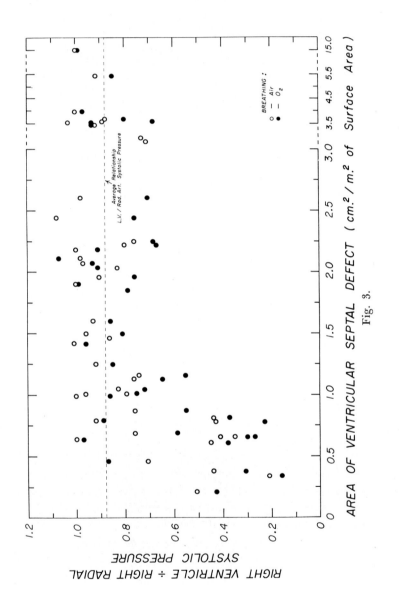

Fig. 3.

matic "defects" illustrated in this figure have been drawn as ellipses whose minor axes are 80% of their major axes. Examination of this plot reveals that a defect with an area of 1 cm² does not appear to be a very large hole and that an error of 1 or 2 mm in the measurement of the dimensions of such a defect would produce a relatively large error in the calculated area for the defect. The broken line included in Fig. 2 is a rectangular hyperbola. The fact that these data can be roughly fitted to a line expressing such a relationship is in harmony with the hydraulic formula relating the area of an orifice to the resistance to blood flow across it.

The relationship of the estimated areas of these ventricular septal defects to the ratio of the systolic pressures recorded simultaneously in the pulmonary and systemic arterial circulations in these patients is shown in Fig. 3. This systolic pressure ratio has been expressed as the systolic pressure in the right ventricle divided by the systolic pressure recorded simultaneously from the radial or femoral artery. Since in normal individuals the systolic pressure in the radial and femoral arteries exceeds the systolic pressure in the thoracic aorta by approximately 14% (8), it would be expected that this ratio would approach an average value of 0.88 for patients in whom the systolic pressures in the right and the left ventricles were equal. This average ratio of 0.88 is shown in Fig. 3 as a horizontal broken line.

The data included in Fig. 3 indicate that as the area of a ventricular defect increases toward 1 cm²/m² there is a progressive increase in

---

Fig. 3. Relationship between the systolic pressures in the pulmonary and systemic circulations and the size (area) of ventricular septal defects. Horizontal broken line indicates the average relationship between systolic pressure in the left ventricle and that in the radial artery in normal persons. It would be anticipated that in patients with equal systolic pressures in the left and right ventricles the values for right ventricular/radial-artery systolic pressures would cluster along this line. Note that for patients with defects with an area of more than 1 cm²/m² the values for systolic pressure do scatter along this line, indicating that in this situation the systolic pressures in the right and left ventricles were closely similar or equal. Note also that the ratios obtained when the patients were breathing air (open circles) nearly always exceeded those obtained when breathing oxygen. This finding is a consequence of the reduction of pulmonary vascular resistance associated with oxygen breathing and indicates that in the presence of a lowered pulmonary resistance a larger ventricular septal defect is required to elevate the right ventricular systolic pressure toward the level being maintained by the left ventricle.

the systolic pressure ratio (that is, decrease in pressure gradient) across the defect, and that as the area of the defect approaches and exceeds 1 cm²/m² this ratio approaches 0.88. In other words, in patients with ventricular septal defects with an area of more than 1 cm²/m² the systolic pressures in the right and left ventricles tend to approach equality. These findings harmonize well with the relationship obtained between the estimated relative resistances to blood flow across such defects and the areas of the defects (Fig. 2). Since the resistance to blood flow across defects of sizes larger than 1 cm² was found to decrease to very low figures, it would be expected that such defects would tend to equalize the pressures between the right and left ventricles and thus decrease the systolic pressure gradient across the defect toward zero. In this regard, however, it should be kept in mind that the systolic pressure in the right ventricle is determined both by the quantity of blood flow and the resistance (pulmonary vascular resistance) against which the ventricle empties. Therefore, if the pulmonary vascular resistance is low (normal), a very large blood flow across the defect will be required to equalize left and right ventricular systolic pressures and still maintain a left ventricular systolic pressure compatible with life. Since the capacity of the left ventricle to maintain a very high flow is limited, a low (normal) pulmonary vascular resistance is incompatible with prolonged survival in the presence of a large ventricular septal defect. Therefore, all surviving patients with very large ventricular septal defects by necessity have an increased resistance to outflow from the right ventricle either due to pulmonary stenosis or increased pulmonary vascular resistance.

Since the magnitude of the blood flow across a ventricular septal defect required to equalize pressures between the right and left ventricles decreases as pulmonary vascular resistance increases, it would be expected that in the presence of defects in the intermediate-size range of approximately 0.5 to 2 cm²/m² the pressure gradient between the left and right ventricles would vary from zero to a relatively large value, depending upon resistance to outflow from the right ventricle, that is, pulmonary vascular resistance and the area of the defect. That this is indeed the case is illustrated in Fig. 4, which shows the effect of a decrease in pulmonary vascular resistance produced by an infusion of acetylcholine on simultaneously recorded systemic and pulmonary-artery pressures. In the control situation, pulmonary and radial-artery and hence presumably right and left ventricular systolic pressures were closely similar in this patient so that the systolic pressure gradient across the ventricular septal defect was zero or nearly so. However, when the pulmonary vascular resistance was decreased, systemic arterial pressure was unchanged while pulmonary-artery pressure decreased in spite of an increase in the left-to-right shunt. As a result, a small but appreciable increase in the systolic pressure gradient between the pulmonary and systemic circulations became apparent. It can be presumed that in this patient the defect was in the intermediate-size range in which the blood flow through the defect was not sufficient to equalize left and right ventricular pressures in the presence of a relatively low pulmonary vascular resistance.

The effect of a striking decrease in pulmonary vascular resistance and consequent large increase in the left-to-right shunt in a patient with a much larger ventricular septal defect in relation to body size is shown in Fig. 5. In the control situation no appreciable gradient was apparent across the defect. Infusion of acetylcholine caused a striking fall in pulmonary-artery systolic pressure from 95 to 65 mm Hg. A concomitant fall from 95 to 80 mm Hg also occurred in systemic arterial systolic pressure, so that this large increase in the pulmonary blood flow and left-to-right shunt was associated with the development of an appreciable pressure gradient of approximately 15 mm Hg across the defect. It can be concluded that, although this was a large defect, its size was not quite sufficient to equalize right and left ventricular systolic pressures in the presence of a large decrease in pulmonary vascular resistance.

Data such as these demonstrate that, as would be expected, the size of a defect capable of producing equalization of right and left ventricular systolic pressures is determined to an important degree by the magnitude of the pulmonary vascular resistance. In actual practice, however, patients with ventricular septal defects larger than 1 cm^2/m^2 have usually been found to have essentially equal systolic pressures in the right and the left ventricles (Fig. 3).

The relationship between the size of the ventricular septal defect and the magnitude of the blood flow across the defect in this series of patients is shown in Fig. 6. Examination of these data reveals no

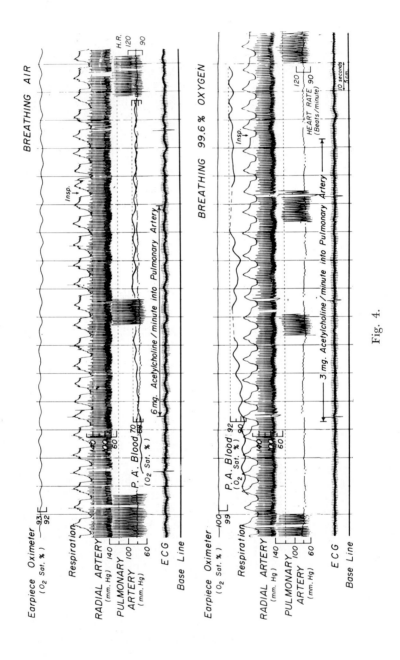

Fig. 4.

apparent relationship between the area of the defect and the blood flow across it. In the interpretation of this finding it should be remembered that this series of patients represents a group that is highly selected on the basis of whether or not their clinical and hemodynamic data were interpreted to indicate them to be suitable candidates for surgical closure of their defects (9). During the period in which these data were collected, only patients with relatively severe disability due to the defects were operated upon with the consequence that only patients with relatively large defects were included in this study. These data suggest, therefore, that in patients with large ventricular septal defects factors other than the area of the defect are of importance in determining the magnitude of the blood flow across such a defect.

In order to obtain data relating the area of small ventricular septal defects to the flow across these defects it is necessary at the present time to utilize data obtained from patients who have not been operated on for this condition. Since the previous data have illustrated that there is a reasonably good relationship between the size of the ventricular septal defect and the systolic pressure ratio across the defect, it is possible to use this systolic pressure ratio as an indirect measure of the size of the defect in a series of patients. The relationship between the pulmonary blood flow and the systolic pressure ratio across

Fig. 4.   The effect of a continuous infusion of acetylcholine into the pulmonary artery on systemic and pulmonary arterial pressures and other variables in a 43-year-old man with a ventricular septal defect, when breathing air (top) and oxygen (bottom). Note that, when air was breathed, the systolic pressures in the right and left ventricles were equal and were maintained so during the infusion of acetylcholine in spite of the fact that the pulmonary vascular resistance dropped from 1860 to 1600 dynes sec cm^{-5}. The increased pulmonary blood flow (left-to-right shunt) consequent to the decreased resistance caused by the acetylcholine is evidenced by the increase in oxygen saturation of pulmonary-artery blood from 67 to 70% during the infusion. When the infusion was repeated during the breathing of oxygen, the estimated pulmonary vascular resistance decreased from 960 to 700 dynes sec cm^{-5} while the systemic arterial resistance was approximately 1600 dynes sec cm^{-5}. In this situation an appreciable systolic pressure gradient of 15 mm Hg became apparent between the radial and pulmonary arteries, indicating that in the face of a decrease in pulmonary vascular resistance of this magnitude the area of the ventricular septal defect was insufficient to maintain equality between the right and left ventricular systolic pressures. The fact that heart rate, systemic arterial pressure, and respiratory rate were unchanged during infusions indicates that the effect of the acetylcholine was confined to the pulmonary circulation.

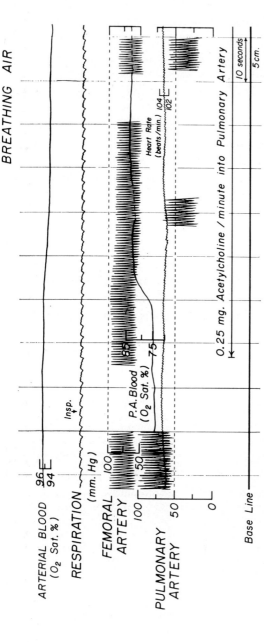

Fig. 5. Effect of a continuous infusion of acetylcholine into the pulmonary artery on systemic and pulmonary arterial pressures and other variables in an 8-year-old boy with a large ventricular septal defect. Note that in the control period the pressures in the femoral and pulmonary arteries were closely similar so that right and left ventricular pressures were essentially equal. The infusion caused a striking decrease in the estimated pulmonary vascular resistance from 1620 to 510 dynes sec cm⁻⁵. This was associated with a decrease of systolic pressure in the pulmonary artery from 95 to 65 while the systolic pressure in the femoral artery decreased to 80 mm Hg. The fact that the heart and respiratory rates were unchanged during the infusion indicates that the acetylcholine was inactivated before reaching the systemic arterial vessels. The area of this defect was sufficient to equalize right and left ventricular systolic pressures in the control period and was such as to compromise the ability of the left ventricle to maintain the systemic arterial pressure during the infusion because of the very large runoff through the ventricular septal defect consequent to the large decrease in pulmonary vascular resistance caused by the acetylcholine. In this situation a small pressure gradient of approximately 15 mm Hg across the defect did develop. [Reproduced with permission from J. T. Shepherd, H. J. Semler, H. F. Helmholz, Jr., and E. H. Wood. Effects of infusions of acetylcholine on pulmonary vascular resistance in patients with pulmonary hypertension and congenital heart disease. *Circulation* **20:** 381–390 (1959).]

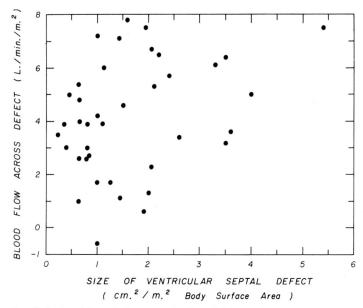

Fig. 6. Relationship of the magnitude of blood flow across a ventricular septal defect to the size (area) of the defect in 39 patients breathing air. Note that in this group of patients, most of whom had large ventricular septal defects, no relationship is apparent between these two parameters. See text for discussion.

the defect in a series of 72 patients with a ventricular septal defect is shown in Fig. 7. On the basis of the data shown in Fig. 3 it has been assumed that patients with systolic pressure ratios across the defect of less than 0.6 have small ventricular septal defects. The data illustrated in Fig. 7 demonstrate that for defects with a ratio of less than 0.6 there is a direct relationship between the magnitude of this ratio and the magnitude of the blood flow across the defect, suggesting, as would be expected, that for small ventricular septal defects there is a direct relationship between these two parameters. However, for defects associated with a systolic pressure ratio of more than 0.8 (that is, large ventricular septal defects) no relationship between the blood flow and the systolic pressure ratio is evident. The findings for this group confirm, therefore, the data from the group of patients selected for surgical closure of ventricular septal defects presented in Fig. 6.

The relationship between the blood flow through a small ventricular septal defect and the apparent size of the ventricular septal

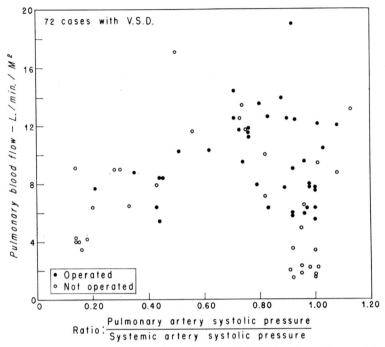

Fig. 7.   Relationship between the pulmonary blood flow in patients with ventricular septal defects and the ratio of the systolic pressure in the pulmonary artery to the systolic pressure in a systemic artery. This ratio is used as a rough index of the area of the defects. Patients with ratios of less than 0.6 can be assumed to have small defects (area less than 1.0 cm²/m²) (Fig. 3). Note that there is a positive correlation between the magnitude of the pulmonary blood flow and the systolic pressure ratio (defect area) in the patients with small defects and that this correlation disappears in the patients presumed to have large defects (ratios greater than 0.60).

defect is shown more clearly in Fig. 8, in which only the data for the 19 patients with small ventricular septal defects, that is, with systolic pressure ratios of less than 0.6, have been included. In this selected group of cases a clear-cut positive correlation is demonstrable between these two parameters.

On the basis of these data it can be concluded that in the presence of a large ventricular septal defect the flow through the defect is not determined primarily by the size of the defect but rather by the relationship of the systemic to the pulmonary vascular resistance. Since as stated previously the systemic vascular resistance is maintained essentially normal in the presence of a ventricular septal defect, it

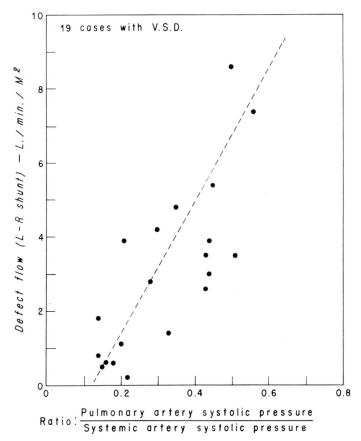

Fig. 8. Relationship of the blood flow across a ventricular septal defect to the pulmonary/systemic arterial systolic pressure ratio in patients presumed to have small defects. This chart supports the concept that in such patients there is a positive correlation between the size (area) of the defect and the magnitude of the blood flow across it. See text for discussion.

follows that in this situation the blood flow across a large ventricular septal defect is determined primarily by the pulmonary vascular resistance. The important question, therefore, arises as to what determines the pulmonary vascular resistance in patients with a large ventricular septal defect.

The relationship between the size of the ventricular septal defect and the ratio of pulmonary vascular resistance to systemic vascular resistance is shown in Fig. 9. The ratio of systemic to pulmonary vascular resistance has been used in preference to the absolute magnitude

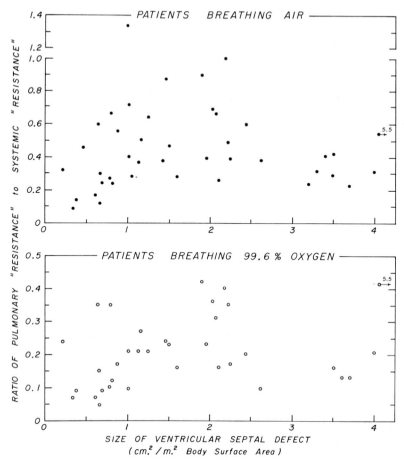

Fig. 9.   Relationship of the ratio of pulmonary/systemic vascular resistance to the size (area) of the ventricular septal defect. Note that no relationship is apparent between these two parameters in this group of patients whose ages varied from less than 1 to more than 40 years and most of whom had large ventricular septal defects. See text for discussion.

of the pulmonary vascular resistance in order to avoid the complicating effect of body size on the absolute magnitude of the vascular resistances in this group of patients who varied from infants to fully developed adults. Since the absolute magnitudes of the pulmonary and systemic vascular resistances are greatly affected by body size but to a closely similar degree, it would be expected that calculation of the ratio of these resistances would largely eliminate the effect of body size on the absolute magnitude of these two parameters. For this series of surgically treated patients no apparent relationship was found between the area of the ventricular septal defect and the ratio of pulmonary to systemic vascular resistance (Fig. 9). Interpretation of these data again should be carried out in the light of the fact that this series of patients selected for surgical closure of their ventricular septal defects is restricted largely to those with large defects and, furthermore, that the series includes patients who range from less than 1 to more than 40 years of age.

Figure 10 has been constructed in an effort to take into account the effect of both the size of the defect and the age of the patient on the pulmonary vascular resistance. The relationship of the systemic and pulmonary systolic pressures has again been used as an index of the size of the defect in order to make possible the inclusion of a large series of patients, including nonsurgically treated patients with small ventricular septal defects. Patients with systolic gradients across the defect of less than 20 mm Hg have been assumed to have large ventricular septal defects, and patients with gradients of more than 20 mm Hg have been assumed to have small ventricular defects. The data plotted in this fashion (Fig. 10) suggest that in patients with large ventricular septal defects there is a positive correlation between the age of the patient and the magnitude of the pulmonary vascular resistance. All patients with large ventricular septal defects as classified in this manner who were older than 10 years of age had significantly elevated pulmonary vascular resistances. In the patients classified as having small ventricular septal defects, however, no apparent relationship was found between the age of the patient and the pulmonary vascular resistance, the pulmonary vascular resistance remaining essentially in the normal range for patients of all age groups. These data suggest, therefore, that both the size of the defect and the age of the patient are important factors in the development of an increase in pulmonary vascular resistance in patients with ventricular septal defect.

Hence it seems logical to conclude that the changes in pulmonary vascular resistance in patients with congenital ventricular septal defect is largely determined by the size of the defect. If the defect is small, the pulmonary vasculature is protected because the ventricular septum still provides an effective (high resistance) although incomplete barrier to blood flow from the left ventricle into the pulmonary

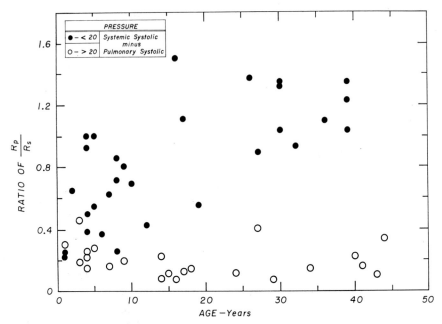

Fig. 10.   Relationship of the ratio of pulmonary/systemic vascular resistance to age in 53 patients with ventricular septal defect. Patients in whom the systemic exceeded the pulmonary systolic pressure by more than 20 mm Hg are presumed to have small ventricular septal defects. In these patients (open circles) this ratio remains low, that is, the vascular resistance is normal or only slightly elevated, and there is no apparent tendency for the pulmonary vascular resistance to increase with age. Patients with closely similar systolic pressures in the pulmonary and systemic arteries are presumed to have large ventricular septal defects. In these patients (solid circles) there is a significant tendency for the ratio of pulmonary/systemic vascular resistance to increase with age. Note that the pulmonary vascular resistance was greatly elevated to values closely similar to or in excess of those for systemic vascular resistance in all patients in this group who were more than 20 years in age.

circulation, and no increase in vascular resistance ordinarily occurs in the pulmonary circulation irrespective of the age of the patient. On the other hand, if the defect is large so that the ventricular septum provides an ineffective (low resistance) barrier to blood flow from the left ventricle into the pulmonary circulation, the pulmonary vasculature is subjected to the systemic arterial pressures generated in the left ventricle and an increase in pulmonary vascular resistance occurs which usually attains or approaches the level of systemic vascular resistance by the age of 20 years or before.

A certain answer as to what is the actual cause or causes for the increase in pulmonary vascular resistance that occurs in patients with a large ventricular septal defect is not available. It would appear almost certain that the increase in systolic pressure in the right ventricle and pulmonary arteries which is inescapably associated with the presence of a large ventricular septal defect is an important inciting cause for the development of increased pulmonary vascular resistance. It also appears highly probable that the magnitude of the increase in blood flow through the pulmonary vasculature associated with a large ventricular septal defect also may be an important factor in the development of an increase in pulmonary vascular resistance.

The increase in blood flow associated with a ventricular septal defect may produce an increase in pulmonary vascular resistance by two mechanisms, namely (*a*) by a direct effect on the pulmonary vasculature and (*b*) by a secondary effect resulting indirectly from the increased work load imposed on the left ventricle. If this work load is very high, as would be expected in the presence of a large ventricular septal defect, some degree of left ventricular incompetence and a consequent increase in the left atrial pressure may develop. On the basis of studies carried out in patients with increased left atrial pressure due to left ventricular failure or mitral stenosis, it is now a conceded fact that an elevated pulmonary venous pressure is a potent stimulus for the development of an increase in pulmonary vascular resistance (10). It would be expected, therefore, that if left atrial pressure were increased as a result of the heavy work load imposed on the left ventricle because of the left-to-right shunt via the ventricular septal defect, this increase in pulmonary venous pressure might in itself provoke the development of an increase in pulmonary vascular resistance.

Figure 11 provides direct evidence that the left atrial pressure does indeed tend to be increased in the presence of large ventricular septal defects. Left atrial pressures were measured directly during operation in 36 patients before and after closure of a ventricular septal defect. The data demonstrate that the left atrial pressure was, in the large majority of cases, significantly reduced after closure of the ventricular septal defect, suggesting that the presence of a ventricular septal defect does indeed produce an appreciable increase in the level of left atrial pressure. The possibility that an increase in left atrial pressure may be of importance in the development of the increase in vascular

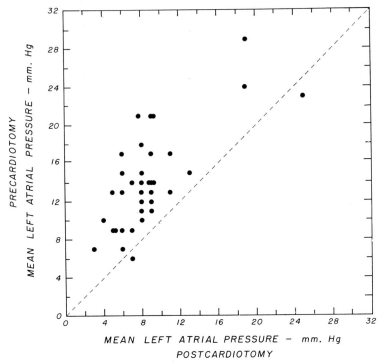

Fig. 11. Comparison of left atrial pressures recorded at operation before and after cardiotomy for closure of ventricular septal defects in 36 patients. Diagonal broken line is line of identity for preclosure and postclosure values. The fact that the left atrial pressure is nearly always reduced after closure of the ventricular septal defect suggests that the increased left ventricular work load associated with the defect had resulted in an increase in left atrial pressure. An increase in left atrial pressure may be a causal factor in the development of pulmonary hypertension in these patients.

resistance associated with a large ventricular septal defect therefore cannot be ignored.

It is now generally recognized that there are two main mechanisms responsible for the increased pulmonary vascular resistance associated with a ventricular septal defect. The first of these mechanisms is related to the histologic changes in the small vessels of the lungs which produce obstructive anatomic lesions in the pulmonary vasculature. This aspect of the problem is discussed in detail by Dr. Edwards in another paper (p. 165), and will not be touched on further here. The second mechanism responsible for the increased pulmonary vascular resistance in this condition is an increase in the vasomotor tone in the small vessels of the lungs. This aspect of the increase in vascular resistance is of particular physiologic interest since it is a dynamic process. It is also of considerable practical medical and surgical importance since the increase in smooth muscle tone responsible for this effect would be expected to be a potentially reversible phenomenon.

The conclusion that a significant component of the increase in vascular resistance associated with a ventricular septal defect is due to vasomotor tone is based on the demonstration of the capability of the pulmonary vessels to dilate in such patients. The studies of Marshall and co-workers (11) have demonstrated that breathing of mixtures high in oxygen content results in a significant decrease in pulmonary-artery pressure and pulmonary vascular resistance in such patients, as illustrated in Fig. 12. Several groups of workers have also demonstrated that infusion of acetylcholine into the pulmonary artery produces a significant dilatation of the pulmonary vasculature in such patients, as illustrated in Figs. 4 and 5.

Summary

These data support the conclusion that the two primary factors that determine the hemodynamic alterations associated with a ventricular septal defect are (*a*) the size, that is, the area, of the ventricular septal defect, and (*b*) the reaction of the pulmonary vasculature to the increase in pulmonary-artery pressure and blood flow that may be associated with such a ventricular septal defect.

The data indicate that the resistance to blood flow through ventricular septal defects whose cross-sectional area is less than 1 cm² is high and increases rapidly with a further decrease in size. Defects with areas of less than 1 cm²/m² have been classified as small, since in this situation the ventricular septum still maintains an effective, albeit incomplete, barrier to blood flow from the left to the right ventricle. In patients with small ventricular septal defects the pressure relationship between the right and left ventricles is usually maintained at an approximately normal range, and the magnitude of the blood flow across the defect is directly related to the area of the defect. The pulmonary-artery pressure remains normal or slightly in excess of the normal range, and little or no tendency for an increase in pulmonary vascular resistance with age is apparent.

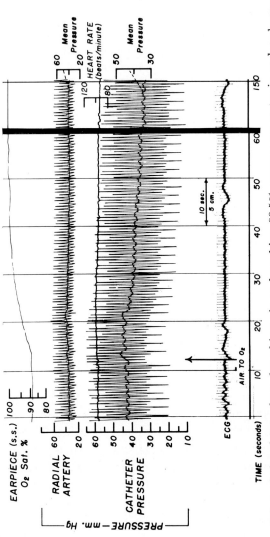

Fig. 12. Effect of the change from breathing air to breathing 99.5% oxygen on systemic and pulmonary-artery pressures, heart rate, and arterial oxygen saturation in an 8-month-old boy with a ventricular septal defect (area 1.3 cm²/m²). Note that the arterial oxygen saturation began to increase within 3 sec and the pulmonary-artery pressure to decrease within 10 sec after the change from breathing air to breathing 99.5% oxygen. The pulse and mean pressures were recorded simultaneously by means of double galvanometer assemblies. The decrease in pulmonary-artery pressure associated with oxygen breathing has been shown to be associated with an increase in pulmonary blood flow (left-to-right shunt) and a decrease in pulmonary vascular resistance (see Edwards, p. 165).

The resistance to blood flow through ventricular septal defects with areas of more than 1 cm^2 decreases to very low values. Defects with areas of more than 1 cm^2/m^2 have been classified as large, since in this situation the ventricular septum provides an ineffectual barrier to blood flow across it, and the pressures in the left and right ventricles tend to be equalized. In patients with large ventricular septal defects the right ventricular pressure must be increased in order to maintain a left ventricular pressure that is sufficient to sustain the systemic circulation. The magnitude of the blood flow across the defect in this situation is not determined solely by the size of the defect but rather by the reaction of the pulmonary vasculature. The volume of blood flow across the defect is directly dependent on the relationship of the systemic to the pulmonary vascular resistance. If the pulmonary vascular resistance remains considerably below systemic vascular resistance, the blood flow through the defect is in the left-to-right direction and is of large magnitude. In this situation there are almost uniformly a significant increase in pulmonary vascular resistance and a tendency for this resistance to increase progressively with the age of the patient.

The causes for this increased pulmonary vascular resistance have not been demonstrated with certainty. However, they are believed to be related almost unquestionably to the high pulmonary-artery pressure that is a necessary accompaniment of large ventricular septal defects and also to the increase in blood flow through the pulmonary vasculature in such a circumstance. This increased flow imposes a proportionate increase in the work load of the left ventricle which may be associated with a demonstrable increase in the left atrial pressure in such patients. It appears possible that an increase in left atrial and pulmonary venous pressure in the early stages of the disease may constitute one of the significant stimuli for the development of an increase in pulmonary vascular resistance, which in turn protects the left ventricle.

The increase in pulmonary vascular resistance associated with large ventricular septal defects is produced by two mechanisms, namely (*a*) by obstructive anatomic changes in the vasculature of the lung, which result in an increase in resistance to blood flow through these vessels, and (*b*) by active vasomotor tone in these vessels. The demonstration that a significant component of the increase in pulmonary vascular resistance associated with ventricular septal defect is due to vasomotor tone is of practical medical and surgical importance since it suggests that a portion of this increased resistance is potentially reversible and, hence, under some circumstances amenable to improvement following surgical closure of the defect.

REFERENCES

1. Selzer, Arthur. Defects of the cardiac septums. *J. Am. Med. Assoc.* **154**:129–135 (1954).
2. Wood, Paul, Magidson, O., and Wilson, P. A. O. Ventricular septal defect: With a note on acyanotic Fallot's tetralogy. *Brit. Heart J.* **16**:387–406 (1954).
3. Blount, S. G., Jr., Mueller, Helmut, and McCord, M. C. Ventricular septal defect: Clinical and hemodynamic patterns. *Am. J. Med.* **18**:871–882 (1955).
4. Brotmacher, L., and Campbell, Maurice. The natural history of ventricular septal defect. *Brit. Heart J.* **20**:97–116 (1958).
5. Grosse-Brockhoff, Von F. Der Phasenwandel im Erscheinungsbild der angebornen Herzfehler mit hohem pulmonalem Stromvolumen. *Verhandl. deut. Ges. Kreislauff* **23**:201–215 (1957).
6. Wood, E. H., and Swan, H. J. C. Right heart catheterization. *Cardiology: An Encyclopedia of the Cardiovascular System*, A. A. Luisada, Editor. Blakiston Publishing Division, McGraw-Hill, New York, Vol. 2, 1959, Pt. 4, pp. 292–322.
7. Wood, E. H., Sutterer, W. F., and Donald, D. E. The monitoring and recording of physiologic variables during closure of ventricular septal defects using extracorporeal circulation. In R. Hegglin, *Advances in Cardiology*. S. Karger, Basel, 1959, Vol. 2, pp. 61–74.
8. Kroeker, E. J., and Wood, E. H. Comparison of simultaneously recorded central and peripheral arterial pressure pulses during rest, exercise and tilted position in man. *Circulation Research* **3**:623–632 (1955).
9. DuShane, J. W., Kirklin, J. W., Patrick, R. T., Donald, D. E., Terry, H. R., Jr., Burchell, H. B., and Wood, E. H. Ventricular septal defects with pulmonary hypertension: Surgical treatment by means of a mechanical pump-oxygenator. *J. Am. Med. Assoc.* **160**:950–953 (1956).
10. Semler, H. J., Shepherd, J. T., and Wood, E. H. The role of vessel tone in maintaining pulmonary vascular resistance in patients with mitral stenosis. *Circulation* **19**:386–394 (1959).
11. Marshall, H. W., Swan, H. J. C., and Wood, E. H. Effect of breathing oxygen and pulmonary vascular resistance in patients with acyanotic congenital heart disease. (Abstr.) *Federation Proc.* **16**:84 (1957).

Pathologic Anatomy of Obstructive Cardiac Anomalies and of Pulmonary Hypertension*

JESSE E. EDWARDS

Section of Pathologic Anatomy, Mayo Clinic and Mayo Foundation†
Rochester, Minnesota

The majority of the malformations of the heart or great vessels are characterized by either an abnormal communication between the two sides of the heart or an obstruction at some region in the heart or great vessels. Some afflicted patients possess only one or the other type of malformation, while others exhibit both.

Dr. Lev has covered the anatomic features of those malformations representing abnormal communications. I have been assigned the subjects of congenital obstructive lesions and of pulmonary hypertension. Superficially, these may appear to be two unrelated entities, but on closer inspection they are intimately related.

Common Sites of Obstruction

On the right side of the heart, congenital obstructive lesions only rarely occur at the tricuspid valve, in the atrium, or in the inflow part of the ventricle. Common types of right-sided obstruction are in the pulmonary valve, the outflow tract of the right ventricle (the right ventricular infundibulum), or in these two regions concomitantly. Although obstruction beyond the pulmonary valve is extremely rare on a congenital basis, it is common for obstruction to develop in the pulmonary vascular bed as a complication of certain communications between the two sides of the heart.

* This investigation was supported in part by research grant H-4014 from the National Heart Institute, Public Health Service.

† The Mayo Foundation, Rochester, Minnesota, is a part of the Graduate School of the University of Minnesota.

On the left side of the circulation, there are many congenital lesions that are obstructive in nature. These may be placed in two major groups, namely (1) those which primarily cause obstruction to pulmonary venous flow and (2) those which primarily are barriers to emptying of the left ventricle. The second group also may be responsible for an impediment to pulmonary venous flow when the primary lesion has been responsible for left ventricular failure.

Obstruction to Right Ventricular Outflow

To understand the functional consequences of obstruction to right ventricular outflow, it is convenient to classify this condition primarily on an anatomico-functional basis as follows: (1) with intact septa; (2) with interatrial communication and intact ventricular septum; (3) with interventricular communication.

OBSTRUCTION TO RIGHT VENTRICULAR OUTFLOW WITH INTACT SEPTA

The commonest form of obstruction to right ventricular outflow when the cardiac septa are intact is represented by the condition often called "isolated pulmonary stenosis" or "pulmonary stenosis with intact ventricular septum." In this condition, the leaflets of the pulmonary valve are fused to form a dome-shaped structure with a narrow central aperture, the latter representing the obstructive focus (Fig. 1a). In such hearts, as a complicating lesion, a secondary zone of obstruction may develop in the outflow tract of the right ventricle.

Less common than primary obstruction at the pulmonary valve is primary stenosis of the outflow tract of the right ventricle, the condition variously termed "right ventricular infundibular stenosis" or "stenosis of the ostium infundibuli."

Regardless of the anatomic detail of the cause of obstruction to right ventricular outflow, the volume of blood flow may be normal when the cardiac septa are intact. This is accomplished by a pronounced increase of right ventricular pressure, which causes the blood from the obstructed ventricle to pass through the narrow orifice at an extremely high velocity. This right ventricular hypertension is associated with pronounced right ventricular hypertrophy, the thickness of the right ventricle often equaling or exceeding that of the left ventricle.

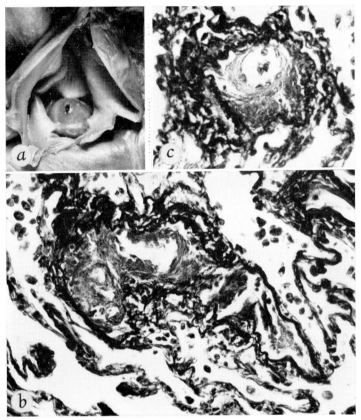

Fig. 1. (*a*) Congenital pulmonary valvular stenosis. The pulmonary trunk has been incised anteriorly and the unopened, stenotic, dome-shaped pulmonary valve is viewed from above. (*b*) Lung in atrial septal defect and pulmonary hypertension, showing intimal fibrous thickening of two arterioles causing severe luminal narrowing (elastic-tissue stain; ×250). (*c*) Small muscular artery in the lung in atrial septal defect and pulmonary hypertension, showing pronounced narrowing of the lumen by intimal fibrous thickening (elastic-tissue stain; ×330).

OBSTRUCTION TO RIGHT VENTRICULAR OUTFLOW WITH INTERATRIAL
COMMUNICATION AND INTACT VENTRICULAR SEPTUM

Obstruction on a Congenital Basis.   Some hearts with the same anatomic types of congenital obstruction to right ventricular outflow as in those just described also may have an associated interatrial communication. This usually takes the form simply of a valvular-competent patent foramen ovale. Less commonly, a true atrial septal defect is present. Regardless of the anatomic type of interatrial communication, a transatrial right-to-left shunt is possible. Whether or not such a shunt occurs apparently depends on the relative resistance to filling of the right ventricle as compared with that of the left ventricle. If the resistance to filling of the right ventricle exceeds that of the left ventricle, a right-to-left shunt occurs. Factors that cause the right ventricle to offer a high degree of resistance to filling are (1) the large mass of the hypertrophied right ventricle, (2) right ventricular failure, and (3) a combination of these two conditions.

Obstruction on an Acquired Basis. Pulmonary stenosis with a right-to-left shunt at the atrial level bears functional similarity to certain stages of atrial septal defect without associated pulmonary valvular or right ventricular infundibular stenosis. In the usual example of atrial septal defect, many years elapse during which the pulmonary flow is high and, because of low pulmonary vascular resistance, the pulmonary pressure is normal. At this stage, abnormal obstruction to right ventricular outflow is absent. The right ventricular chamber is large but the wall is only slightly hypertrophied, if at all. The wall of the right ventricle, being considerably thinner than the left, offers less resistance to filling than does the left ventricle. The flow across the atrial septal defect is primarily in a left-to-right direction. Pulmonary hypertension tends to develop ultimately in such patients, however; this phenomenon has been emphasized for many years by Dr. Lewis Dexter (1), chairman of this session.

In atrial septal defect, development of pulmonary hypertension depends on the appearance of a complicating increased pulmonary vascular resistance. Observations of my colleagues and me have indicated that this functional disturbance depends primarily on the appearance of occlusive intimal fibrotic lesions in the small pulmonary arteries and arterioles (2). These lesions are particularly localized to the origins of the arterioles from the small muscular arteries and in the terminal portions of the latter (Fig. 1*b*, *c*).

The occlusive lesions in the tiny vessels of the lungs may be said to operate collectively as an obstruction to right ventricular outflow. From a functional viewpoint, similarities exist between the resistance offered to right ventricular outflow by pulmonary valvular stenosis with intact ventricular septum and interatrial communication and that offered by the complicating occlusive pulmonary vascular lesions in patients having atrial septal defect without pulmonary valvular or right ventricular infundibular stenosis. In either case, the resistance to right ventricular filling may exceed the resistance to filling of the left ventricle. This change may result in a right-to-left shunt at the interatrial communication.

OBSTRUCTION TO RIGHT VENTRICULAR OUTFLOW WITH INTERVENTRICU-
  LAR COMMUNICATION

Under ordinary circumstances, when obstruction to right ventricular outflow is associated with an interventricular communication, the latter is large. For this reason, the immediately following discussion will concern itself only with those conditions in which the communication is of this type. Functionally, the large defect between the two ventricles allows free and unobstructive communication between the two chambers (3). For this reason, the two ventricles operate as a single pump. The systolic pressure in each is similar.

Many anatomic varieties of malformations are present in which obstruction to right ventricular outflow is associated with free interventricular communication. The two common varieties may be employed as prototypes. The first variety is the so-called tetralogy of Fallot, and the second is the ordinary ventricular septal defect without pulmonary stenosis.

In the tetralogy of Fallot, the aorta arises from both ventricles above a large ventricular septal defect. Obstruction is present at one or several places between the right ventricle and the pulmonary trunk (Fig. 2). The obstruction often exists both in the right ventricular infundibulum and at the pulmonary valve; less commonly, it is in the pulmonary trunk itself. The right ventricular infundibulum is the most common site of the severest obstruction, but the point of greatest obstruction varies from patient to patient. An occasional patient has no tract whatever between the right ventricle and the pulmonary trunk. Usually, however, there is an opening, but this varies considerably in its caliber, ranging from a slight opening representing severe obstruction to a relatively wide opening causing only the slightest degree of stenosis.

When the two ventricles operate as a single pump, as in the tetral-

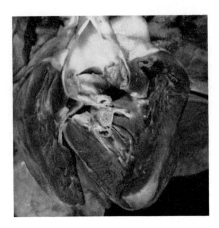

Fig. 2. Tetralogy of Fallot, showing interior of right ventricle and partial origin of aorta from this chamber. The ventricular septal defect is of the classic variety seen in this condition, being of the "large" type. The tract within the right ventricle leading to the pulmonary artery (right side of illustration) shows stenosis, which constituted the major point of obstruction in the pathway to the pulmonary vessels in this case.

ogy of Fallot, the proportional distribution of blood from the single ventricle into the aorta and into the pulmonary trunk depends on the resistance offered to the flow of blood into one arterial system as compared to the other. If the systemic peripheral resistance is constant, the determining factor in the distribution of blood will be the degree of obstruction to pulmonary flow offered by the congenital obstruction in the pathway from the right ventricle to the pulmonary trunk (2) (Fig. 3). This may be demonstrated readily by observing that all the left ventricular blood and a considerable portion of the right ventricular blood are delivered to the aorta in patients who have severe obstruction in this pathway (severe pulmonary stenosis). At the other extreme, when the pulmonary stenosis is mild, in general, all the right ventricular blood and a considerable amount of the left ventricular blood are delivered to the pulmonary trunk. Between these two extremes in degrees of pulmonary stenosis are many variations. Depending on these are the direction and magnitudes of shunts according to the principle, already stated, that the direction of major blood flow will be into that system offering the lesser resistance to flow through it.

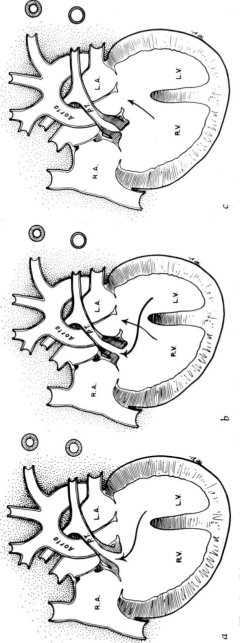

Fig. 3. Diagrammatic representation of mild (*a*), moderate (*b*), and severe (*c*) pulmonary stenosis in the tetralogy of Fallot. The direction of the shunt depends on the degree of resistance offered by the pulmonary stenosis. When the stenosis is severe, the shunt is entirely right to left. When the stenosis is mild, the shunt is entirely left to right. In moderate pulmonary stenosis, a bidirectional shunt is present. [Reproduced with permission of the publishers from J. E. Edwards, Recent concepts of the functional pathology in ventricular septal defect. *Wisconsin Med. J.* **56**:481–485 (Dec. 1957).]

172   *J. E. Edwards*

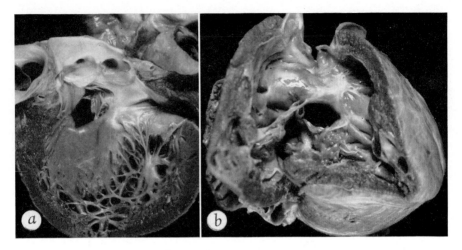

Fig. 4. Typical large ventricular septal defect without pulmonary stenosis. (*a*) Left ventricular aspect. (*b*) Right ventricular aspect.

The second prototype of conditions characterized by obstruction to right ventricular outflow associated with a large interventricular communication is the ordinary type of large ventricular septal defect (Fig. 4). Large ventricular septal defects of the classic variety do not cause obstruction to blood flow within the heart. Moreover, in the early months and years after birth, the pulmonary vascular resistance (4) is significantly less than the systemic vascular resistance. Despite this, however, the pulmonary systolic pressure may approach the systemic arterial pressure on the basis of large volumes of pulmonary flow resulting from the left-to-right shunt (Fig. 5a). Later, a right-to-left shunt may appear as pulmonary resistance increases (Fig. 5b).

With time (rarely before 3 years of age but commonly by adolescence), chronic pulmonary hypertension is responsible for the presence of complicating occlusive lesions in the large muscular arteries of the lungs (Fig. 6a, b). These lesions functionally eliminate substantial segments of the pulmonary arterial bed, and the reduction in its capacity may be termed "high pulmonary vascular resistance" (2). As the pulmonary vascular resistance increases, and with the assumption that the systemic vascular resistance remains constant, the difference between the resistance in the two systems becomes less. The left-to-right shunt becomes smaller (5). As the pulmonary resistance

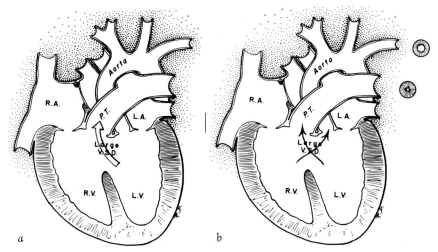

Fig. 5. (*a*) Diagrammatic representation of large ventricular septal defect with pulmonary resistance less than systemic resistance. As the result of this relationship, the shunt is entirely in a left-to-right direction, and it may be huge. (*b*) Diagrammatic representation of large ventricular septal defect with pulmonary resistance greater than systemic resistance. As a result of this relationship, a right-to-left shunt exists. In some instances, as portrayed in this diagram, a coexistent left-to-right shunt also may be present. [Reproduced with permission of the publishers from J. E. Edwards (2).]

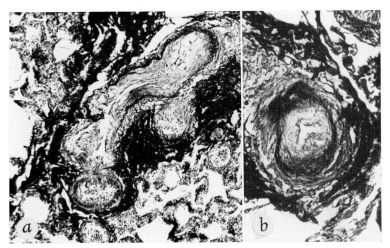

Fig. 6. Small pulmonary arteries in a patient with a large ventricular septal defect, showing intimal lesions causing profound luminal narrowing or occlusion [both, elastic-tissue stain; (*a*) ×120; (*b*) ×200].

increases to levels that equal or exceed the systemic resistance, a right-to-left shunt occurs (Fig. 5b).

At this stage, the functional nature of the simple ventricular septal defect becomes similar to that of the tetralogy of Fallot with severe pulmonary stenosis (Fig. 3c).

In ventricular septal defect, despite a change in direction of the shunt, the systolic pressures remain equalized across the large ventricular septal defect. If the ventricular septal defect is closed, the right-to-left shunt is eliminated and all of the right ventricular blood is directed to the pulmonary trunk. If the cardiac output remains constant after closure of the ventricular septal defect in a case with a net right-to-left shunt, the pulmonary pressure increases.

Left-Sided Obstructive Anomalies

Congenital malformations of the left side of the heart or the aorta may be associated with abnormal communications. Nevertheless, such combinations are comparatively uncommon and thus will not be considered further in this presentation. The significant component, or at least one component, of the functional disturbance is the fact that left-sided obstructive lesions are responsible for obstruction to pulmonary venous flow and thus for hypertension in the pulmonary circuit. In this way, left-sided obstructive lesions ultimately have an obstructive effect on the right ventricle as well.

Left-sided obstructive lesions may be classified anatomically depending on whether obstruction to pulmonary venous flow is a primary effect or whether this functional derangement is secondary to left ventricular failure. The two classes are (1) anomalies primarily responsible for obstruction to pulmonary venous flow and (2) anomalies secondarily responsible for obstruction to pulmonary venous flow.

PRIMARY OBSTRUCTION TO PULMONARY VENOUS FLOW

Lesions in this category lie in the pulmonary veins, the mitral valve, or the left ventricle.

Pulmonary venous obstruction on a congenital basis may involve each of the pulmonary veins as it joins the left atrium. The basis for obstruction is nonspecific fibrous thickening of the venous intima at

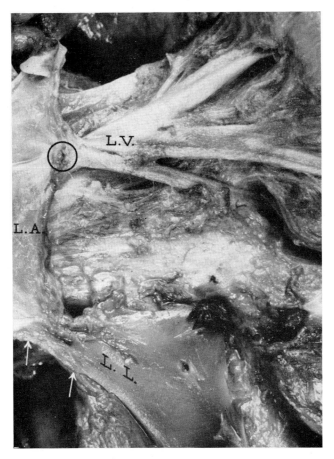

Fig. 7.   Portion of left atrium and ostia of left pulmonary veins in a patient in whom each of the four definitive pulmonary veins was severely stenotic at the left atrial junction. L. A., left atrium; L. L., left lower pulmonary vein opened longitudinally; L. V., left upper pulmonary vein. The unopened ostium of the latter is enclosed in a circle.

the point of obstruction. Such lesions rarely may involve each of the pulmonary veins, as in one case that I have observed (Fig. 7). More commonly, some of the pulmonary veins are uninvolved, whereas others are severely obstructed at the left atrial junction.

More common than obstructive lesions involving the individual pulmonary veins is obstruction in the primordial outgrowth of the sinoatrial region of the embryo, an outgrowth that connects with the

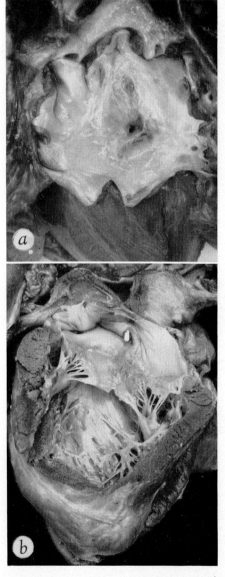

Fig. 8. Cor triatriatum. (*a*) The accessory chamber viewed from above. The chamber receives the definitive pulmonary veins and communicates by a small opening (center of illustration) with the normal left atrium below. (*b*) The left atrium and left ventricle. The left atrium is normal and communicates with the accessory left atrial chamber through a small opening (probe). The accessory chamber itself is not shown in this view. The mitral valve is normal.

capillary plexus of the developing lung. As a result of obstruction in this region, an accessory chamber develops that connects above with the pulmonary veins (Fig. 8*a*) and connects below by a narrow opening with the left atrium (Fig. 8*b*). This accessory chamber has been termed

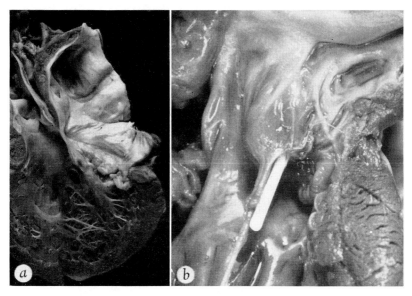

Fig. 9. Congenital mitral stenosis. (*a*) Sagittal section of a heart with congenital mitral stenosis. The leaflets and chordae are short and thickened. Although this lesion is believed to be congenital, it is difficult to distinguish the pathologic picture from that of rheumatic mitral stenosis. (*b*) Left ventricular aspect of a congenitally stenotic mitral valve in which the valvular leaflets are fused to form a funnel-shaped structure with a central perforation (probe).

an "accessory left atrium"; hence, the term "triatrial heart" or "cor triatriatum" is used for hearts with this malformation.

Anomalies of the mitral valve that cause obstruction to pulmonary venous flow are mitral stenosis and mitral insufficiency. Congenital mitral stenosis is comparatively rare (6). The valve leaflets usually are thickened and fused, changes that are associated with a single narrow orifice (Fig. 9). It is difficult or impossible to distinguish such valves from those affected by rheumatic mitral stenosis when only structural alterations are taken into account. Rarely, the mitral orifice is represented by a sievelike accumulation of several narrow openings. Such valves are more readily identified as representing congenital disease.

While mitral insufficiency does not represent pulmonary venous obstruction during ventricular diastole, the regurgitation during ventricular systole does have this effect. In the aggregate, there is increase

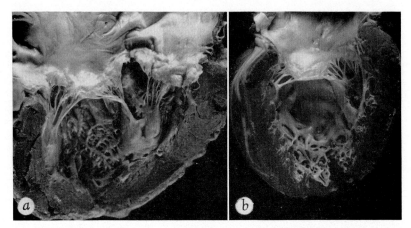

Fig. 10.   (*a*) Congenital mitral insufficiency. The chordae related to the posteromedial papillary muscles and commissure are inserted eccentrically. The insufficiency apparently results from improper tension on the related portions of the leaflets, allowing them to balloon upward and be responsible for incompetence of the valve. (*b*) Left atrium and ventricle of heart with primary endocardial sclerosis of the left ventricle. This shows the characteristic picture of pronounced fibrous thickening of the left ventricular endocardium.

of left atrial pressure, thereby making it proper to include congenital mitral insufficiency along with those lesions that cause obstruction to pulmonary venous flow as a primary disturbance.

Several anatomic bases exist for congenital incompetence of the mitral valve in the absence of septal defects (7, 8). These alterations include a deficiency of valvular tissue in the form of either a cleft in a leaflet or an accessory opening in it (the so-called double orifice of the mitral valve). Anomalous insertion of chordae tendineae may offer an undue restraining effect on the involved portion of the leaflet and prevent closure at this region (Fig. 10*a*).

For unknown reasons, the endocardium of the left ventricle may develop as a grossly visible, thick, rigid, fibroelastic layer, a condition called "fibroelastosis" or "endocardial sclerosis" (Fig. 10*b*). The binding quality of this layer prevents normal distention of the left ventricle during diastole and perhaps causes incomplete emptying during systole (9). The altered dynamics of the ventricle are reflected as obstruction to pulmonary venous flow (10, 11).

SECONDARY OBSTRUCTION TO PULMONARY VENOUS FLOW

When lesions in this category cause obstruction to pulmonary venous flow, they do so by first causing left ventricular failure. The pertinent manifestation of the latter is an increase of left ventricular diastolic pressure.

Congenital obstructive lesions that may cause left ventricular failure are situated at or near the aortic valve or in the aorta.

In relationship to the aortic valve, the obstruction may be at the level of the valve itself and may be a result of maldevelopment of the leaflets. The leaflets usually are represented by a dome-shaped structure that, with its narrow orifice, protrudes into the aorta. There are two main varieties of this type of congenitally stenotic aortic valve (7). In one, the valvular tissue is attached to the aorta only at the base of the dome, there being no lateral attachment of the cuspid tissue to the aortic wall. In the other variety, the cuspid tissue is attached laterally at only one zone, yielding one commissure instead of the three commissures characteristic of the normal structure.

In obstruction just below the aortic valve, or subaortic stenosis, it is common for a fibrous ring to encircle the outflow tract of the left ventricle (Fig. 11). This is attached to the anterior leaflet of the mitral valve, to the anterior wall of the left ventricle, and to the muscular part of the ventricular septum, structures that are not closely related developmentally. While this ring of fibrous tissue may contribute to the obstruction, it is probably not the primary basis for the obstruction. I share the opinion of those who believe that the primary disturbance is in the muscular structure of the left ventricular outflow tract. In hearts with subaortic obstruction, there is an uncommon bulge of the base of the ventricular septum into the left ventricular outflow tract.

A rare lesion that has received some attention recently is one characterized by obstruction of the aorta just above the aortic valve, the so-called supravalvular obstruction of the aorta (12). From the functional point of view, this lesion is similar to aortic or subaortic stenosis.

Obstruction of the aorta remote from the aortic valve most com-

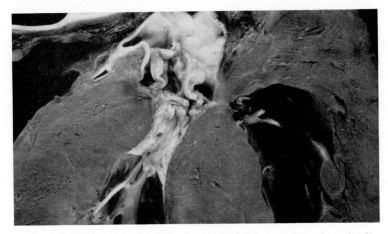

Fig. 11. Subaortic stenosis. The heart has been sectioned sagittally and viewed from behind. A zone of fibrous thickening in the wall of the outflow tract of the left ventricle lies just beneath the aortic valve. Although the fibrous tissue contributes to the obstruction, the basic cause of the obstruction appears to be a greater deviation of the ventricular septum into the left ventricular chamber (left side of illustration) than is normal. The cavity of the right ventricle is in the right side of this illustration.

monly occurs at the junction of the arch and the descending aorta, the well-known coarctation of the aorta. This lesion has a characteristic appearance in which the anterior, superior, and posterior walls of the aortic media are folded in toward the aortic lumen, creating an eccentric and narrowed aortic channel. Individual patients with this lesion vary in their ability to compensate for the obstruction. Left ventricular failure sometimes occurs during infancy, whereas this complication does not develop until later in life in other patients. In still other patients, left ventricular competence is maintained, while important complications in the form of rupture of the aorta, rupture of a cerebral aneurysm, or infection of the aortic valve appear. Obstruction in the aorta beyond the typical site for coarctation occurs on rare occasions. Obstruction in the abdominal aorta usually is sufficiently distal that it does not directly cause any significant embarrassment of the left ventricle. However, it may be responsible for renal hypertension if the obstruction lies proximal to the renal arteries.

When the obstruction lies in the lowermost part of the thoracic aorta, it may be responsible for obstructive phenomena as in typical coarctation.

As has been indicated, obstructive anomalies involving the left side of the heart may be responsible for obstruction to the pulmonary venous flow as a primary functional effect, or they may cause this phenomenon indirectly if they are responsible for left ventricular failure. If the latter condition occurs, and in instances of the former anomalies, the pulmonary venous and capillary pressures are increased. The pulmonary arteriolar pressure is greater than the pulmonary capillary pressure, indicating that a zone of obstruction exists between the pulmonary arterioles and the pulmonary capillaries. The most likely explanation for this secondary obstructive phenomenon is

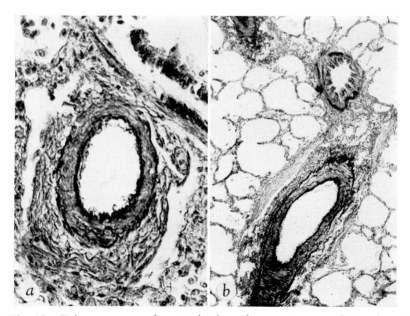

Fig. 12. Pulmonary muscular arteries in pulmonary venous obstruction. (*a*) Medial hypertrophy in cor triatriatum, a condition primarily causing obstruction to pulmonary venous flow (elastic-tissue stain; ×305). (*b*) Medial hypertrophy in congenital aortic stenosis, a condition in which pulmonary venous obstruction depends on the interposition of left ventricular failure (elastic-tissue stain; ×60).

arteriolar spasm. Structurally, this is manifested by hypertrophy of the medial layers of the smaller arteries (Fig. 12) and the arterioles. There is also a suggestion that muscles from the proximal portion of the arteriole extend into the more distal parts of the arteriole, which normally is devoid of identifiable layers of muscle. The additional changes in the pulmonary vascular bed when obstruction of pulmonary venous flow is present include hypertrophy of the medial layers of the veins and intimal fibrous thickening of the veins and venules. Nonspecific fibrous thickening of the intima may be added to the medial hypertrophic changes in the arteries and arterioles.

The structural changes in the pulmonary vascular bed in cases of obstruction to pulmonary venous flow correspond to the functional derangements in these conditions. These structural changes, however, are only rarely responsible for permanent impairment to pulmonary flow if the underlying cause of the obstructed pulmonary venous flow is eliminated. Among patients who have mitral stenosis, this point is frequently emphasized by a significant decrease in pulmonary arterial pressure after adequate surgical relief of the mitral stenosis.

Summary

Congenital anomalies responsible for obstruction in the right side of the heart are mainly in the right ventricle or pulmonary valve. These anomalies include pulmonary valvular stenosis with an intact ventricular septum and large ventricular septal defects with or without pulmonary stenosis. Regardless of the presence or absence of pulmonary stenosis, the large ventricular septal defect allows free communication between the right ventricle and the systemic arterial circulation. In the presence of a large ventricular septal defect associated with pulmonary stenosis, the pulmonary arterial pressure is not increased. In the absence of pulmonary stenosis, the pulmonary arterial systolic pressure approaches the systemic arterial systolic pressure.

The increased pulmonary pressure is responsible for the appearance of occlusive pulmonary vascular lesions and increased resistance.

This does not change the pulmonary or right ventricular pressure but does change the direction of the shunt. Before occlusive lesions appear, the shunt usually is exclusively in a left-to-right direction. When occlusive lesions are extensive, a right-to-left shunt appears and may even be the dominant one.

Obstructive lesions in the left side of the heart primarily or secondarily cause obstruction to pulmonary venous flow and thus are responsible for pulmonary hypertension. The latter lesions cause pulmonary hypertension by first producing left ventricular failure. The former conditions include stenotic lesions of the pulmonary veins or mitral valve, mitral insufficiency, and endocardial sclerosis of the left ventricle. The latter anomalies include obstructive lesions of or in relation to the aortic valve or obstruction in the thoracic aorta.

REFERENCES

1. Dexter, Lewis. Atrial septal defect. *Brit. Heart J.* **18**:209–225 (1956).
2. Edwards, J. E. The Lewis A. Conner Memorial Lecture. Functional pathology of the pulmonary vascular tree in congenital cardiac disease. *Circulation* **15**:164–196 (1957).
3. Blount, S. G., Jr., Mueller, Helmut, and McCord, M. C. Ventricular septal defect: Clinical and hemodynamic patterns. *Am. J. Med.* **18**:871–882 (1955).
4. Dammann, J. F., Jr., and Ferencz, Charlotte. The significance of the pulmonary vascular bed in congenital heart disease. III. Defects between the ventricles or great vessels in which both increased pressure and blood flow may act upon the lungs and in which there is a common ejectile force. *Am. Heart J.* **52**:210–231 (1956).
5. Heath, Donald, Helmholz, H. F., Jr., Burchell, H. B., DuShane, J. W., and Edwards, J. E. Graded pulmonary vascular changes and hemodynamic findings in cases of atrial and ventricular septal defect and patent ductus arteriosus. *Circulation* **18**:1155–1166 (1958).
6. Ferencz, Charlotte, Johnson, A. L., and Wiglesworth, F. W. Congenital mitral stenosis. *Circulation* **9**:161–179 (1954).
7. Edwards, J. E. Pathologic aspects of cardiac valvular insufficiencies. *A.M.A. Arch. Surg.* **77**:634–649 (1958).
8. Edwards, J. E., and Burchell, H. B. Pathologic anatomy of mitral insufficiency. *Proc. Staff Meetings Mayo Clin.* **33**:497–509 (1958).
9. Linde, L. M., Adams, F. H., and O'Loughlin, B. J. Endocardial fibroelastosis. Angiocardiographic studies. *Circulation* **17**:40–45 (1958).

10. Mannheimer, E., Bengtsson, E., and Winberg, J. Pure congenital mitral stenosis due to fibro-elastosis. *Cardiologia* 21:574–582 (1952).
11. Maxwell, G. M., and Young, W. P. Isolated mitral stenosis in an infant of three months. Report of a case treated surgically. *Am. Heart J.* 48:787–791 (1954).
12. Denie, J. J., and Verheugt, A. P. Supravalvular aortic stenosis. *Circulation* 18:902–908 (1958).

Pathophysiology Associated with Congenital Obstructive Defects

S. GILBERT BLOUNT, JR.

University of Colorado Medical Center, Denver, Colorado

Defects that give rise to the obstruction of blood flow into the heart, through the heart, or from the heart, are probably the most common form of abnormalities found in congenital heart disease. Such defects might be considered under the following headings:

1. Defects resulting in the obstruction of blood flow into the heart: stenosis of pulmonary veins or the common pulmonary vein at entrance into the left atrium.

2. Defects resulting in the obstruction of blood flow through the heart: stenosis of the atrioventricular valves.

3. Defects resulting in the obstruction of blood flow from the heart or in the great vessels that lead from the heart: (*a*) stenosis of the semilunar valves, (*b*) stenosis at subvalvular levels, (*c*) stenosis at supravalvular levels, and (*d*) diffuse obstructive lesions distal in pulmonary vascular bed.

Limitations of time make it impossible to discuss all these entities. Thus, only two common and important forms of obstruction will be considered, namely valvular pulmonary stenosis and pulmonary vascular obstruction.

The hemodynamic alterations attending valvular pulmonary stenosis are in general similar to all lesions affecting the free egress of blood from the ventricles. The nature of accompanying defects of course would modify the response to some extent. It might be questioned as to why the hemodynamic response to pulmonary vascular obstruction is being considered. Certainly, in the opinion of this observer, pulmonary vascular obstruction giving rise to pulmonary hypertension is rarely, if ever, of a basic congenital origin. Nevertheless, inasmuch

185

as it is so frequently a concomitant finding and the limiting factor in
the natural history of various congenital cardiac defects and exists
from birth in many individuals, it is considered reasonable to include
it in this discussion.

Certain fundamental points might be mentioned at this time
relative to the hemodynamic responses common to all obstructive
lesions. If the forward flow across the obstructed site is to be maintained at the normal level, the pressure proximal to the obstruction
must rise. As the degree of obstruction increases, the pressure level
proximal to the narrowed area must continue to increase. The blood
flow is usually maintained at relatively normal values until the myocardium begins to fail. At this point, the cardiac output falls, as does
the proximal pressure and gradient across the obstruction. The major
factor limiting the compensation of the myocardium is probably the
metabolic support as derived from the coronary flow.

Much of our knowledge of the dynamics of obstructing vascular
defects has been derived from acute animal experiments. The conditions of such experiments of course differ vastly from those of patients with congenital defects in whom the abnormality has existed
from birth or actually prior to birth.

A second basic point is that the natural history of the defect and the
symptomatology experienced by the patient is dependent upon the
site of the obstruction within the heart and the nature of the vascular
structures distal to and proximal to the site of the obstruction. Thus,
obstruction at the level of the aortic valve is well tolerated, as the left
ventricle is proximal to the obstruction, and as long as this chamber
retains compensation, cardiac output is adequate and there is but little
elevation of pressure in the left atrial-pulmonary venous-capillary
bed. However, when the obstruction is at the level of the mitral valve,
the left atrium is the proximal chamber. This is a thin wall chamber
without valves, and as soon as a rise in pressure develops, it is immediately transmitted backward into the pulmonary capillary bed and
symptoms of pulmonary capillary congestion ensue. The cardiac
output also tends to be low with marked obstruction because of the
characteristics of the proximal chamber. Because of these differences
the critical degree of stenosis will be much smaller in aortic than in
mitral stenosis.

Valvular Pulmonary Stenosis with Intact Septa

Let us now consider the response of the circulation to valvular pulmonary stenosis with intact septa.

The degree of stenosis may vary from slight to severe, and while the systolic pressure gradient across the valve offers some indication of the severity of the obstruction, a true evaluation of the significance of the stenosis must allow for the blood flow across the valve at the time the pressure gradient is determined. Under conditions of a great pulmonary artery blood flow it is possible for a normal valve to be relatively stenotic and a significant pressure gradient be manifest. Also, a small gradient may be noted in the face of severe stenosis when the existing blood flow is low. Dividing the pressure gradient in millimeters of mercury by the pulmonary index gives a rough evaluation of the stenosis. However, Gorlin, by applying hydraulic principles and formulas of fixed orifices, has derived a formula that will calculate with some accuracy the valve area and thus, better evaluate the degree of obstruction.

The demonstration on the withdrawl of the cardiac catheter from the pulmonary artery into the right ventricle of a sharply demarcated pressure change, high at the area of pulmonary valve from a low or normal pulmonary artery pressure to a high right ventricular systolic pressure is the physiologic proof of the existing stenosis. The pulmonary artery pressure is normal or low, the contour varies, dependent upon the severity of the stenosis and the resistance of the pulmonary vascular bed.

Conversion of the great potential energy developed by the right ventricle into velocity energy, as blood is expelled through the small orifice, results in negative systolic pressure waves, when the catheter tip is in the immediate area of the stenotic orifice. These are so-called Venturi curves. In the case of infundibular stenosis, an entirely different pressure curve may be noted on withdrawal of the catheter into the right ventricle. Variations are dependent upon the anatomy of the outflow area of the right ventricle and the pulmonary valve. Venturi curves are rarely noted in patients with infundibular stenosis, but we have noted this effect in several instances.

The range of stenosis, we have noted, is wide and varies from a right ventricular systolic pressure of 40 to 240 mm Hg, although higher right ventricular systolic pressures have been recorded. When septa are intact, the cardiac output usually remains roughly within normal limits, despite the severity of the stenosis, until cardiac failure ensues. The arteriovenous (a-v) oxygen difference, however, in patients with moderately severe valvular pulmonary stenosis but not in failure has usually been increased, which suggests some inadequacy of the existing output.

Severe stenosis is accompanied by a relatively fixed output and right ventricular systolic pressure, as evaluated by the response to exercise. Just as in the case of severe aortic stenosis, great increases in ventricular systolic pressures are necessary in order to elevate, even slightly, the cardiac output in the face of severe stenosis. Because of the inability of coronary blood flow to increase in proportion to the demands of ventricular work, ventricular systolic pressures seldom exceed 250 mm Hg. Thus, a relatively fixed stroke volume in a patient with pure pulmonary stenosis or aortic stenosis in the absence of failure and often in the absence of symptoms indicates a very severe obstructive lesion. The cardiac output does not increase with exercise in these patients, but the a-v difference widens. The work of the right ventricle is greatly increased, and the total work of course does not equal the effective work as a great proportion of the total work is used in overcoming the stenosis.

The architecture of the right ventricle is of such design that it is able to eject large volumes of blood with relatively slight degrees of myocardial shortening. However, it is not prepared to withstand the sudden development of outflow obstruction. This is certainly born out by acute animal experiments which reveal that slight degrees of constriction of the pulmonary artery result in an elevation of right ventricular pressure. Increasing the degree of constriction, further elevates the right ventricular systolic pressure until at about a 60% constriction: the right ventricular diastolic pressure rises, the right atrial pressure rises, the right ventricular systolic pressure declines, and the cardiac output falls. This occurs when the constriction has resulted in a right ventricular systolic pressure of about 90 mm Hg.

As previously stated, these are acute experiments and differ greatly from the status of the patient with congenital pulmonary valvular stenosis. A right ventricular systolic pressure of 90 mm Hg is a relatively mild degree of stenosis: the heart is of normal size, right ventricular hypertrophy is, however, present. The patient is asymptomatic and the valve orifice is at least 60% narrowed.

Severe degrees of stenosis with right ventricular systolic pressure over 150 mm Hg and valve orifices restricted to 80% or more of normal are well tolerated for long periods of time in patients with congenital pulmonary valvular stenosis.

Under the conditions of a defect existing from birth or with the gradual development of the obstruction, the architecture of the right ventricle comes to resemble that of the left and is better able to handle a high-resistance type work load. According to Rushmer the architecture of the ventricles reflects the type of work load that they bear, and that, in accordance with the law of LaPlace, their structure better enables them from a mechanical standpoint to handle their particular type work load.

What factors other than change in architecture determine the ability of the right ventricle to handle for many years this greatly elevated work load? Certainly, if we consider the normal pressure relationships within the right and left ventricles, a right ventricular systolic pressure of 200 mm Hg is a fantastic pressure level and might be compared with a left ventricular systolic pressure of 1000 mm Hg for a similar degree of obstruction. It is of interest that we have never recorded a left ventricular systolic pressure in congenital aortic stenosis significantly higher than our highest right ventricular pressure with severe valvular pulmonary stenosis. This provokes speculation relative to the ability and the manner by which the right ventricle is able to perform this greatly increased work load. The pressure within the ventricles is about equal at the time of birth, as is the muscular development. Is it possible that an increase in the work load of the right ventricle from birth, or actually prior to birth, may lead to a true proliferation as well as an increase in the size of the muscle fibers? This has been stated by some observers, although relatively few studies have been published pertaining to his problem. Certainly, it is hard to conceive the right ventricle compensating for this greatly increased work load and performing adequately for years with the same number of fibers present as in a normal right ventricle. There must be an actual increase in the number of fibers as well as hypertrophy. Little is known about the coronary blood supply to the right ventricle under these circumstances, but it is considered that there is an actual increase in the volume of coronary artery blood and possibly a variation in the anatomy of the coronary circulation.

What is the limiting factor to the ventricular compensation? From the work of Wiggers, Sarnoff, Guyton, and others, it would seem that decreased metabolic support due to inadequate oxygenation of the myocardium is probably the most important limiting factor. The onset of failure results in a further elevation of the end distolic and elevation of the mean diastolic pressure and an increased right atrial filling pressure. Despite this the cardiac output falls, and the patient might be said to be on the descending limb of the Starling curve.

The finding, however, of an elevated right ventricular end diastolic pressure in a patient with severe valvular pulmonary stenosis does not necessarily indicate failure, but may merely reflect the elevated pressure occurring with atrial systole and transmitted to the ventricle. The changes in the right ventricle accompanying hypertrophy result in an increased resistance to the filling of this chamber. With the normal low pressure in the right atrium, filling of the less distensible hypertrophied right ventricle is incomplete, and a residual volume of blood remains in the right atrium. Hypertrophy of the right atrium occurs as a consequence, and the increased force of contraction is manifested by development of an elevated pressure at the time of atrial contraction. This increased effective filling pressure enhances the strength of ventricular contraction. Failure of the right ventricle results in elevation of pressure throughout diastole, and the right atrial pressure tracing reveals evidence of insufficiency of the tricuspid valve with a prominent *c* wave.

Under conditions of intact septa, regardless of the volume of pulmonary blood flow, the peripheral arterial oxygen saturation is full, although with failure and greatly reduced cardiac output, cyanosis might become apparent, a stasis form of cyanosis due to increased oxygen extraction by peripheral tissues.

Results Following Surgery

The technical aspects of the surgery is being presented by Dr. Henry Swan in another paper at this meeting. The gradient across the valve is markedly decreased or obliterated, and the right ventricular systolic pressure returns toward normal or to normal levels. There is an increase in the pulmonary arterial pressure and a change in the contour and pulse pressure of the pulmonary artery pressure curve. Persistence of some gradient due to hypertrophy of muscular structures in the area of the outflow tract of the right ventricle may be noted. The finding of pulmonary hypertension following the removal of obstruction has been noted in some patients and reflects changes in the pulmonary vascular bed giving rise to elevated resistance, although the possibility of distal localized stenosis must be considered. When the valvular stenosis is removed, the increased pulmonary artery blood flow may be reflected by an abnormal increase in the pulmonary artery pressure in the face of a reduced area of the pulmonary vascular bed.

The level of the pressure developed with atrial systole decreases and reflects a decrease in the resistance to the filling of the right ventricle. When failure has existed for some time and the heart is greatly dilated, removal of the obstruction will not always return cardiac function to normal.

Valvular Pulmonary Stenosis with Defect in Atrial Septum

It is difficult, if not impossible, to determine whether a patent foramen ovale is present or true secundum type of defect. However, when a left-to-right shunt exists, then one can be reasonably certain that a true atrial septal defect is present. This, however, is a reasonably rare occurrence and we have encountered this but twice in a group of 225 patients operated upon for either atrial septal defect or valvular pulmonary stenosis. Certainly, the degree of stenosis must be mild, and the atrial septal defect is the more significant lesion. Should severe stenosis be present, the resistance to filling of the right ventricle would be greater than the left, and a right-to-left shunt (the usual state) would exist. When a left-to-right shunt exists the atrial septal defect should be closed first or both defects corrected at the same time. Removal of the stenosis, which in effect acts as a governor relative to the volume of the left-to-right shunt, could be disastrous. We have encountered one such situation. The fact that some observers have stated that pulmonary stenosis exists in about

10% of patients with atrial septal defect is considered to be due to failure to recognize the presence of a functional stenosis.

A right-to-left shunt and peripheral arterial unsaturation and at times cyanosis are the usual findings in this combination of defects. In the 20 patients that we have evaluated and operated upon with this combination (trilogy of Fallot), the defect at the time of surgery has been small and given the appearance of a patent foramen ovale and not a true atrial septal defect, although this is difficult to be certain of. The reason for the patency is certainly not entirely clear to this observer. Certainly, if the reason for the failure to close is the presence of a higher pressure in the right than in the left atrium, then one would expect such to occur in all cases of severe valvular stenosis. Yet, this does not seem to be the case. Many of the more severe degrees of stenosis, if the gradient is any indication of severity, are found in patients with intact atrial septum.

The explanation offered for the right-to-left shunt at times is not completely satisfying. The finding of a relatively low right ventricular systolic pressure and a small gradient in a patient with a right-to-left shunt and not in failure is disturbing, for it would certainly not seem that the right ventricular musculature was sufficiently hypertrophied to offer a greater resistance to filling than the left ventricle. The volume of right-to-left shunt is usually slight with peripheral arterial saturations of the order from 80 to 90%. However, large right-to-left shunts have been encountered in infants with peripheral arterial saturations as low as 35%. Our highest gradients have not been noted in cyanotic patients and this is, at least in part, accounted for by the decreased volume of the pulmonary blood flow, because of the right-to-left shunt present in these cases. The operative approach has been repair of both defects at the same time and results have been excellent.

Pulmonary Hypertension

Normal pulmonary artery pressure is dependent upon the maintenance of a physiologic relationship between the volume of blood flow into the pulmonary vascular bed and a normal cross-sectional area or capacity of this bed. The derangement of either of these factors can lead to elevated pulmonary arterial pressure. Elevated left atrial pressure by retrograde transmission will also lead to an increase of pulmonary artery pressure, but this does not often play a major role in the development of the pulmonary hypertension of congenital heart disease. When a normal pulmonary vasculature exists, it requires maximum increases in pulmonary blood flow to give rise to slight increases in pulmonary artery pressure. Thus, maximal treadmill exercise of normal young males has revealed a mean pulmonary artery pressure of 28 mm Hg with systolic peak swings of 40–45 mm Hg and diastolic levels of 6–10 mm Hg, and a cardiac index of from 9 to 10 liters. This exercise consists of 18% grade at 3.5 miles per hour for six minutes.

Patients with atrial septal defects may have higher pulmonary artery blood flows and entirely normal pulmonary artery blood pressure, suggesting maximum dilatation of the pulmonary vascular bed. However, in the face of a slight reduction of the normal capacity of the pulmonary vasculature, significant elevations of pulmonary artery pressure may be noted with increased pulmonary blood flows. Clear-cut elevation of pulmonary artery pressure in the patient with congenital heart disease indicates definite reduction in the overall capacity of the pulmonary vascular bed.

The pulmonary artery resistance, a function of the flow and pressure, is of great importance in the evaluation of the patient with increased pulmonary artery pressure. While it is certainly true that our determinations of pulmonary vascular resistance are crude estimates, nevertheless, this knowledge is of much greater value than the level of the pulmonary artery pressure itself in the evaluation of the status of the pulmonary vascular bed. The resistance is determined by dividing the mean pulmonary arterial pressure by the pulmonary blood flow. This may be expressed in arbitrary units and is of as much practical value as the more elaborate but no more accurate formula that is generally employed.

The pathologic changes that develop and decrease the cross-sectional area of the pulmonary vascular bed and give rise to pulmonary hypertension have been brilliantly discussed by the preceding speaker, Dr. Jesse Edwards. As the area is progressively decreased, either by various morphologic changes or possibly in addition by neurogenic effects, the pulmonary artery pressure rises. We also believe that the pulmonary hypertension that exists from birth to be due largely, if not completely, to an increase in the thickness of the media, so-called persistence of the fetal pattern with but little intimal involvement. The elevated pressure and resistance in these patients can at times be affected by drugs altering the neurogenic balance. This is much less likely to be noted in other patients usually older in whom intimal cellular proliferation and fibrosis play the prominent role in the pathologic process.

The finding of pulmonary blood pressure levels and resistance of systemic magnitude during the first two decades of life usually indicates that this situation has existed from birth. These are patients with large ventricular septal defects in whom the resistance limiting the pulmonary blood flow is not at the level of the ventricular septum but in the pulmonary vascular bed. This would also occur with any defect in which the pulmonary vasculature was exposed to systemic artery pressure from birth. There are, of course, exceptions when pulmonary vascular changes of sufficient severity to give rise to pulmonary vascular resistance of systemic order may develop during this period. These changes may be concomitant with defects giving rise to high pulmonary artery blood flows, but it is doubtful that they are secondary to the increased flow alone.

As the area of the pulmonary vascular bed progressively decreases, pulmonary hypertension may exist with normal or decreased pulmonary artery blood flow. Thus, in patients with so-called idiopathic pulmonary artery hypertension, marked elevated pulmonary artery pressure may exist with decreased pulmonary blood flow.

It is apparent that when severe pulmonary hypertension exists from birth, that the right ventricle is able to hypertrophy and adequately handle the greatly increased work load for many years. Thus, once again, the ability of the right ventricle to handle such increased work loads brings forth much interesting speculation. The response of the ventricle is somewhat similar to that in valvular pulmonary stenosis, although it is altered by the presence of the defect in the ventricular septum. The main difference is the site of the obstruction. In the one, it is localized at the outflow area from the right ventricle into the pulmonary artery, while in the present instance, it is diffuse, distal in the pulmonary vasculature. The right ventricular hypertrophy may be massive as is the case of severe valvular pulmonary stenosis, although, because of the presence of the defect in the ventricular septum, the systolic pressure generated within the right ventricle is limited by the systemic resistance and left ventricular systolic pressure. However, in the patient with idiopathic pulmonary hypertension, the right ventricular systolic pressure may greatly exceed the left. Resistance to filling the right ventricle develops and an elevated right atrial pressure follows. Large *a* waves are noted, however, in the right atrial pressure tracing only when the ventricular septum is intact and the pulmonary artery pressure exceeds the systemic.

When severe pulmonary hypertension develops later in life, the right ventricle would seem to be less able to handle the increased work load, and failure supervenes. The rate of development of the increased pulmonary vascular resistance and pressure is most important in determining the ability of the right ventricle to hypertrophy and handle the increased work load. The capillary pressure, a reflection of left atrial pressure, is within normal limits in most patients not in failure with congenital heart disease. The cardiac output is low normal or decreased and relatively fixed, again as in the case of the patient with severe valvular pulmonary stenosis. The natural history of the patient with pulmonary hypertension ends in congestive failure and death or at times sudden death without preceding failure. The development of failure again is probably in large part due to the failure of the metabolic support of the myocardium, secondary to the development of inadequate coronary blood flow.

III

DIAGNOSIS

Cardiac Catheterization Techniques Using Pressure, Flow, and Oxygen Analysis

LEWIS DEXTER

Departments of Medicine, Peter Bent Brigham Hospital and Harvard Medical School, Boston, Massachusetts

Venous catheterization consists of directing a catheter into various parts of the venous system of the body, including the chambers of the right side of the heart and pulmonary artery. Pressures may be recorded through the catheter and blood samples may be withdrawn for blood gas analysis. The position of the catheter, which is radio-opaque, may be identified roentgenographically. The methods for detecting a variety of types of congenital heart disease have been described in detail by many (1–5) and are widely used. Being common knowledge, they will not be discussed here. Instead, an appraisal of some of the methods will be discussed.

Left-to-Right Shunts

Shunts from left to right are recognized by the appearance of arterialized blood in some chamber of the right side of the heart—pulmonary artery for patent ductus arteriosus, right ventricle for ventricular septal defect, right atrium for atrial septal defect. The differential diagnosis of such a finding and some of the shortcomings and errors of this method of evaluation have been previously described (6). The sensitivity of determining left-to-right shunts by analysis of the oxygen content or saturation of blood samples depends partly on the number of samples withdrawn from each chamber and also on the normal variations in oxygen content of blood from the various chambers. Table I shows differences reported by Dexter *et*

TABLE I[a]

	Variation of Maximal O$_2$ Content (vol. %) between		
	PA-RV	RV-RA	RA-SVC
Average	+0.1	+0.2	+0.8
Range	−0.4 to +0.5	−0.8 to +0.9	−0.2 to +1.9
St. deviation	±0.3	±0.5	±0.6
95% probability of left-to-right shunt	>+0.2	>+0.4	>1.8+

[a] From reference 7.

al. (7) for consecutive sampling from the various chambers. It is seen that on multiple sampling, there is normally only slight variation in the maximal oxygen content of blood withdrawn from right atrium, right ventricle, and pulmonary artery, so that the recognition of patent ductus arteriosus and ventricular septal defect is rather good. The variation of oxygen content between superior vena cava and right atrium is, however, great, so that there is a 95% probability of an atrial septal defect only when the maximal value in the right atrium exceeds that in the superior vena cava by more than 1.8 vol. %.

Barratt-Boyes and Wood (8) found much the same variations in oxygen saturation (Table II) in the pulmonary artery, right ventricle, and right atrium, but they improved the sensitivity of detecting an atrial septal defect by averaging the oxygen saturation from superior vena cava and inferior vena cava and showed that there was a 95% likelihood of significant arterialization in the right atrium if the oxygen saturation of a blood sample withdrawn from the right atrium exceeded the average saturation of samples withdrawn from the inferior and superior venae cavae by more than 4% saturation (a content of 0.8 vol. %, assuming an oxygen capacity of 20.0 vol. %). If three or more *series* of samples were withdrawn in rapid succession from the inferior vena cava, superior vena cava and mid-right atrium, this variation was reduced to 2% saturation (or a content of 0.4 vol. %). With this improvement in recognizing arterialization in the right atrium, left-to-right shunts into the right atrium, right ventricle, or pulmonary artery amounting to more than 10 to 15% of the pulmonary blood flow (greater than about 0.5 liter/minute in the average adult) can usually be discovered by this method. Smaller shunts will usually not be detected.

TABLE II[a]

	Variation of O_2 Saturation (%) between			
	PA-High RV	Low RV-RA	RA-SVC	RA-IVC
Average	0	0	+2.9	−2.2
Range	−3 to +2	−9 to +10	−3 to +12	−11 to +6
St. deviation	±1.4	±2.9	±3.0	±4.3
95% probability of L–R shunt	>2	>3	>4 3 series >2	

	Variation of O_2 Content (vol.%) between			
	PA-High RV	Low RV-RA	RA-SVC	RA-IVC
Average	0	0	0.6	−0.4
Range	−0.6 to +0.4	−1.8 to +2.0	−0.6 to +2.4	−2.2 to +1.2
St. deviation	±0.3	±0.6	±0.6	±0.9
95% probability of L–R shunt	>0.4	>0.6	>0.8 3 series >0.4	

[a] Adapted from reference 8.

Further refinement by use of a rapid-response polarograph on the tip of the catheter remains to be evaluated (9).

Right-to-Left Shunts

Right-to-left shunts produce arterial oxygen unsaturation, but oxygen unsaturation may be due to other causes, specifically pulmonary disease, which not infrequently is associated with congenital heart disease. It might be thought that the administration of 100% oxygen would produce full arterial oxygen saturation when unsaturation is on a pulmonary basis and less than complete saturation when on the basis of a right-to-left shunt. Although this is usually true, there are exceptions. As Wood (10) has nicely demonstrated by indicator-dilution techniques, the administration of 100% oxygen may, in certain cases, reverse the shunt. Indicator-dilution techniques are more accurate than oxygen methods in detecting the existence and location of right-to-left shunts.

Flows

The standard method of measuring flow in congenital heart disease is the Fick method:

$$\text{Cardiac output (l/min)} = \frac{\text{O}_2 \text{ consumption (cc/min)}}{\text{a-v O}_2 \text{ difference (cc/l)}}$$

The built-in error of this method is ±5% at normal flow rates, due to the errors inherent in measuring oxygen consumption and in oxygen analysis by the Van Slyke or spectrophotometric methods. At high flow rates across the lung, as in patients with large left-to-right shunts, the error becomes progressively greater approaching infinity, due to the narrow a-v oxygen difference in the denominator. The following example illustrates this point.

R. R., Atrial Septal Defect, Age 22

Oxygen content	
Brachial artery	187 cc/l (98%)
Pulmonary artery	185 cc/l
Pulmonary a-v O$_2$ difference	2 cc/l
Oxygen consumption	210 cc/min
Pulmonary blood flow (210 ÷ 2)	105 l/min

All that one can say is that the pulmonary blood flow and shunt were enormous, but certainly not of the order of 105 liters/minute or even more than a fraction thereof. The Fick method does not lend itself to the accurate determination of flow when flows are high and when the arteriovenous oxygen difference approaches 1.0 vol. %, and serious question may be raised as to its use at all in such cases (11). The use of the nitrous oxide method as recently reported by Sanders and Morrow (12) avoids this difficulty. With the patient breathing relatively high concentrations of nitrous oxide (50%), the arteriovenous nitrous oxide difference is large, and the calculation of pulmonary blood flow in relation to systemic blood flow is apparently more sensitive and accurate than by oxygen methods.

Pressures

It is usually stated, and rightly so, that pressure recording with modern, small displacement, critically damped manometers is very accurate. This applies especially to pressures recorded through nee-

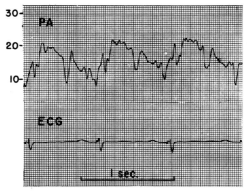

Fig. 1. Catheter artifacts. Distortion of wave form of pressures recorded through a catheter.

dles. When registration is made through a catheter, movement of the catheter in a cardiac chamber during systole and diastole not infrequently produces gross distortion of the wave form of the systolic and of the diastolic pressures (Fig. 1). There is no way of testing the frequency or square wave response of a manometer recording pressure through a catheter. A small air bubble or clot in the catheter may dampen the pressure sufficiently to disprove, apparently, Newton's second law of gravity (Fig. 2).

Wave form, systolic peaks, and diastolic dips are subject, therefore, to considerable distortion when recorded through a catheter. Current evidence indicates that mean pressure is the one really valid measurement, the others sometimes being accurate and at other times inaccurate. Therefore, the interpretation of pressures contains a certain element of subjective appraisal which is undesirable.

The attachment of a high-frequency micromanometer on the tip of the catheter, such as that of Allard and Laurens as reported by Soulié *et al.* (13), obviates damping and distortion difficulties and gives faithful recordings of the wave form, peaks, and diastolic levels of intracavity pressures.

Valvular Stenosis

Stenosis of a valve is indicated by a pressure difference on the two sides of the valve. Pulmonic stenosis is the commonest congenital valvular lesion and may be valvular, infundibular, or both. Examples

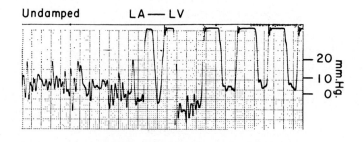

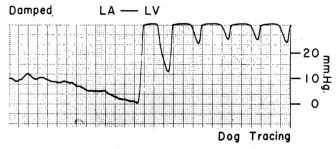

Fig. 2.   Effect of damping on pressure tracing. The lower tracing seems to indicate that the diastolic pressure in the left ventricle is higher than that in the left
atrium. A more faithful recording is shown in the upper tracing, where it is seen
that these two pressures are approximately the same.

of findings are shown in Fig. 3 (14). The approximate length of the
infundibular stenosis, a point of surgical significance, can be estimated by the distance fluoroscopically over which the infundibular
type of pressure extends while the catheter is withdrawn (15). Such
measurements are qualitatively useful but quantitatively lack precision due to dispersion of the x-rays.

In our experience, a pressure difference over 4 mm Hg between
right ventricle and pulmonary artery in systole is not a normal finding, even in atrial septal defect with high flows (Fig. 4). Higher gradients may, of course, disappear after the large flow has been eliminated by surgical correction of the defect.

The severity of stenosis may be evaluated by the Gorlin formula
(16)

$$A = \frac{F}{K\Delta P}$$

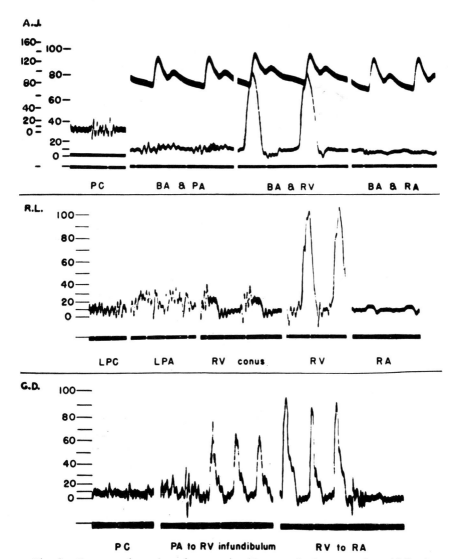

Fig. 3. Pressures in pulmonic stenosis: Above, valvular stenosis; middle, in-fundibular stenosis; below, valvular and infundibular stenosis (14).

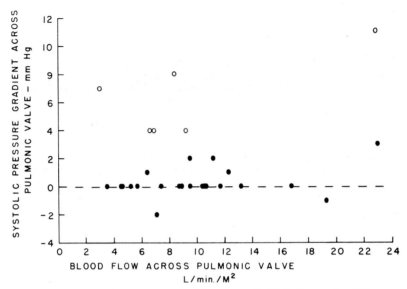

Fig. 4.   Note that in many cases with extremely high flows, the difference of systolic pressures across the pulmonic valve is usually less than 4 mm Hg.

This calculation is not valid if regurgitation exists or if the stenosis is too mild to produce a significant pressure difference.

Pulmonary Vascular Resistance

For evaluation of pulmonary vascular disease, resistance to blood flow through a vascular bed is calculated by using the Poiseuille equation, $R = \Delta P/F$. This is the best one can currently use, but it has two serious handicaps. First, it assumes a linear relationship between pressure and flow. This holds true for glass tubes but not for a vascular bed (17, 18). The interpretation of minor changes in calculated resistance is therefore of doubtful value and only when there is a considerable change is interpretation possible. Secondly, no changes of pressure or flow, and therefore of calculated resistance, occur in the pulmonary circuit until the cross-sectional area of the pulmonary artery is reduced by at least two-thirds (18). In other words, changes in calculated pulmonary vascular resistance are late to appear and occur only at an advanced stage of pulmonary vascular disease. There is currently no good way of detecting early changes.

Summary

In summary, no attempt has been made to describe the findings in individual types of congenital heart disease, since these are well known to this audience, but rather some of the problems which arise and some of the limitations involved in measuring pressures, determining flows by the Fick method, and detecting shunts by oxygen analysis of blood samples. These are the techniques which have so impressively advanced the subject of congenital heart disease in the last decade and a half. The remainder of this program is largely concerned with the use of other methods which have been devised to enhance accuracy of measurement or to elucidate other aspects of congenital heart disease not revealed by the approach described.

REFERENCES

1. Dexter, L., Haynes, F. W., Burwell, C. S., Eppinger, E. C., Sosman, M. C., and Evans, J. M. Studies of congenital heart disease. III. Venous catheterization as a diagnostic aid in patent ductus arteriosus, tetralogy of Fallot, ventricular septal defect, and auricular septal defect. *J. Clin. Invest.* **26:**561 (1947).
2. Cournand, A., Baldwin, J. S., and Himmelstein, A. *Cardiac Catheterization in Congenital Heart Disease.* Commonwealth Fund, New York, 1949.
3. Soulié, P. *Cardiopathies Congénitales.* Expansion Scientifique Française, Paris, 1956.
4. Heim de Balsac, R., Métianu, C., Durand, M., and Dubost, Ch. *Traité des Cardiopathies Congénitales.* Masson et Cie., Paris, 1954.
5. Wood, P. *Diseases of the Heart and Circulation.* Eyre & Spottiswoode, London, 1956.
6. Dexter, L. Cardiac catheterization in the diagnosis of congenital heart disease. *Minn. Med.* **37:**116 (1954).
7. Dexter, L., Haynes, F. W., Burwell, C. S., Eppinger, E. C., Sagerson, R. P., and Evans, J. M. Studies of congenital heart disease. II. The pressure and oxygen content of blood in the right auricle, right ventricle, and pulmonary artery in control patients, with observations on the oxygen saturation and source of pulmonary "capillary" blood. *J. Clin. Invest.* **26:**554 (1947).
8. Barratt-Boyes, B. G., and Wood, E. H. The oxygen saturation of blood in the venae cavae, right heart chambers and pulmonary vessels of healthy subjects. *J. Lab. Clin. Med.* **50:**93 (1957).
9. Kreuzer, F., and Nessler, C. G., Jr. Method of polarographic *in vivo* continuous recording of blood oxygen tension. *Science* **128:**1005 (1958).

10. Burchell, H. B., Swan, H. J. C., and Wood, E. H. Demonstration of differential effects on pulmonary and systemic arterial pressure by variation in oxygen content of inspired air in patients with patent ductus arteriosus and pulmonary hypertension. *Circulation* 8:681 (1953).
11. Dexter, L., Haynes, F. W., Burwell, C. S., Eppinger, E. C., Seibel, R. E., and Evans, J. M. Studies of congenital heart disease. I. Technique of venous catheterization as a diagnostic procedure. *J. Clin. Invest.* 26:547 (1947).
12. Sanders, R. J., and Morrow, A. G. The diagnosis of circulatory shunts by the nitrous oxide test. Improvements in technic and methods for quantification of the shunt. *Circulation* 18:856 (1958).
13. Soulié, P., Laurens, P., Bouchard, F., Cornu, C., and Brial, E. Enrégistrement des pressions et des bruits intracardiaques à l'aide d'un micromanomètre. *Soc. Méd. Hôp. Paris* 73:713 (1957).
14. Dow, J. W., Levine, H. D., Elkin, M., Haynes, F. W., Hellems, H. K., Wittenberger, J. W., Ferris, B. G., Goodale, W. T., Harvey, W. P., Eppinger, E. C., and Dexter, L. Studies in congenital heart disease. IV. Uncomplicated pulmonic stenosis. *Circulation* 1:267 (1950).
15. Connolly, D. C., Lev, R., Kirklin, J. W., and Wood, E. The problem of isolated valvular versus infundibular pulmonic stenosis with particular reference to cardiac catheterization data on records obtained at the time of operation. *Proc. Staff Meetings Mayo Clin.* 28:65 (1953).
16. Gorlin, R., and Gorlin, S. G. Hydraulic formula for calculation of the area of the stenotic mitral valve, other cardiac valves, and central circulatory shunts. *Am. Heart J.* 41:1 (1951).
17. Green, H. D. Shock. *Anesthesiology*, 3:611 (1942).
18. Burton, A. The relation between pressure and flow in the pulmonary bed. *Pulmonary Circulation*. Grune and Stratton, New York, 1959, pp. 26–35.
19. Gibbon, J. H., Jr., Hopkinson, M., and Churchill, E. D. Changes in the circulation produced by gradual occlusion of the pulmonary artery. *J. Clin. Invest.* 11:543 (1932).

Use of Indicator-Dilution Technics*

EARL H. WOOD

Section of Physiology, Mayo Clinic and Mayo Foundation,† Rochester, Minnesota

An indicator-dilution curve can be defined as a recording of the concentration of an indicator with time at a site in the circulation after injection of this indicator at another site in the circulation.

For the purposes of this presentation, dilution curves are separated into arterial dilution curves and venous dilution curves. An arterial dilution curve is defined as a recording of the concentration of an indicator from any site in the arterial circulation or from the left side of the heart (1).

A venous dilution curve is defined as a recording of the concentration of an indicator at any site in the right heart or the venous circulation (2).

General Considerations

General considerations concerning indicator-dilution curves can be facilitated by reference to Fig. 1. This is a schematic representation of a circulation which could be considered to represent, for instance, the pulmonary circulation with the indicator being injected into the pulmonary artery at the site marked *A*. In most indicator-dilution technics, the indicator is injected as rapidly as possible as a single bolus at the injection site. As the indicator traverses the circulation, it is dispersed along the circulatory system by the action of two main factors. First, owing to the effect of laminar flow through single vessels, the central axial stream of the dye-blood mixture travels at a much higher rate of speed than does the dye-blood mixture

* This study was supported in part by Research Grant No. H-3532 from the National Institutes of Health, Public Health Service.

† The Mayo Foundation, Rochester, Minnesota, is a part of the Graduate School of the University of Minnesota.

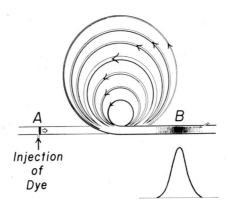

A   B

Injection
of
Dye

Fig. 1.   Effect of paths of different traversal times such as would occur in the lungs on the distribution of a miscible substance introduced into a flowing stream at point *A* and observed at *B*. Duration of the curve on the time axis represents the interval required for the blood in which the indicator is dispersed to pass the sampling site at point *B*.

at the periphery of the vessel; therefore, the dye in the central axial stream tends to arrive more quickly at the sampling site than does the dye traveling in proximity to the vessel walls (3). Second, when the dye-blood mixture enters a complex capillary circulation, such as that in the lungs, it is further dispersed by the fact that the circulatory pathway divides into many paths of varying lengths through which, if the velocity of the dye-blood mixture is approximately the same, the portions which pass through short pathways will reach the sampling site in a much shorter period than will the portion of the dye-blood mixture which traversed longer circulatory pathways (4). As a result of these two effects, when the dye-blood mixture reaches the sampling site marked by point *B* on Fig. 1, the dye is dispersed over a considerable length of the circulatory system so that the concentration of indicator as recorded against time increases more or less rapidly to a peak concentration and then decreases slightly more slowly, and if the circulatory system is such that no recirculation of the indicator occurs, it approaches zero concentration.

As is well known, considerable information concerning the status and characteristics of the circulatory system between the injection and the sampling sites can be derived from such an indicator-dilution curve. Such a curve, for instance, can be used to calculate the volume rate of blood flow between injection and sampling sites (5, 6), the volume of the vascular system between injection and sampling sites (7), the rapidity or velocity of such a circulation, and the presence or absence of abnormal circulatory pathways or abnormally functioning valves in this circulatory system (1, 2).

The importance of indicator-dilution curves of this type in cardiovascular physiology and diagnosis perhaps can be emphasized properly by the statement that more information concerning the status of the circulatory system can be obtained from such an indicator-dilution curve than can be obtained from a recording of any other single physiologic variable.

Before discussing the various parameters of the circulation about which information can be obtained by means of indicator-dilution curves, it is of value to have clearly in mind the factors which are known and the factors which must be measured for the various applications of this technic. The things which are known are (1) the dose of the dye, (2) the site of injection, and (3) the site of sampling of the resulting dye-blood mixture from the circulatory system. The factors which are measured from such a curve are (1) the time at which the indicator is injected and (2) the concentration of the indicator at the sampling site at any time during the inscription of the curve.

The time of arrival of indicator particles at the sampling site is determined by two factors: (1) the length of the path, that is, the distance traversed by the dye-blood mixture between the injection and sampling site; (2) the velocity of blood flow through this segment of the circulatory system. The velocity of the blood flow through this segment of the circulatory system is determined, in turn, by the volume of blood contained in this segment of the circulatory system and the volume rate of blood flow through this circulation.

The concentration of indicator at the sampling site at any time during the recording of an indicator-dilution curve is affected by the volume rate of blood flow through this segment of the circulatory system, the volume of blood contained between the injection and sampling sites, the anatomy of this circulatory segment, and the nature of the blood flow through it.

It is evident, therefore, that many factors may have a striking effect on the contour of an indicator-dilution curve. For instance, an increase in the volume rate of blood flow through a given segment of the circulation would tend to decrease the time components of the indicator-dilution curve as well as the concentrations, since the velocity of blood flow would be increased and the indicator would be diluted in a greater volume of blood. Similarly, an increase in the volume of blood contained in this segment of the circulation which was associated with no change in the volume rate of flow would be expected not only to increase the time components of the curve but also to decrease the concentrations since, again, the indicator would be diluted in a greater volume of blood. Likewise, it would be expected that any abnormal communication or short cut in the circulatory system would produce specific effects on the contour of the dilution curve (8). The effects of abnormal communications in the central circulation on indicator-dilution curves can perhaps be most readily understood by reference to Fig. 2. Abnormal communications, that is, intracardiac or great-vessel defects, are usually the result of congenital heart disease and are usually associated with abnormal circulatory shunts, either in the right-to-left or the left-to-right direction. Figure 2 illustrates from above downward a schema of the normal circulation, the circulation associated with a left-to-right shunt and the circulation associated with a right-to-left shunt. The typical contours of the dilution curves associated with these three conditions are shown on the left.

A left-to-right shunt, such as usually would occur through a ventricular or atrial septal defect, results in an increase in volume of blood flow through the pulmonary circulation so that, in this situation, the dye is diluted in the greater volume of blood and, hence, the deflection or the concentration of the indicator-dilution curve is reduced below that usually encountered in normals. Due to the presence of the left-to-right shunt, the dye-blood mixture continues to recirculate through the lungs so that the clearance of the dye from the central circulation is delayed, thus producing the characteristic disproportionate prolongation of the disappearance phase of the dilution curve associated with a left-to-right shunt (9).

In the presence of a right-to-left shunt, a portion of the dye-blood mixture gains direct access from the right to the left side of the heart,

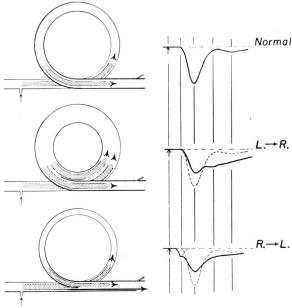

Fig. 2. Major differences from normal of dilution curves characteristic of left-to-right and right-to-left shunts. The distribution of paths of differing traversal times (Fig. 1) has been simplified (upper panel) to a single circuit representing the normal pathway from the venous to the systemic arterial circulation. Normal dilution curve obtained from such a circulation, when the indicator is injected rapidly into the venous circulation (at the arrow) and the resultant dye-blood mixture is sampled from a systemic artery, is shown at the right. In middle panel the circulation is characterized by increased pulmonary blood flow due to a large left-to-right shunt. Indicator is not cleared rapidly but recirculates via the defect through the central circulation. A constant fraction (dependent on the relative magnitudes of the left-to-right shunt and the pulmonary blood flow) leaves this central pool on each circulation. Dilution curve at right reflects this situation and may be contrasted to the normal (broken line). The maximal deflection is reduced, because the indicator is dispersed and diluted in the large volume of the central circulation and the high pulmonary flow. The disappearance phase is prolonged owing to the slow clearance of dye from the central pool. In bottom panel is shown the circulation in cases of a right-to-left shunt, which is usually associated with a reduced pulmonary flow. A portion of the indicator passes directly to the arterial circulation via the defect without traversing the longer normal circulatory pathway through the lungs and arrives at the arterial sampling site before the portion which traverses the central circulation. Dilution curve to right demonstrates this early arrival of the portion of the indicator shunted right to left by the shortened appearance time and the abnormal initial deflection superimposed on the buildup portion of the curve.

thus bypassing the longer and normal pulmonary circulation and hence arriving at the sampling site in an abnormally short time. This results in the characteristic abnormal initial deflection in the buildup phase of the dilution curve which is characteristic of a right-to-left shunt (10).

Since left-to-right and right-to-left shunts are two of the most important manifestations of the presence of congenital heart disease, the association of typical contours of dilution curves with these circulatory shunts is of evident diagnostic importance (1).

The importance of various applications of indicator-dilution technics in the diagnosis and study of congenital heart disease perhaps can be properly emphasized by the following two statements: (1) Recordings of arterial indicator-dilution curves obtained after injections of the indicator at selected sites on the right side of the heart provide the most sensitive practical method currently available for the detection, localization, and quantitation of right-to-left shunts (10, 11). (2) Venous dilution curves recorded from selected sites on the right side of the heart provide the most sensitive practical method currently available for the detection, localization, and quantitation of left-to-right shunts (2, 12). Although the indicator-dilution technic is of considerable diagnostic value as an independent method, it attains by far its greatest value when used in conjunction with cardiac catheterization.

Role of Indicator-Dilution Technics in Cardiac Catheterization

The procedure of diagnostic cardiac catheterization, when carried out in an adequate fashion, is based on the integration and the judicious selection of several technics. The most important technics include the recording of pressures in selected sites in the cardiac chambers and great vessels and the measurement of the blood-oxygen content of blood withdrawn from these sites as discussed previously by Dexter (13). In relation to the determination of blood-oxygen content, it is of paramount importance that a method be available for the immediate determination of blood-oxygen content or saturation if the highest possible degree of accuracy is to be obtained from diagnostic cardiac catheterization (14–17). The third technic is selective indicator-dilution studies (1, 2), and the fourth, selective angiocardiography (18–20). Each of these four technics is indispensable for the performance of the best possible type of diagnostic cardiac catheterization, and none of the technics should be used to the exclusion of the others. Since angiocardiography carries a slight, but unquestionably the greatest, inherent danger to the patient, in my opinion, it should not be used unless the data required cannot be obtained by any of the other safer methods. However, the extensive experiences of Sones (19) and of Campbell (20) with the selective, multiple injection, cine-angiographic technic have demonstrated that the risk of this procedure is apparently almost negligible in relation to the valuable diagnostic information which can be obtained.

A multitude of diagnostic and investigative applications of selective arterial and venous indicator-dilution technics has been described previously (1, 2). Rather than attempt to review all these various applications, this discussion will be restricted to a small number of specific applications which may serve to give the reader some indication of the diagnostic value of the various applications of indicator-dilution technics.

First to be considered will be specific applications of arterial indicator-dilution technics.

Diagnostic Applications of Arterial Dilution Curves

One of the earliest and most important applications of arterial indicator-dilution technics is their use for the detection, localization, and quantitation of right-to-left shunts (8, 10) (Fig. 3). If, in the presence of a right-to-left shunt, the cardiac catheter is advanced so that its tip lies distal to the site of the shunt and indicator is injected, the recording of the concentration of this indicator at an arterial sampling site may approach that of normal. However, if the tip of the cardiac catheter is then withdrawn to a site at or upstream to the right-to-left shunt, and a second injection of indicator is carried out, the dilution curve recorded at the arterial sampling site will show the typical abnormal initial deflection associated with the right-to-left shunt and, thus, demonstrate and localize the site of the right-to-left shunt to the site in the circulatory system at which the indicator was injected. By equations which have been described previously by Swan and co-workers (10), it is possible, from such an indicator-dilu-

Injection into :

Pulmonary artery   Right ventricle

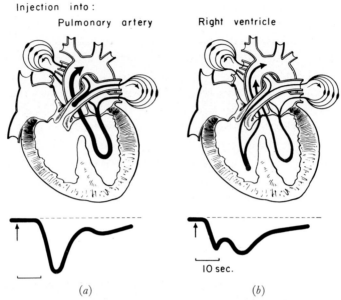

IO sec.

(a)   (b)

Fig. 3.   Method of localizing the site of a right-to-left shunt by means of indicator-dilution curves. There is pulmonary stenosis and a right-to-left shunt via a ventricular septal defect. Below are shown the arterial dilution curves recorded after injections (at arrows) into the pulmonary artery and the right ventricle. When the dye is injected downstream to the shunt, that is, into the pulmonary artery (a), a nearly normal dye curve results; when the dye is injected upstream to the shunt (b), part of it escapes to the left side of the heart via the ventricular septal defect and appears prematurely in the systemic artery to produce an early abnormal initial deflection of the curve. The dye traversing a normal pathway appears later, and the characteristic double-humped curve results. The difference in these two curves localizes the site of the shunt to the right ventricle.

tion curve, to calculate the magnitude of the right-to-left shunt with reasonable accuracy. This technic has its greatest value in localizing the site of large right-to-left shunts and in the detection and quantitation of the magnitude of relatively small right-to-left shunts some of which cannot be detected by the slight decrease in the oxygen saturation of arterial blood which they may cause. By means of this technic, it is possible to detect and obtain some idea of the magnitude of shunts of less than 5% of the systemic blood flow. In the presence of balanced pressures between the cardiac chambers or extremely small defects, the detection of right-to-left shunts by this method frequently may be the only evidence obtained at cardiac catheterization of the presence and location of the defect in question.

Left-to-right shunts usually are studied best by means of venous dilution curves since left-to-right shunts of less than 20% of pulmonary blood flow may not produce a significant alteration in the contour of arterial indicator-dilution curves (9, 21). However, in certain instances, the pattern of left-to-right shunt of arterial dilution curves may be of considerable importance in elucidating a complex cardiac abnormality. Such an application is illustrated in Fig. 4 in which a cardiac catheter has traversed an atrial septal defect and entered the left ventricle. In the presence of an atrial septal defect, it is often difficult to be certain whether or not there is a co-existing communication between the ventricles. Such a communication be-

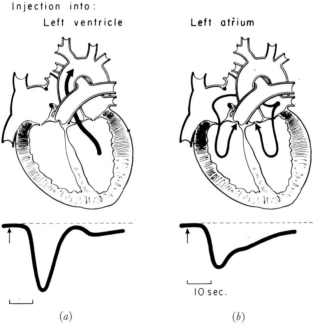

Injection into:

Left ventricle   Left atrium

10 sec.

(a)   (b)

Fig. 4. Localization of left-to-right shunt via an atrial septal defect. (a) An injection is made into the left ventricle which is guarded by a competent valve and from which no left-to-right shunt occurs. A normal dilution curve results. (b) The catheter tip is withdrawn to the left atrium from which there is a left-to-right shunt through an atrial septal defect. The abnormal dilution curve demonstrates the presence of a left-to-right shunt from this chamber.

tween the ventricles may be of considerable practical importance in selecting the method to be used for surgical correction of the defect in question. Also, in this situation, it may be of considerable practical importance to obtain information as to the possible presence of mitral regurgitation. If dye is injected via the catheter into the left ventricle and a completely normal dilution curve is recorded at a systemic artery, one can be relatively certain that there is no left-to-right shunt at or distal to the left ventricle, and that a severe degree of mitral regurgitation is not present. In this situation, when the catheter tip is withdrawn into the left atrium, and the injection repeated, the typical pattern of the left-to-right shunt will be obtained at the systemic artery, thus localizing the site of the left-to-right shunt to the atrial septum.

A third important diagnostic application of arterial indicator-dilution technics is their use for identification of the drainage pathway of a pulmonary vein. When a cardiac catheter passes from the cardiac silhouette into a pulmonary vein in the right lung field, it is often difficult or impossible, by ordinary fluoroscopic or roentgenologic technics, to be certain whether or not this vein is connected normally to the left atrium, the catheter passing to it via an atrial septal defect, or whether this vein connects directly and abnormally to the right atrium. The drainage pathway of such a vein entered by the catheter can be identified with ease and certainty by means of indicator-dilution technics as illustrated in Fig. 5. If an injection of indicator is carried out into the pulmonary vein via the catheter, and its concentration is recorded at a systemic artery in a case of a normally connected vein (Fig. 5), an indicator-dilution curve will be obtained that shows an early appearance time and a large initial deflection due to the large quantity of dye which passes directly into the left ventricle and out to the arterial sampling site. A second abnormal deflection will be present on the disappearance phase of this curve if an appreciable left-to-right shunt is present via the atrial septal defect traversed by the catheter.

If the catheter tip is then withdrawn into the superior or inferior vena cava, and the injection is repeated, the contour of the dilution curve recorded at a systemic artery will be strikingly different from that recorded after the injection into the pulmonary vein owing to

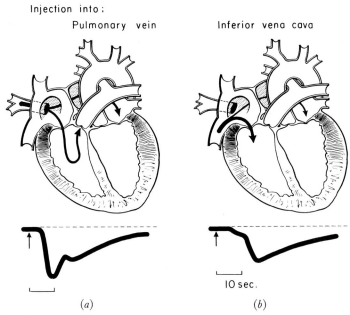

Injection into:

Pulmonary vein   Inferior vena cava

10 sec.

(a)   (b)

Fig. 5.   Schematic diagram of heart and circulation in atrial septal defect. The right pulmonary vein passes behind the right atrium to connect normally to the left atrium. The circulatory path (solid line) from the pulmonary vein (a) is fundamentally different from that from the inferior vena cava (b). Indicator-dilution curves (below) recorded at a systemic artery show dissimilar contours because of the differences in circulatory paths. In (a) a considerable proportion of the blood-dye mixture passes to the left ventricle, giving rise to an initial deflection of moderate magnitude. Remainder of the blood-dye mixture is shunted left to right, entering the right ventricle and pulmonary circulation and producing distortion of the disappearance phase of the curve. In (b) a very small proportion of the blood-dye mixture passes across the interatrial communication, and the remainder recirculates through the lungs. The resulting dilution curve is characterized by a small initial deflection, while the main portion of the curve shows the reduced deflection and prolonged disappearance phase associated with pulmonary recirculation. This demonstration of differing drainage from each of these sites indicates that the pulmonary vein is normally connected to the left atrium.

the fact that this dye-blood mixture drains into the right atrium and all or a major portion of it passes through the normal pulmonary circulation before entering the left side of the heart. This striking difference in the contour of the dilution curves recorded after these two injections demonstrates that the drainage pathway of the pul-

Injection into :

Pulmonary vein   Inferior vena cava

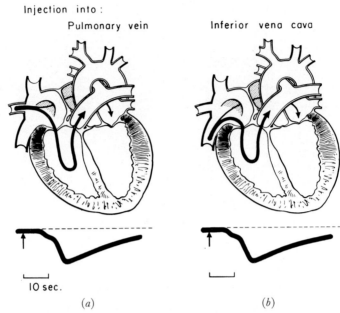

10 sec.

(a)   (b)

Fig. 6. Schematic diagram of heart and circulation in a case of atrial septal defect with anomalous connection of the right pulmonary vein to the right atrium. Since blood from the pulmonary vein and that from the venae cavae mix freely in the right atrium, the dilution curves recorded after injection into the right pulmonary vein (a) and inferior vena cava (b) were nearly identical. This feature demonstrates that all the blood from the right pulmonary vein drains anomalously, that is, in the same manner as the caval blood, permitting the diagnosis of anomalous pulmonary venous connection. The small initial deflection is caused by a small right-to-left shunt through the defect, and the prolongation of the disappearance slope is due to the much larger left-to-right shunt through this same defect.

monary vein entered by the catheter is different from that of the systemic veins and, therefore, that the pulmonary vein is almost certainly normally connected to the left atrium.

In the case of an abnormally connected pulmonary vein such as that illustrated in Fig. 6, the pattern of the dilution curve recorded after injection of indicator into the pulmonary vein and into the superior and inferior venae cavae will be closely similar. This indicates that the drainage pathway of blood from this pulmonary vein and the systemic veins is practically identical and, therefore, that the pulmonary vein is abnormally connected to the right atrium.

Another specific application of arterial indicator-dilution curves is in the identification of a central arterial vessel which may be entered by the catheter.

In some instances of relatively complex congenital heart disease, the situation may obtain in which the pressure and the oxygen content of blood withdrawn from the pulmonary artery and the aorta are closely similar. If in such a situation, as sometimes occurs, it is impossible to advance the catheter peripherally in the central arterial vessel, it may be extremely difficult to be certain whether the catheter has entered the pulmonary artery or the aorta. The site of the catheter tip, however, can be easily and accurately determined by the characteristics of the dilution curve recorded at a systemic artery after injection of indicator into the vessel entered by the catheter (Fig. 7). If the injection is made into the aorta (left panels, Fig. 7), a dilution curve characteristic of an aortic injection is obtained; that is, there are a rapid appearance of the dye and a large initial deflection that thus identify the vessel as the aorta. If, however, the injection is carried out into the pulmonary artery, a dilution curve characteristic of this injection site will be obtained, showing a longer appearance time and a smaller deflection as a result of the dye passing through the pulmonary circulation before entering the left ventricular and arterial circulation. The application of this technic to the identification of the central arterial vessels entered by the catheter in a 27-year-old man with transposition of the great vessels and single ventricle is illustrated in Fig. 8. In this patient, the oxygen saturation and pressure of blood in the aorta and pulmonary artery were similar. A central arterial vessel was entered in a position which, by roentgenography and fluoroscopy, was typical of that for the pulmonary artery. However, injection of indicator into this vessel indicated that it was indeed the aorta. Subsequently, the catheter was introduced into a second arterial vessel whose position, as evidenced by an anteroposterior roentgenogram of the thorax, was characteristic of the aorta, but injection of indicator into this central arterial vessel indicated that this vessel was the pulmonary artery. Thus, the diagnosis of transposition of the great vessels was established with certainty and, in conjunction with the other data obtained by the cardiac catheterization procedure, the diagnosis of transposed origin

222   E. H. Wood

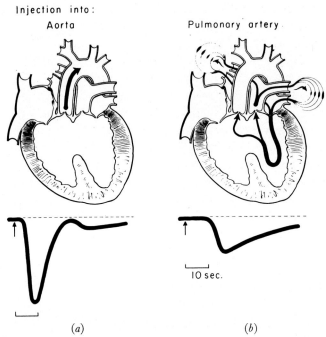

Injection into:
Aorta   Pulmonary artery

10 sec.

(a)   (b)

Fig. 7.   Schematic diagram of heart and great vessels and dilution curves
obtained in a case of transposition of the central great vessels with a single
ventricle. The aorta arises from the position usually occupied by the pulmonary
artery, and in the absence of another major interatrial or aortopulmonary communication, the presence of the ventricular defect is essential to survival, for
through it alone can systemic venous blood enter the lungs and pulmonary
venous blood enter the arterial system. (a) Injection of the dye into the aorta
and the characteristic short appearance time and large sharp deflection of the
dilution curve obtained. (b) Injection of the dye into the pulmonary artery. The
longer pathway taken by the dyed blood through the lungs and pulmonary recirculation produces the dilution curve (below) characteristic for this injection.

of the great vessels from the cardiac silhouette in association with a
single ventricle was established.

Many other applications of arterial indicator-dilution technics will
not be discussed at this time. These include demonstration of whether
or not there are two ejection pathways from a ventricular cavity (22);
that is, whether or not blood gains access to both the pulmonary artery
and aorta from this ventricle and the relative magnitude of blood
ejected from this ventricle into these two pathways. The important
applications of dilution curves to the study and localization of valve

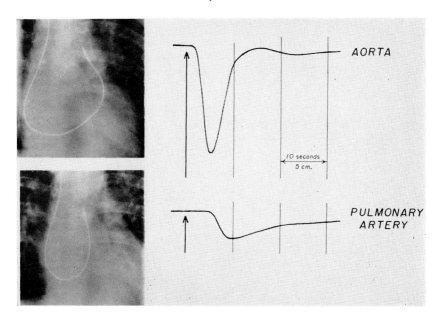

Fig. 8. Identification of central arterial vessels by means of dilution curves recorded at the radial artery after injection of indicator through a catheter at positions in the heart shown by the accompanying roentgenograms. (Top) Catheter lying in the position usually occupied by the pulmonary artery, but the short appearance time and the sharp deflection of the associated dilution curve demonstrated this vessel to be the aorta. (Bottom) Catheter in a position suggestive of the aorta but the longer appearance time, smaller deflection and evidence for recirculation through the lungs shown by the dilution curve identify this vessel as the pulmonary artery.

regurgitation (2, 23–25) will not be discussed. Important applications in the demonstration of total anomalous pulmonary venous connection (26, 27) and anomalous connection of systemic veins (27), the diagnosis of tricuspid atresia (28), and other variants and combinations of congenital heart disease (29–31) frequently make possible the establishment of a definite diagnosis at cardiac catheterization which otherwise would yield inconclusive or confusing results.

Diagnostic Applications of Venous Dilution Curves

The recording of venous dilution curves requires two routes of ingress or egress to the right heart, one for the injection of indicator and the other for the sampling of the resulting dye-blood mixture.

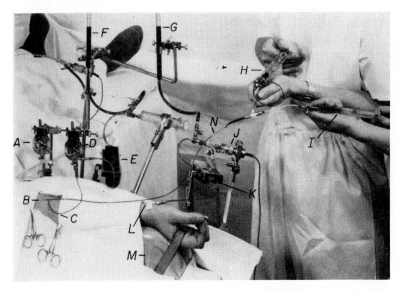

Fig. 9.   Instrument assembly used during catheterization of the right side of the heart, incorporating two cardiac catheters introduced by percutaneous puncture of a medial and a lateral antecubital vein for simultaneous injection of indicator and recording of its concentration from selected sites in the central circulation. Assembly for recording dilution curves from the radial artery also is shown. *A,* strain-gage manometer records pressures transmitted via a catheter, *B,* in the right side of the heart, which has been disconnected temporarily for injection of the indicator contained in the syringe, *H. C,* catheter to the right side of the heart is connected to a two-way stopcock for interchangeable connection of the lumen of the catheter to a strain-gage manometer, *D,* for recording pressure, or to a cuvette oximeter, *E,* for recording of oxygen saturation or dye concentration in blood being withdrawn via the catheter from selected sites in the heart or great vessels. Rate of blood flow from the catheter during the recording of dilution curves is measured by signaling each milliliter of blood collected in a buret, *F.* Upper end of the buret is connected to a source of constant vacuum (not shown). *L,* an indwelling needle in the radial artery is connected via a cuvette oximeter, *K,* to a two-way stopcock that allows interchangeable connection of the arterial needle to a strain-gage manometer, *J,* for recording of systemic arterial pressure, or to a buret, *G,* for measurement of the rate of blood flow through the cuvette during recording of dilution curves. Blood withdrawn into burets is maintained sterile and is reinfused into the patient by applying air pressure to top ends of the burets immediately after inscription of each dilution curve. By this technic it is possible to record multiple dilution curves even from small infants without serious loss of blood. With an especially designed and calibrated syringe, *H,* 1 ml of the indicator solution is injected as rapidly as possible into selected sites in the heart or great vessels, and the residual indicator in the lumen of the catheter is flushed into the site of injection

These two routes may be provided by the use of conventional types of double-lumen catheters or concentric catheter assemblies, as described previously, or by simultaneous use of two conventional type cardiac catheters (32). The latter technic is usually preferred in this laboratory due to the great flexibility of possible combinations of sampling and injection sites which can be used as required to obtain specific information necessary to establish a definite diagnosis in the various congenital conditions which may be encountered. The assembly of equipment used for simultaneous recording of arterial and venous dilution curves is illustrated in Fig. 9. Diagnosis and measurement of blood flow and shunts by means of venous dilution curves obtain the highest degree of accuracy when an arterial dilution curve is recorded simultaneously with the recording of the venous dilution curve.

The characteristic normal patterns of dilution curves recorded from various sites in the right side of the heart in a patient without a right-to-left shunt and in a normal dog are illustrated in Fig. 10. The "mixed venous" dilution curve recorded from the right ventricle after an injection downstream to this site is a badly damped version of the dilution curve recorded from the systemic artery. The dilution curve recorded from the coronary sinus, owing to the rapidity and relatively small volume of this circulation, is similar to an arterial dilution curve. Note that, as would be expected, the dye does not appear at the right ventricular sampling site until after its appearance at the systemic artery.

In the presence of a left-to-right shunt at or upstream to the right ventricle, it would be expected that dye would appear in the right ventricle in an abnormally short period because of the shunt of dyed blood from the left to the right side of the heart. The rapid arrival of dyed blood in the right side of the heart in the presence of a left-to-right shunt after injection of the dye downstream from the site of the shunt can be used as a method for detection and localization

by an immediate subsequent injection of 5 ml of sterile Ringer's solution contained in another syringe, *I. M,* a special armboard, is used to fix the hand in a dorsiflexed position and thus to facilitate puncture of the radial artery. *N,* the needle, is used for percutaneous introduction of catheter *B* which has been withdrawn from the vein to the hub of the catheter during subsequent manipulation of the catheter.

226   **E. H. Wood**

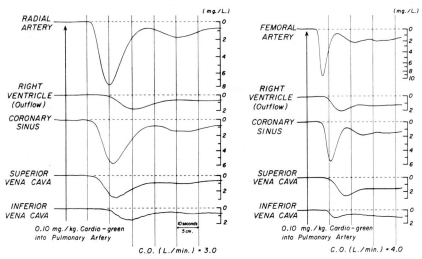

Fig. 10.   Comparison of systemic arterial and venous dilution curves recorded from various sites on the right side of the heart in a patient without arterio-venous shunt (left) and a normal anesthetized dog (right). The sites in the vascular systems from which the respective dilution curves were recorded are indicated on the left of the panels, and the instant and site of dye injection are specified by the vertical arrow. Note that curves recorded from the coronary sinus of both patient and dog are similar to curves recorded from a systemic artery. In contrast, curves recorded from the other venous sites resemble badly damped versions of the "parent" arterial curve. Also note that the right ventricular "mixed venous curve" resembles a composite of the superior and inferior caval curves and that, as a result of the relatively much smaller blood flow from this site, the effect of the coronary sinus curve on the "mixed venous curve" is not apparent. Dilution curves in this and subsequent figures are photographs of photostats of the original photographic records which were cut out and re-aligned, correcting for the effect of the dead space of the sampling systems, so that the true time relationships of the dilution curves recorded at the various sampling sites are illustrated.

of a left-to-right shunt (Fig. 11) (33). If dye is injected into a distal pulmonary artery, and its concentration is recorded from the right ventricle and pulmonary artery in a patient with a left-to-right shunt via, for example, a ventricular septal defect, the dilution curve re-corded from the right ventricle will exhibit an abnormal initial de-flection (Fig. 11). If the sampling catheter is then withdrawn to a site on the right side of the heart which is upstream to the site of the defect, in this instance the right atrium, and the pulmonary ar-tery injection is repeated, the dilution curve recorded from this site

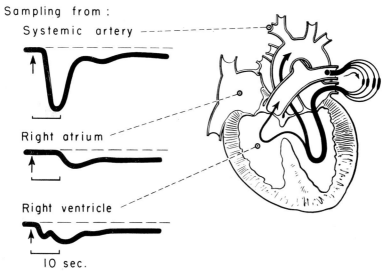

Injection into distal pulmonary artery

Sampling from :

Systemic artery

Right atrium

Right ventricle

10 sec.

Fig. 11. Schematic illustration of a method for localizing a left-to-right shunt by dilution curves recorded from selected sites in the right side of the heart. Indicator is injected at a site in the right or left side of the heart which is downstream to the sampling site, but upstream to the site of origin of the left-to-right shunt. Dye curves (left) of the circulation in the presence of ventricular septal defect were recorded from a systemic artery, the right ventricle, and the right atrium after injections into a distal pulmonary artery. Note (1) that dye was detected in the right ventricle before it appeared in the systemic artery, thus demonstrating the presence of a left-to-right shunt, and (2) that early appearing dye was not detected from the right atrium, thus localizing the site of the left-to-right shunt to the right ventricle.

will not show the abnormal initial deflection. This demonstrates and localizes the site of the left-to-right shunt to the next chamber downstream to the site at which no left-to-right shunt was detected (33), that is, in this example to the right ventricle.

The use of this technic to demonstrate and localize a left-to-right shunt in a dog before and after creation of a ventricular septal defect is illustrated in Fig. 12. In this dog, before the creation of the ventricular septal defect, the dilution curves recorded simultaneously from the pulmonary artery and from the femoral artery, after injection into the distal pulmonary artery, were normal in contour. After creation of the ventricular septal defect by the technic of Griffin and

228   E. H. Wood

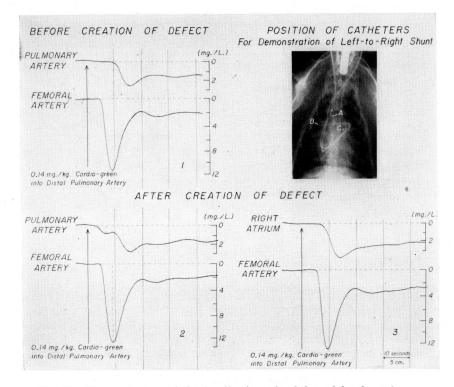

Fig. 12.   Demonstration of the localization of a left-to-right shunt by means of dilution curves recorded simultaneously from the right side of the heart and a systemic artery during operation for creation of a ventricular septal defect in a dog. Roentgenogram shows positions of the tips of the catheters during recording of these dilution curves: *A*, in right atrium; *B* in a distal right pulmonary artery; *C*, in the main pulmonary artery. Cardio-green was injected into the distal right pulmonary artery, with sampling from the main pulmonary artery and femoral artery immediately before and after creation of the defect (panels 1 and 2 respectively) and from the right atrium and femoral artery after creation of the defect (panel 3). The instant of injection of dye is shown by vertical arrows. Note abnormally early appearance of dye in the curve recorded from the main pulmonary artery after creation of the defect; this is caused by dyed blood that has shunted left to right through the defect. The fact that no abnormally early appearing dye was detected from the curve recorded from the right atrium indicates that the shunt is downstream to this site. The magnitude of the shunt calculated from these dilution curves from the measurements of the areas of the "forward triangles" indicated by the vertical broken lines (panel 2) was 9% of pulmonary blood flow. Note that a shunt of this size does not produce apparent distortion of the systemic arterial (femoral artery) dilution curve.

Essex (34), the dilution curves recorded in a similar fashion show a small abnormal initial deflection on the curve recorded from the pulmonary artery and thus demonstrate the presence of a left-to-right shunt. Since this abnormal initial deflection was absent from the right atrial curve, the left-to-right shunt was localized to the right ventricle. It is of interest that the magnitude of this left-to-right shunt was too small to be detected by ordinary repetitive determinations of blood-oxygen saturations from various sites in the right heart, when a cuvette oximeter was utilized, and that the contour of the dilution curve recorded from the femoral artery in the presence of this small left-to-right shunt was not appreciably different from normal.

Dilution curves recorded simultaneously from the right side of the heart and from a systemic artery in the presence of a left-to-right shunt can be used for simultaneous determinations of the systemic blood flow, the pulmonary blood flow, and the magnitude of the left-to-right shunt by methods which have been previously described (32). The four measurements which are necessary from the dilution curve to make these calculations (Fig. 13) can be made directly from the simultaneously recorded systemic artery and pulmonary artery dilution curves, and they consist of the determination of the buildup time and the peak deflections of the systemic artery curve, and of these same parameters for the initial portion, that is, the left-to-right portion of the pulmonary artery curve. That it is indeed possible to obtain reasonably accurate simultaneous measurements of the pulmonary and the systemic blood flow and the left-to-right shunt by means of this indicator-dilution technic is demonstrated by the data shown in Fig. 14. Estimations of the pulmonary and systemic blood flows and the left-to-right shunt determined by the conventional Fick method have been compared with data obtained by utilizing indicator-dilution technics in the same series of patients with the left-to-right shunts and in dogs with ventricular septal defects. No systematic difference between the values derived by these two separate technics is evident, and the scattering of the values determined by the two technics is no greater than what would be expected from the error which is inherent in the Fick determinations of flow and the determinations by the dye-dilution technic.

Certain distinct advantages of indicator-dilution technics in the

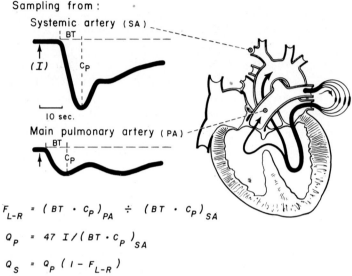

Injection into distal pulmonary artery

Sampling from :

Systemic artery (SA)

Main pulmonary artery (PA)

$$F_{L-R} = (BT \cdot C_p)_{PA} \div (BT \cdot C_p)_{SA}$$

$$Q_p = 47\ I / (BT \cdot C_p)_{SA}$$

$$Q_s = Q_p (1 - F_{L-R})$$

Fig. 13. Measurements and equations required for calculation of pulmonary blood flow, magnitude of left-to-right shunt, and systemic blood flow from dilution curves recorded simultaneously from a systemic artery (example: the radial artery) and the main pulmonary artery after injection of indicator into a distal pulmonary artery in a patient with a left-to-right shunt via a ventricular septal defect. Pulmonary flow (Q_p) is calculated from the initial forward-triangle portion of the systemic arterial curve as described by Ramirez de Arellano and co-workers (35). The fraction of the pulmonary flow composed of shunted blood (F_{L-R}) is the ratio of the area of the forward triangle of the pulmonary artery curve $(BT \cdot C_p)_{PA}$, to that of the forward triangle of the curve recorded simultaneously at the systemic artery, $(BT \cdot C_p)_{SA}$. Systemic flow (Q_s) is calculated by multiplying the pulmonary flow (Q_p) times the fraction of unshunted blood $(1 — F_{L-R})$.

measurement of these parameters should be emphasized. The measurements required for the indicator-dilution values are recorded simultaneously over less than 60 seconds. Therefore, the values obtained provide an accurate comparison of the hemodynamics of the pulmonary and systemic circulations, information which may be of considerable practical value in selecting patients with intracardiac defects for possible surgical repair. The dye-dilution technics do not require blood-gas analyses or active cooperation by the patient. The

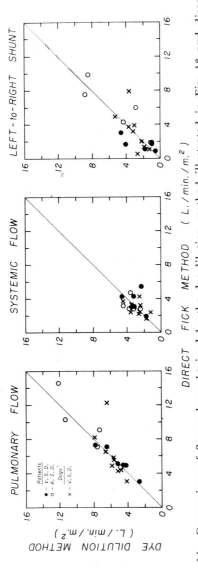

Fig. 14. Comparison of flow values obtained by the dye-dilution method illustrated in Fig. 13 and direct Fick method in twelve patients and nine dogs with intracardiac shunts. Note that there is no systematic difference in the values obtained by these methods and that the magnitude of the differences between the two methods is within the margin of error for the Fick method when applied to measurement of pulmonary and systemic blood flows in the presence of a left-to-right shunt.

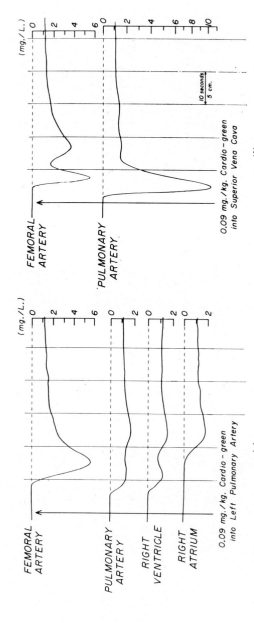

Fig. 15. Demonstration of left-to-right and right-to-left shunts by dilution curves recorded simultaneously from the right side of the heart and from a systemic artery. See Fig. 10 legend for additional details. (a) The presence of a left-to-right shunt is demonstrated by abnormally early initial deflection in curves recorded from main pulmonary artery and right ventricle, and the site of this shunt is localized to the right ventricle by the absence of this initial deflection in the curve recorded from the right atrium. (b) The presence of a coexisting right-to-left shunt was demonstrated by abnormally early initial deflection on the dilution curve recorded from the femoral artery when indicator was injected into the superior vena cava, a site which therefore was upstream to the defect. The absence of this initial deflection from the femoral artery curve recorded after injection into the left pulmonary artery demonstrates that this site is downstream to the defect. Demonstration of an abnormal initial deflection in the femoral artery curve after an injection into the right ventricle (curve not shown) allowed the site of the right-to-left shunt to be localized at ventricular level.

indicator-dilution method is not interfered with by the presence of foreign gases in the blood so that the technics can be applied readily during anesthesia and during clinical surgical measures. No accessory determinations or respiratory gas exchange is required.

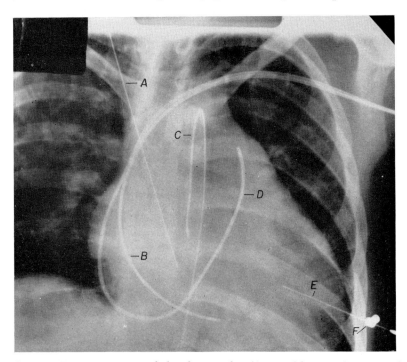

Fig. 16.   Roentgenogram of the thorax of a 40-year-old man, demonstrating the positions of needles and catheters during combined puncture of the left atrium and the left ventricle and catheterization of the aorta and the right side of the heart. *A*, 21T-gage needle, 23 cm long, outside diameter 0.8 mm, internal diameter 0.6 mm, has been inserted via the suprasternal route, and its tip has been advanced until it lies in the left atrium. *B*, No. 6-F cardiac catheter, introduced by percutaneous needle puncture of a vein in the left arm, has been advanced until its tip lies in the right ventricle. *D*, second catheter, No. 7 F, introduced similarly via a second vein in the same arm, has been advanced so that its tip is positioned in the pulmonary artery. *C*, No. 5-F. aortic catheter, introduced by percutaneous needle puncture of the right femoral artery, has been advanced so that its tip lies above the aortic valve. *E*, 21T-gage needle, has been inserted into the left side of the thorax at the position of maximal cardiac impulse and its tip has been advanced until it has entered the left ventricular cavity. *F*, the needle stop, maintains the position of the needle in relation to the skin surface.

In addition to the use of venous indicator-dilution technics for the detection and quantitation of relatively simple cardiac defects, these technics also are applicable to the elucidation of multiple or complicated congenital or acquired cardiac defects. Their use for the demonstration of a bidirectional shunt through a ventricular septal defect is illustrated in Fig. 15.

The technics may have particular application in congenital or acquired lesions affecting the left side of the heart, not ordinarily

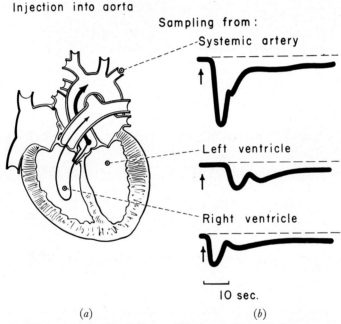

Fig. 17.   Demonstration by indicator-dilution technics of rupture of an aortic-sinus aneurysm into the right ventricle. (*a*) The central circulation in the presence of an aortic-sinus aneurysm opening into the right ventricle, and (*b*) dilution curves recorded from a systemic artery, left ventricle, and right ventricle after injection of indicator just distal to a competent aortic valve. Vertical arrows indicate the instant of injection of indicator. The almost instantaneous appearance of dye in the right ventricle, before it is recorded from the left ventricle and systemic artery, is indicative of an abnormal communication between the aortic root and the right ventricle. The curve recorded from the systemic artery shows an abnormal deflection on the disappearance slope indicative of a left-to-right shunt originating at or distal to the aortic valve. The abnormal initial deflection on the left ventricular curve is due to this left-to-right shunt.

accessible to study by conventional right heart catheterization. By means of technics which have been developed in recent years, it is now possible to gain access to any chamber of the heart or great vessels for either the injection of indicator or withdrawal of the resulting dye-blood mixture. When the need arises in the case of complicated or multiple cardiac defects involving the left side of the heart, it is possible to utilize these technics in conjunction with one another with an acceptable degree of safety.

The assembly of needles and catheters which can be used for study of any of the four heart valves or cardiac chambers during one procedure is illustrated by means of a roentgenogram of the thorax of a patient undergoing combined right heart and aortic catheterization and left ventricular and left atrial puncture (Fig. 16). This type of procedure is carried out only in a small number of specially selected patients with multiple lesions of the left side of the heart and perhaps also with involvement of the right side of the heart in whom the information required to establish a diagnosis and determine the feasibility of surgical repair cannot be obtained with certainty by simpler technics.

An example of the use of technics of this type for the demonstration and estimation of the severity of a ruptured aortic sinus aneurysm is shown in Fig. 17. In the presence of an aortic sinus aneurysm ruptured into the right ventricle, if dye is injected into the aorta just above the aortic valve and a dilution curve is recorded from the right ventricle and the left ventricle, immediately appearing dye will be detected in the right ventricle, and at a later period, abnormally early appearing dye will be detected in the left ventricle because of the left-to-right shunt via the aortic sinus aneurysm. Actual dilution curves recorded from a patient with an aortic sinus aneurysm communicating with the right ventricle are illustrated in Fig. 18.

Summary

In summarizing the diagnostic value of indicator-dilution technics in the study and investigation of congenital heart disease, perhaps a simple listing of the advantages and disadvantages of the technics will suffice.

The advantages are as follows: (1) The technic has a high degree

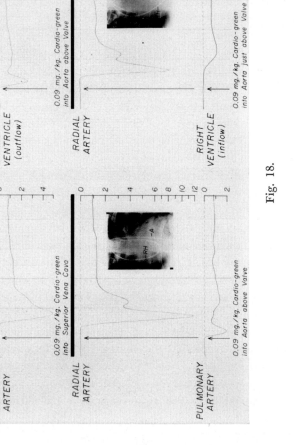

Fig. 18.

of safety. In the more than one thousand cardiac patients in whom it has been utilized, there is no record of mortality and little or no morbidity. (2) The sensitivity of the technics for the detection and localization of right-to-left and left-to-right shunts is much superior to the conventional blood-gas methods and is equal or superior to the foreign gas methods. (3) Quantitative determinations of systemic and pulmonary blood flow and intrathoracic shunts by indicator-dilution methods can be made simultaneously over less than 1 minute, they do not require manometric analyses, accessory respiratory exchange studies, or active cooperation of the patient, and they are independent of foreign (anesthetic) gases in the blood. (4) The technic is versatile and can be extremely useful for the detection and diagnosis of either minimal relatively simple defects or for the elucidation of extremely complex types of congenital malformations. (5) The information obtained is of both a qualitative and quantitative nature; that is, the nature and location of defects can be determined and, in addition, the magnitude and direction of flow through the defects in question as well as systemic and pulmonary blood flows can be estimated.

The disadvantages of the technic are as follows: (1) Rather complicated and sensitive recording equipment is required. (2) Consider-

Fig. 18. Demonstration by dilution curves of a shunt from the aorta to the right ventricle in a 33-year-old woman with a ruptured aortic-sinus aneurysm. The sites in the vascular system from which the respective dilution curves were recorded are indicated to the left of each panel, and the instants and sites of dye injections are specified by arrows. The roentgenograms show positions of catheters in the right side of the heart (*RH*) and the aorta (*A*) that were used for injection and sampling of dye from the central circulation. Note: (1) Dye curves recorded at the radial and pulmonary arteries after injection of dye into the superior vena cava (left upper panel) show the disproportionate prolongation of the disappearance slope, diminished peak concentration, and absence of a systemic recirculation peak characteristically associated with a left-to-right shunt. (2) Curves recorded at the pulmonary artery (left lower panel) and the outflow tract of the right ventricle (right upper panel) after injection of indicator into the aorta above the valve show abnormally early appearing indicator in approximately equal amounts, while the curve recorded from the inflow tract of the right ventricle (right lower panel) after injection into the same site shows only dye that has traversed the normal circulatory pathway, thus localizing the site of rupture to the right ventricular outflow tract. (3) Curves recorded at the radial artery after injection into the aorta above the valve show an abnormal disappearance slope, which is also indicative of a left-to-right shunt at or distal to the aortic valve.

able technical skill is required of the persons carrying out the procedure in the placement of the necessary needles and catheters and in the proper selection of multiple possible injection and sampling sites reached by these instruments in order to obtain the information needed to establish the diagnosis in question. (3) Correct interpretation of the diagnostic significance of the dilution curves obtained requires careful study and considerable experience by the person responsible for this phase of the investigation. In other words, the technic entails relatively little discomfort and little danger for the patient, but it requires good equipment and, more important, considerable time, effort, and skill on the part of the investigator and his assistants in order to attain highly successful results.

ACKNOWLEDGMENT

The studies on which this report is based were carried out in collaboration with my colleagues in the sections of medicine, surgery, anesthesiology, engineering, and physiology. In the last group Drs. H. J. C. Swan and J. T. Shepherd, Miss Lucille Cronin, Mrs. Jean Frank, and Mr. William Sutterer are deserving of particular commendation.

REFERENCES

1. Symposium on diagnostic applications of indicator-dilution technics. *Proc. Staff Meetings Mayo Clin.* **32:** 463–508; 509–553 (1957).
2. Symposium on diagnostic applications of indicator-dilution curves recorded from the right and left sides of the heart. *Proc. Staff Meetings Mayo Clin.* **33:** 535–577; 581–610 (1958).
3. Rossi, H. H., Powers, S. H., and Dwork, Bernard. Measurement of flow in straight tubes by means of the dilution technique. *Am. J. Physiol.* **173:** 103–108 (1953).
4. Sheppard, C. W. Mathematical considerations of indicator dilution techniques. *Minn. Med.* **37:** 93–104 (1954).
5. Stewart, G. N. Pulmonary circulation time, quantity of blood in lungs and output of heart. *Am. J. Physiol.* **58:** 20 (1921).
6. Hamilton, W. F., Moore, J .W., Kinsman, J. M., and Spurling, R. G. Simultaneous determination of the pulmonary and systemic circulation times in man and of a figure related to the cardiac output. *Am. J. Physiol.* **84:** 338–344 (1928).
7. Kinsman, J. M., Moore, J. W., and Hamilton, W. F. Studies on the circulation. I. Injection method: Physical and mathematical considerations. *Am. J. Physiol.* **89:** 322–330 (1929).

8. Nicholson, J. W., III, Burchell, H. B., and Wood, E. H. A method for the continuous recording of Evans blue dye curves in arterial blood, and its application to the diagnosis of cardiovascular abnormalities. *J. Lab. Clin. Med.* **37**: 353–364 (1951).

9. Broadbent, J. C., and Wood, E. H. Indicator-dilution curves in acyanotic congenital heart disease. *Circulation* **9**: 890–902 (1954).

10. Swan, H. J. C., Zapata-Diaz, J., and Wood, E. H. Dye dilution curves in cyanotic congenital heart disease. *Circulation* **8**: 70–81 (1953).

11. Swan, H. J. C., Burchell, H. B., and Wood, E. H. The presence of venoarterial shunts in patients with interatrial communications. *Circulation.* **10**: 705–713 (1954).

12. Russell, J. L., Donald, D. E., Moersch, R. N., and Marshall, H. W. Localization and quantitation of left-to-right shunts via experimental cardiac defects. *Proc. Staff Meetings Mayo Clin.* **33**: 553–561 (1958).

13. Dexter, Lewis. Cardiac catheterization techniques using pressure, flow, and oxygen analysis. This volume, p. 199.

14. Groom, Dale, Wood, E. H., Burchell, H. B., and Parker, R. L. The application of an oximeter for whole blood to diagnostic cardiac catheterization. *Proc. Staff Meetings Mayo Clin.* **23**: 601–609 (1948).

15. Wood, E. H., Sutterer, W. F., and Cronin, Lucille. *Medical Physics,* Otto Glasser, Editor. Year Book Publishers, Inc., Chicago, Ill., Vol. 3, Oximetry (in press).

16. Wood, E. H., and Swan, H. J. C. Right-heart catheterization. *Cardiology: An Encyclopedia of the Cardiovascular System*, A. A. Luisada, Editor. Blakiston Publishing Division, McGraw-Hill, New York, Vol. 2, 1959, pp. 292–322.

17. Zijlstra, W. G., and Mook, G. A. Direct measurement of the oxygen saturation of human blood during cardiac catheterization. *Arch. intern. pharmacodynamie* **110**: 344–346 (1957).

18. Kjellberg, S. R., Mannheimer, Edgar, Rudhe, Ulf, and Jansson, Bengt. *Diagnosis of Congenital Heart Disease: A Clinical and Technical Study by the Cardiologic Team of the Pediatric Clinic, Karolinska sjukhuset, Stockholm.* Year Book Publishers, Inc., Chicago, 1955.

19. Sones, F. M. Cinecardioangiography. This volume, p. 251.

20. Campbell, John: Unpublished data.

21. Carter, S. A., Bajec, D. F., Yannicelli, Eduardo, and Wood, E. H. Estimation of left-to-right shunt from arterial dilution curves. *J. Lab. Clin. Med.* **55**: 77–88 (1960).

22. Weil, M. H., and Swan, H. J. C. Demonstration of ejection pathways from the right ventricle. *Proc. Staff Meetings Mayo Clin.* **32**: 502–505 (1957).

23. Korner, P. I., and Shillingford, J. P. The quantitative estimation of valvular incompetence by dye dilution curves. *Clin. Sci.* **14**: 553–573 (1955).

24. Korner, P. I., and Shillingford, J. P. Further observations on the estimation of valvular incompetence from indicator dilution curves. *Clin. Sci.* **15**: 417–431 (1956).

25. Marshall, H. W., Woodward, Edward, Jr., and Wood, E. H. Hemodynamic methods for differentiation of mitral stenosis and regurgitation. *Am. J. Cardiol.* **2**: 24–60 (1958).

26. Swan, H. J. C., Toscano-Barboza, Ely, and Wood, E. H. Hemodynamic findings in total anomalous pulmonary venous drainage. *Proc. Staff Meetings Mayo Clin.* **31**: 177–182 (1956).

27. Swan, H. J. C., and Wood, E. H. Anomalous connection of the pulmonary and systemic veins. *Proc. Staff Meetings Mayo Clin.* **32**: 496–499 (1957).

28. Birkhead, N. C., and Wood, E. H. The diagnosis of tricuspid atresia. *Proc. Staff Meetings Mayo Clin.* **32**: 506–508 (1957).

29. Swan, H. J. C., Burchell, H. B., and Wood, E. H. Special applications of indicator-dilution technics in congenital and acquired heart disease. *Proc. Staff Meetings Mayo Clin.* **32**: 485–486 (1957).

30. Ledbetter, M. K., and Daugherty, G. W. Ventricular septal defect with aortic regurgitation. *Proc. Staff Meetings Mayo Clin.* **33**: 600–603 (1958).

31. Semler, H. J., and Brandenburg, R. O. Demonstration of site of rupture of aortic-sinus aneurysm. *Proc. Staff Meetings Mayo Clin.* **33**: 604–608 (1958).

32. Wood, E. H., Swan, H. J. C., and Marshall, H. W. Technic and Diagnostic applications of dilution curves recorded simultaneously from the right side of the heart and from the arterial circulation. *Proc. Staff Meetings Mayo Clin.* **33**: 536–553 (1958).

33. Fox, I. J., and Wood, E. H. Applications of dilution curves recorded from the right side of the heart or venous circulation with the aid of a new indicator dye. *Proc. Staff Meetings Mayo Clin.* **32**: 541–550 (1957).

34. Griffin, G. D. J., and Essex, H. E. Experimental production of interventricular septal defects: Certain physiologic and pathologic effects. *Surg., Gynecol. Obstet.* **92**: 325–332 (1951).

35. Ramirez de Arellano, A. A., Hetzel, P. S., and Wood, E. H. Measurement of pulmonary blood flow using the indicator-dilution technic in patients with a central arteriovenous shunt. *Circulation Research* **4**: 400–405 (1956).

Characterization of Circulatory Shunts by Foreign Gas Technics

EUGENE BRAUNWALD, ANDREW G. MORROW, RICHARD J. SANDERS, and ROBERT T. L. LONG

Clinic of Surgery, National Heart Institute, Bethesda, Maryland

The detection, precise localization, and quantification of cardiac shunts is fundamental to the physiologic and clinical evaluation of patients with congenital heart disease. The sampling of blood from the venae cavae, the chambers of the right heart, and pulmonary artery and the demonstration of an oxygen stepup between successive chambers has been the standard method for the characterization of left-to-right shunts (1–3). In the majority of patients this method has yielded satisfactory results. However, in a disturbingly large number of patients encountered in most clinical laboratories, this approach has yielded inconclusive results, of little value either to the physician in his management of the patient or to the clinical investigator studying patients with congenital heart disease.

It may, first of all, be of interest to examine the reasons for the limitations of the oxygen method. Since the oxygen content of right heart blood is a function of the cardiac output and of the total peripheral oxygen consumption, it varies markedly among different subjects and in the same subject at different times. Therefore, it becomes necessary to compare in every patient the oxygen content of blood obtained from the chamber proximal to the entry of the suspected shunt to that obtained from the chamber distal to it. During the time required for positioning the catheter and withdrawing several blood samples in each chamber, alterations in the patient's total oxygen consumption and cardiac output may obscure the changes produced by a shunt.

When the oxygen content of blood samples obtained from two different chambers is compared, it is assumed that these samples are entirely representative of the blood within that chamber. However, it has been demonstrated that the blood in the venae cavae and right atrium is incompletely mixed. Laminar flow and streaming occur in these areas and lead to difficulties in the diagnosis of left-to-right shunts, particularly those at the atrial level (4–9). For example, the sampling of a stream of well-oxygenated renal venous blood in the inferior vena cava may mask the presence of an atrial septal defect.

Furthermore, in some patients the catheter cannot be passed into the inferior vena cava. Since it has been conclusively demonstrated that the oxygen content of superior caval blood is generally less than that of inferior caval blood (7, 9), a comparison of superior caval and right atrial blood could lead to the false diagnosis of an atrial septal defect. The use of the oxygen method for the quantification of left-to-right shunts is fraught with many inaccuracies which are well recognized.

Finally, another of the disadvantages of the oxygen method is the relatively large number of blood samples required. The duration of the catheterization procedure is prolonged. In laboratories in which the standard Van Slyke analytic technics are employed, the amount of blood required is substantial, and the technicians' time required for analysis is not inconsiderable. The results are generally not available until after the catheterization has been completed, and for this reason the course of the diagnostic procedure cannot usually be modified by the results. However, the use of a cuvette oximeter for the immediate analysis of the oxygen saturation of blood withdrawn from the cardiac catheter has largely obviated the latter difficulties (10).

The principle of the use of an inert foreign gas such as nitrous oxide (N_2O) or radioactive krypton (Kr^{85}) in the detection of left-to-right shunts has received extensive clinical application at the National Heart Institute since 1954 (9, 11–15). During the first two minutes of inhalation of an inert foreign gas, such as N_2O or Kr^{85}, the concentration in blood in the left side of the heart or in a peripheral artery rises sharply, then it levels off (Fig. 1). Since N_2O is quite soluble in the tissues of the body, the concentration in the systemic veins rises much more slowly. Hence, in the absence of a left-to-right shunt, the content of N_2O or Kr^{85} in the right heart or pulmonary artery blood constitutes a small and relatively constant percentage of the arterial content.

However, in the presence of a left-to-right shunt, blood from the

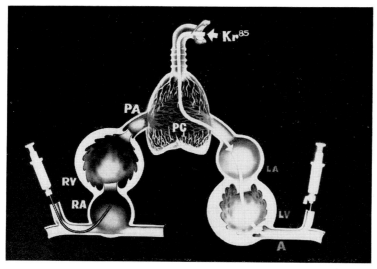

Fig. 1. Diagram illustrating the use of foreign gas technic in the detection of left-to-right shunts. In the absence of a shunt, during the first 30 sec of inhalation of a foreign gas, such as Kr^{85} or N_2O, significant quantities of the gas appear in the arterial blood but not in the right heart blood. RA, right atrium; RV, right ventricle; PA, pulmonary artery; PC, pulmonary capillary bed; LA, left atrium; LV, left ventricle; A, systemic arterial bed.

left side of the heart, rich in foreign gas content, is shunted across to the right side of the heart, thereby elevating the gas content of right heart blood and the ratio of the concentration of right heart to arterial N_2O or Kr^{85} (Fig. 2). The determination of the presence or absence of a shunt therefore may be based simply on the determination of this ratio and requires only two blood samples. The systemic and pulmonary arterial N_2O content during the ten minutes of inhalation in a patient without a cardiac shunt is illustrated in Fig. 3. The marked difference in N_2O content between systemic and pulmonary arterial blood during the first two minutes of inhalation is apparent.

Figure 4 shows the results of 150 N_2O tests performed in 98 patients (14). In these tests 50% N_2O and 21% O_2 in N_2 were inhaled for 30 seconds, and arterial and right heart samples were drawn at a constant rate between the 10th and 30th seconds of inhalation. In all 96 tests performed in patients without shunts, the level of N_2O in the right side of the heart or pulmonary artery was less than 15% of the

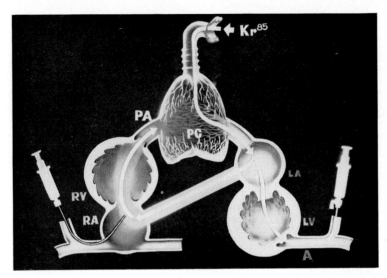

Fig. 2.   Diagram illustrating the use of foreign gas technic in the detection of left-to-right shunts. In the presence of an atrial septal defect, substantial quantities of blood, rich in the foreign gas, appear in the right atrium. The presence of the foreign gas may be detected by analysis of blood sampled from the right atrium. Symbols same as Fig. 1.

arterial level. In 91 of the 96 tests this percentage was less than 10%. Seventy-two N_2O tests were performed in 35 patients with left-to-right shunts. With one exception the N_2O content of blood sampled in or distal to the chamber receiving the shunt exceeded 15% of the arterial N_2O content. Thus, with this one exception, the two groups of patients could be successfully separated.

The use of foreign gas technics may also be employed in the quantification of left-to-right shunts. The N_2O content of blood obtained distal to the entry of a left-to-right shunt reflects the mixing of venous blood, low in N_2O content, with shunted blood, rich in N_2O content. The proportion of pulmonary artery blood derived from shunted blood may then be calculated from a consideration of the gas contents in venous blood, in shunted blood, and in the pulmonary arterial blood. There is little variation in the concentration of gas in the venous blood proximal to any shunt; it has been found to be 6 ± 6% of the arterial level (14). The N_2O content of shunted blood may be considered to be identical to that of arterial blood. The ratio of pulmonary to systemic flow can then be calculated from the follow-

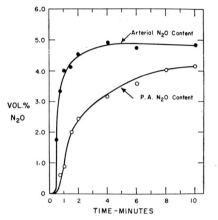

Fig. 3. N_2O levels in the femoral artery and pulmonary artery of a patient without a left-to-right shunt. Fifteen per cent N_2O was inhaled for 10 min. (Reproduced by permission from reference 9.)

ing formula which has been derived elsewhere (14, 16, 17):

$$\frac{\text{Pulmonary flow}}{\text{Systemic flow}} = \frac{100\% - 6\%}{100\% - [(PA/A)(\%)]}$$

where PA/A represents the N_2O or Kr^{85} test in the pulmonary artery. In order to determine the validity of this formula, both the total pulmonary blood flow as well as blood flow through an artificial left-to-right shunt were measured directly in a group of dogs by means of electromagnetic flowmeters (18). N_2O tests were then performed while shunts of various magnitudes were functioning. No systematic difference between the flow ratios determined by the two methods was observed; the coefficient of correlation was 0.96.

In view of the necessity for analyzing N_2O in the Van Slyke manometric apparatus, it was thought that other inert gases might behave in a similar manner, but permit easier and faster analysis (17, 19). Kr^{85} had been evaluated experimentally and found as satisfactory as N_2O in the diagnosis of left-to-right shunts. Arterial and right heart blood samples drawn during the 10th to 30th seconds of Kr^{85} inhalation may be analyzed simply by inserting them into a continuous gas-flow GM tube capable of counting beta emissions. The results with the clinical use of Kr^{85} were essentially identical to those obtained with N_2O (13, 15).

The oxygen and Kr^{85} methods were compared in a group of 54

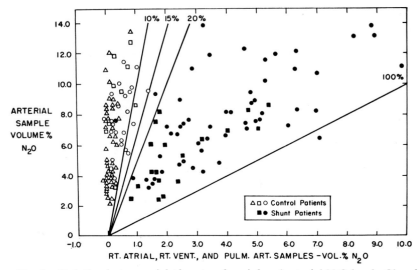

Fig. 4.   Relation between right heart and peripheral arterial N₂O levels. Closed figures represent patients proved to have left-to-right shunts. Open figures represent patients proved not to have left-to-right shunts. (Reproduced by permission from reference 14.)

patients in whom both technics were applied at the same right heart catheterization (15). Among the 32 patients with proved left-to-right shunts, there were six with oxygen stepups less than 1.0 vol % into the chamber receiving the shunt. In the group of 22 patients without a shunt, there was one with an oxygen increase greater than 1.0 vol%. The oxygen method thus would have provided an incorrect diagnosis in 7 of these 54 patients. There were no errors with the Kr[85] method. In all 22 patients proved not to have shunts, the Kr[85] test was less than 15%. It exceeded 15% in all 32 patients, with proved left-to-right shunts.

The relatively poor solubility of Kr[85] in blood suggested a totally different approach to the study of patients with cardiac or intrapulmonary shunts. When Kr[85] dissolved in saline is injected into a peripheral vein or into the right side of the heart, that portion which passes through capillaries perfusing normally ventilated alveoli comes out of solution and immediately appears in the expired gas. Clearance by the lungs is virtually complete during one circulation, and, therefore, the levels of Kr[85] in arterial blood are only slightly above background, following right heart or intravenous injections in the absence of a right-to-left shunt. However, when the injection is made proximal to the origin of a right-to-left shunt, that portion of the Kr^{85} which bypasses the pulmonary capillary bed appears in the arterial blood and leads to an elevated arterial Kr^{85} level. The validity of this concept has recently been demonstrated by Long *et al.* in a group of dogs with experimentally produced right-to-left shunts (20). The arterial count of Kr^{85} in a sample drawn during the 20 seconds following injection exceeded 1500 cpm in 26 injections into 6 dogs with patent right-to-left shunts. However, the highest arterial count after 43 injections into 11 dogs without shunts was only 200 cpm. The method has been applied to 20 patients, and has been found to be of considerable value in the detection of right-to-left shunts. This technic has been compared with cardio-green dye-dilution curves simultaneously recorded from a systemic artery, and appears to be of slightly or even greater sensitivity.

Immediately after the arrival of injected Kr^{85} in the pulmonary artery, it appears in expired gas where it may be readily detected by means of an end-window GM tube inserted directly into the expiratory gas line and its concentration may be recorded continuously with a count rate meter and direct writing recorder (21). This affords a relatively simple method for the detection of the presence of left-to-

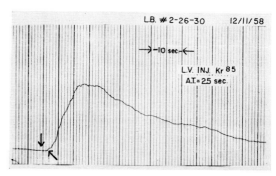

Fig. 5. Expiratory gas Kr^{85} curve obtained from a 22-year-old male with a large atrial septal defect. An indicator-dilution curve using cardio-green dye was performed with a left ventricular injection and arterial sampling. The resultant dye curve was equivocal for a left-to-right shunt originating distal to the mitral valve. The appearance of Kr^{85} in the expired gas 2.5 sec after left ventricular injection clearly indicated that a shunt originated downstream to the mitral valve. A selective angiocardiogram with left ventricular injection demonstrated a small ventricular septal defect.

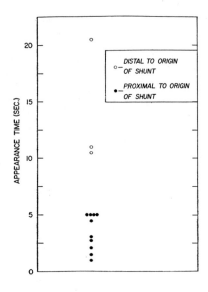

Fig. 6. Scattergram showing appearance times in expired gas following injections of Kr⁸⁵ into the left heart, proximal (closed circles), and distal (open circles) to the origin of a left-to-right shunt.

right cardiac shunts as well as for the localization of their site of origin. Thus, if the Kr^{85} is injected into the right side of the heart, or into the left side of the heart proximal to the origin of a left-to-right shunt, it appears in the expired gas in less than 5 seconds (Fig. 5). However, when the Kr^{85} is injected into the left side of the heart or aorta distal to the origin of a left-to-right shunt it must first traverse the systemic circulation before reaching the pulmonary circulation, and therefore its appearance in the expired gas is delayed and longer than 10 seconds (22).

Figure 6 is a scattergram of the Kr^{85} appearance times in the expired gas. The solid circles represent injections made into the left heart or aorta proximal to a left-to-right shunt. The open circles represent the Kr^{85} appearance times in expired gas after injection into the left side of the heart or aorta distal to the origin of a left-to-right shunt. There is no overlap of values.

This method appears to be capable of detecting even the smallest left-to-right shunts and to be at least as sensitive as any of the dye-dilution technics. Only one catheter need be inserted into the heart; no blood samples are required. The results of the study are available instantaneously and the instrumentation required is not complicated (23).

Summary

A variety of foreign gas technics are employed in the study of patients with cardiac shunts at the National Heart Institute. The detection of inhaled N_2O or Kr^{85} in the right side of the heart permits detection of the site of entry as well as the determination of the magnitude of left-to-right shunts. The determination of the appearance time of Kr^{85} in expired gas after its injection into the left heart serves to localize the site of origin of the left-to-right shunts. Right-to-left shunts may also be detected and localized by the selective injection of Kr^{85} into a peripheral vein and the right heart chambers and its subsequent measurement in systemic arterial blood. These technics have been found to be sensitive, reliable, accurate, and convenient to apply and, in our laboratory, are replacing other methods for the characterization of cardiac shunts.

REFERENCES

1. Cournand, A., Baldwin, J. S., and Himmelstein, A. *Cardiac Catheterization in Congenital Heart Disease.* The Commonwealth Fund, New York, 1949.
2. Dexter, L., Haynes, F. W., Burwell, C. S., Eppinger, E. C., Seibel, R. E., and Evans, J. M. Studies on congenital heart disease. I .Technique of venous catheterization as a diagnostic procedure. *J. Clin. Invest.* **26**:547 (1947).
3. Kjellberg, S. R., Mannheimer, E., Rudhe, U., and Jönsson, B. *Diagnosis of Congenital Heart Disease.* Year Book Publishers, Inc., Chicago, Ill. 1955.
4. Cournand, A., Riley, R. L., Breed, E. S., Baldwin, E. de F., and Richards, D. W. Measurement of cardiac output in man, using the technique of catheterization of the right auricle or ventricle. *J. Clin. Invest.* **24**:106 (1945).
5. Warren, J. V., Stead, E. A., Jr., and Brannon, E. S. The cardiac output in man: A study of some of the errors of right heart catheterization. *Am. .J. Physiol.* **145**:458 (1946).
6. Dexter, L., Haynes, F. W., Burwell, C. S., Eppinger, E. C., Sagerson, R. P., and Evans, J. M. Studies of congenital heart disease. II. *J. Clin. Invest.* **26**:554 (1947).
7. Keith, J. D., Rowe, R. D., and Vlad, P. *Heart Disease in Infancy and Childhood.* The Macmillan Company, New York, 1958, p. 72.
8. Sirota, J. H., and Gordon, A. J. Methods to measure regional contributions to total cardiac output in man with observations on laminar flow in the great veins. *J. Appl. Physiol.* **6**:485 (1954).
9. Morrow, A. G., Sanders, R. J., and Braunwald, E. The nitrous oxide

test: An improved method for the detection of left-to-right shunts. *Circulation* **17**:284 (1958).

10. Groom, D., Wood, E. H., Burchell, H. B., and Parker, R. L. The application of an oximeter for whole blood to diagnostic cardiac catheterization. *Proc. Staff Meetings Mayo Clin.* **23**:601 (1948).

11. Morrow, A. G. New methods in the diagnosis of interatrial septal defects. *Cardiovascular Surgery,* International Symposium at the Henry Ford Hospital. W. B. Saunders Company, Philadelphia, Pa., 1955, p. 345.

12. Grant, R. P., Sanders, R. J., Morrow, A. G., and Braunwald, E. Symposium on diagnostic methods in the study of left-to-right shunts. *Circulation* **16**:791 (1957).

13. Sanders, R. J., and Morrow, A. G. The localization of circulatory shunts with inhaled krypton-85. *Bull. Johns Hopkins Hosp.* **103**:27 (1958).

14. Sanders, R. J., and Morrow, A. G. The diagnosis of circulatory shunts by the nitrous oxide test: Improvements in technic and methods for quantification of the shunt. *Circulation* **18**: 856 (1958).

15. Sanders, R. J., and Morrow, A. G. The identification and quantification of left-to-right circulatory shunts: A new diagnostic method utilizing the inhalation of a radioactive gas, Kr[85]. *Am. J. Med.* **26**:508 (1959).

16. Eppinger, E. C., Burwell, C. S., and Gross, R. E. The effects of the patent ductus arteriosus on the circulation. *J. Clin. Invest.* **20**:127 (1941).

17. Case, R. B., Hurley, H. W., Keating, R. P., Keating, P., Sachs, H. L., and Loeffler, E. D. Detection of circulatory shunts by use of a radioactive gas. *Proc. Soc. Exptl. Biol. Med.* **97**:4 (1958).

18. Sanders, R. J., Cooper, T., and Morrow, A. G. An evaluation of the nitrous oxide method for the quantification of left-to-right shunts. *Circulation* **19**:898 (1959).

19. Sanders, R. J. The inhalation of a radioactive gas (Kr[85]) for the diagnoses of cardiac shunts. *Proc. Soc. Exptl. Biol. Med.* **97**:1 (1958).

20. Long, R. T. L., Waldhausen, J. A., and Cornell, W. P. Use of radioactive gas solutions in the diagnosis of right-to-left shunts. To be published.

21. Long, R. T. L., and Cornell, W. P. Experimental detection of left-to-right circulatory shunts with injections of krypton-85. *Proc. Soc. Exptl. Biol. Med.* **101**:836 (1959).

22. Braunwald, E., Long, R. T. L., and Morrow, A. G. Infections of radioactive krypton (Kr[85]) solutions in the detection and localization of cardiac shunts (Abstract). *J. Clin. Invest.* **39**:990 (1959).

23. Long, R. T. L., Braunwald, E., and Morrow, A. G. The intracardiac injection of radioactive krypton: The clinical applications of new methods for the characterization of circulatory shunts. *Circulation* (in press).

Cinecardioangiography

F. MASON SONES, JR.

Cardiac Laboratory, Cleveland Clinic Foundation, Cleveland, Ohio

The technique of selective cinecardioangiography is essentially a practical combination of cardiac catheterization and angiocardiographic methods, made possible by the development of the fluoroscopic image amplifier. Its purpose is to combine intracardiac pressure and flow measurements with motion picture photography of the passage of contrast media through selected areas of the central circulation, in an attempt to provide exact anatomic diagnosis, in addition to an estimate of the functional stress imposed on the heart by any combination of lesions that may be encountered.

During the past three and one-half years this method has been applied to diagnostic problems presented by patients in whom a congenital heart lesion has been suspected, when exact diagnosis could not be established by routine clinical methods of study.

A 5-in. image amplifier* has been used for fluoroscopy during exploration of the heart and great vessels with the catheter tip, and for motion picture photography of contrast media injected into any desired area of the central circulation. By increasing the brightness of the fluoroscopic image more than one thousand times, this instrument provides an image bright enough to be observed comfortably in a well-lighted room by means of any of several available optical viewing systems. This eliminates the necessity for dark accommodation by the operator, and permits all members of the catheterization team to function with improved efficiency.

Better observation of the patient's functional status makes it possible to attend more adequately to his comfort, reduce his anxiety, and improve the overall safety of the procedure.

X-ray dosage to patients has been reduced to less than 30% of that

---

* North American Philips Co., Inc., 525 West 52nd Street, New York, N.Y.

formally required for equivalent periods of conventional fluoroscopy. In studying the chest of an infant weighing 15 to 20 lb with a chest thickness of 12 cm an excellent "amplified" image is obtained with a tube current of ½ to 1 ma at 65 kv. By using an identical x-ray source with filtration and distance factors constant, conventional fluoroscopic examination of a similar subject in total darkness required from 2 to 3 ma at 65 kv.

With the x-ray factors noted above it has been possible to reproduce the "amplified" fluoroscopic image on a conveniently placed television receiver, connected by coaxial cable to a small television camera, mounted above the image amplifier (Fig. 1). The televised image may be easily observed simultaneously by all members of the catheteriza-

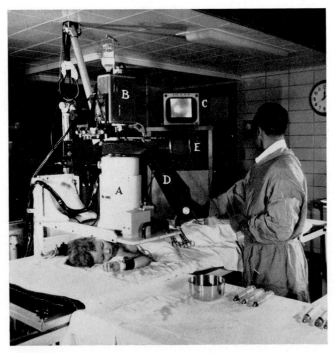

Fig. 1.   The image amplifier (A) produces a fluoroscopic image bright enough to be photographed with a television camera (B), connected by closed circuit to a conveniently placed television receiver (C). An oscilloscope (E) provides simultaneous visualization of the electrocardiogram and intracardiac pressures during catheter manipulation. The fluoroscopic image may also be observed by the operator through the optical periscope (D).

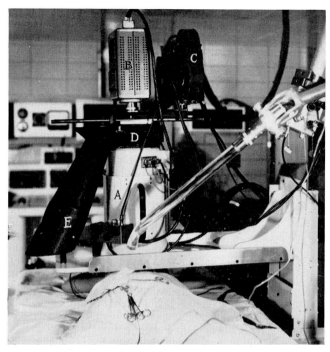

Fig. 2. Television (B) and optical motion picture (C) cameras are fixed on a sliding mount above the image amplifier (A). A pellicle inside the optical periscope at D deflects 7 to 10% of the light beam from the amplifier to a mirror at E, permitting direct observation of the image, while the remaining light is transmitted through the pellicle to the camera lens.

tion team, and has been particularly valuable in teaching physicians the techniques of intracardiac catheter manipulation.

An electrically driven 35-mm motion picture camera equipped with a commercially available F 2.0 lens is used for permanent photographic recording of the image. It is fixed above the image amplifier on a sliding mount in tandem with the television camera (Fig. 2), and may be shifted into position in a few seconds whenever a permanent photographic record is desired during the course of a study. Motion pictures are routinely exposed at a rate of sixty frames per second on Eastman Tri-X negative film, at individual frame exposures of 8.3 msec. Adequate film exposures of this type are made in infants weighing up to 20 lb with x-ray tube currents of 4 to 6 ma at 65 kv in the frontal projection, and from 6 to 10 ma at 65 kv in the lateral or oblique projections. The x-ray dose measured at the skin averages two roentgens per minute for the frontal projection and three roentgens per minute for lateral or oblique projections, in patients of this body mass. The duration of single exposures varies between 4 and 10 sec. The x-ray tube has inherent filtration equivalent to 0.5 mm of aluminum; additional filtration of 1.0 mm of aluminum and 0.1 mm of copper is provided. The standard target to skin distance is 19 in.

The negative 35-mm film is processed in x-ray developer for 5 to 6 min on Nikkor reels of 100-ft capacity at 68°F, and is available for study within an hour of exposure. It may be immediately reviewed by small groups of three or four individuals with a 35-mm editing machine which permits slow-motion analysis, or detailed study of individual frames. A 35-mm projector is used for larger group conferences to provide an image of adequate size for this purpose. The original negative film may be reproduced in the form of 16-mm positive prints for convenient presentation to larger medical groups.

The optical system of the 5-in. image amplifier contains a pellicle, which is interposed in the light path from the amplifier to the camera. This deflects 7 to 10% of the light image from the amplifier into an optical periscope (Fig. 2), allowing the remainder of the light to pass through to the recording camera lens. The small amount of light diverted into the periscope allows the operator to observe the image being photographed. This makes it possible to observe the passage of contrast media through the central circulation at the moment of injection and provides important practical advantages over conventional angiocardiographic techniques which reduce the possibility of diagnostic failure. It is usually possible, during this brief period of observation, for the operator to recognize the most important diagnostic features demonstrated by an injection so that he may intelligently guide the further course of an individual study. Improper placement of the catheter tip or recoil of the catheter to a proximal cardiac chamber during the early phase of an injection is easily recognized, and therefore the injection may be stopped before a full dose of contrast substance has been disadvantageously introduced into the circulation. In other instances it may be recognized that a lesion is inadequately demonstrated because an injection of media has been made too slowly or in insufficient volume to provide adequate contrast at the desired location. Occasionally the planes of the cardiac septa are abnormally related to external body landmarks, and repeated injections in unusual projections are required before the best possible demonstration of intracardiac structure is obtained. When multiple defects coexist, a single injection may adequately reveal them all, but more often serial injections into different areas of the circulation are necessary to define precisely all the anatomic components involved.

With increasing experience anxiety regarding the use of multiple doses of contrast media during the course of a single study has been dispelled. In nearly every patient studied at least two injections are made. In more than one hundred patients three or four serial injections have been made during the course of a single procedure.

During the past two years 90% Hypaque has been the sole contrast substance employed. Individual doses are limited to from 0.3 to 0.5 cc per pound of body weight up to maximal individual doses of 30 cc. In the presence of normal blood flows, the former dose has been adequate. When large volume shunts, which cause very rapid dilution of media, have been encountered, the higher dose has been used. In the latter group of patients larger individual doses appear to be safe, because very rapid dispersal of media prevents its prolonged retention in high concentration in the capillary bed of any organ through which it is distributed, and the possibility of specific tissue injury is minimized.

Selective injections of contrast media in the doses noted above have been made into all areas of the central circulation except into a "wedged" coronary sinus. This is avoided because of the risk of rupturing the thin-walled sinus, which may lead to the rapid occurrence of cardiac tamponade. More than five hundred injections have been made directly into the left atrium, left ventricle, or ascending aorta without evidence of central nervous system or renal injury and without the occurrence of significant cardiac arrhythmias.

Venous catheterization by way of the saphenous or superficial femoral veins is routinely employed because in the majority of patients with congenital lesions this approach permits direct access to the left side of the heart by way of a patent foramen ovale or an atrial septal defect. Pressure measurements and blood oxygen determinations are made in the right heart chambers and pulmonary arteries. When access to the left side of the heart is possible, similar measurements are made in the left atrium, pulmonary veins, and left ventricle.

Immediate appraisal of these measurements provides a basis for

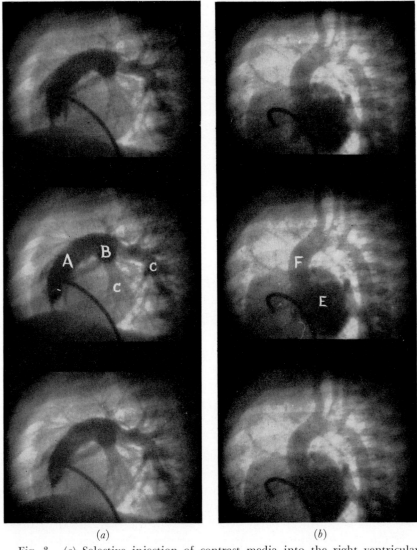

(a)   (b)

Fig. 3. (a) Selective injection of contrast media into the right ventricular
apex of a normal child (L.O.A. projection) shows a normal right ventricular outflow tract during systole (A). There is no obstruction at the pulmonary valve or
in the right ventricular outflow tract. There is no right-to-left shunt. The pulmonary artery (B) is normal in size and position and divides into right and left
branches (C) of normal size and distribution. (b) After passage through the lungs,
the diluted media opacifies the left atrium and ventricle, superimposed at E. There
is no intracardiac left-to-right shunt. The ascending aorta (F) arises normally from
the left ventricular outflow tract. The thoracic aorta and its major branches are
faintly but adequately visualized.

selecting sites for the injection of contrast media which will most adequately demonstrate the anatomic structures capable of producing any physiologic abnormalities which are recognized. In each instance *the objective should be to provide maximal concentration of media in the area of the suspected lesion with the least possible loss of detail by simultaneous opacification of overlapping structures.*

If preliminary catheter exploration reveals normal intracardiac pressures and fails to demonstrate an intracardiac shunt or a direct communication that may be crossed by the catheter at the atrial, ventricular, or pulmonary artery levels, a single injection of contrast media is made into the right ventricular apex with the patient in the left anterior oblique position. This usually provides the best overall "photographic survey" of the central circulation that can be obtained with a single injection (Fig. 3). It provides an effective check in confirming the absence of a left-to-right shunt, and occasionally has demonstrated such shunts when they were not recognized by blood oxygen determinations. It will rule out the presence of an obstruction in the right ventricular outflow tract or in the proximal pulmonary arteries, and will demonstrate the presence or absence of left atrial or ventricular enlargement. When a large left-to-right shunt or severe cardiomegaly is not present, the thoracic aorta is seen well enough to permit recognition of segmental dilatation, hypoplasia, or coarctation and to demonstrate the origin of its major branches.

When right ventricular pressure is elevated, an injection into the apex of the chamber with the patient in the left anterior oblique position will demonstrate the anatomic characteristics of obstructive lesions in its outflow tract or at the pulmonary valve (Figs. 4 and 5). Some of the anatomic variants encountered have been described in detail in a previous communication (1). They are of considerable practical surgical and prognostic importance, and have not, in our experience been differentiated consistently by physiologic studies.

Segmental hypoplasia of the pulmonary arteries may involve the main trunk (Fig. 5) or the major vessels beyond its bifurcation. The latter problem is best demonstrated by injection into the right ventricle with the patient in frontal projection (Fig. 6).

When a left-to-right shunt is present at the ventricular level with normal or only moderately elevated right ventricular pressures, dem-

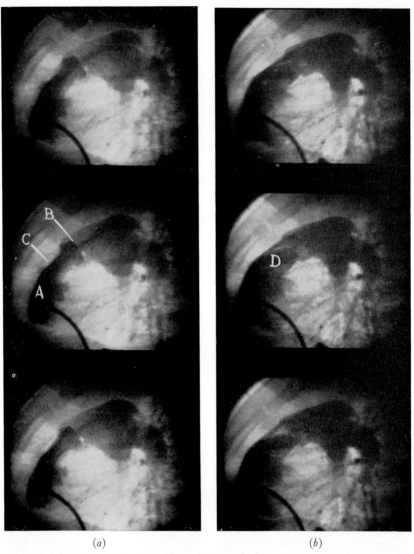

(a)   (b)

Fig. 4. (a) Severe valvular pulmonic stenosis demonstrated by right ventricular cardioangiogram (L.O.A. projection). Injection is made into right ventricular apex (A). The jet of media is seen crossing the thickened pulmonary valve (B) into the large pulmonary artery during systole. The right ventricular outflow tract below the valve (C) is narrowed by moderately severe concentric hypertrophy during maximal systolic ejection. (b) In diastole the outflow tract widens to a normal diameter (D), demonstrating the absence of a fixed infundibular obstruction below the valve. This type of functional obstruction often causes a significant pressure gradient to persist after effective pulmonary valvulotomy for as long as twelve months, but ultimately it disappears if adequate relief of valvular obstruction has been achieved.

258

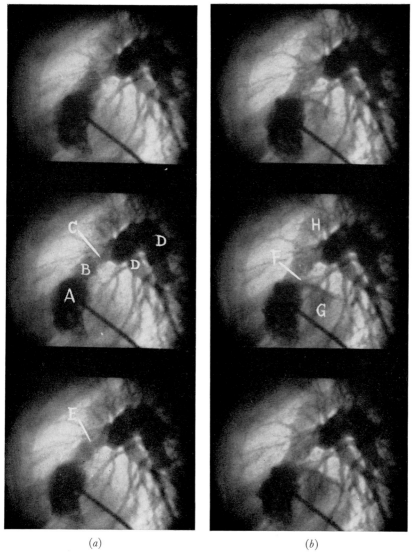

(a)   (b)

Fig. 5. (a) A tetralogy of Fallot is demonstrated by right ventricular cardioangiogram in the L.O.A. projection. The right ventricular inflow tract (A) is moderately dilated. Immediately above this, a fixed muscular obstruction separates the
outflow tract from a small "third ventricle" (B), which is bounded above by a
stenotic pulmonary valve (E). The short main pulmonary artery trunk (C) above
the valve is hypoplastic. The pulmonary vessels (D) beyond the bifurcation are of
large size. (b) In the succeeding early diastole, a small defect in the ventricular septum (F) permits faint opacification of the left ventricle (G). The ascending aorta
(H) is faintly visualized.

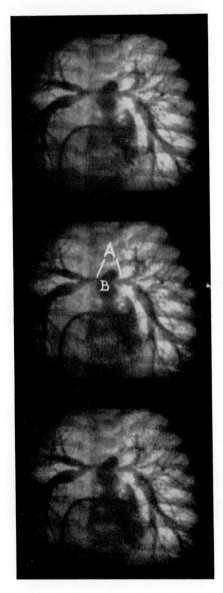

Fig. 6. Segmental hypoplasia of the pulmonary arteries (A) beyond the main trunk of the vessel (B) is demonstrated by right ventricular injection in the P.A. projection. Note the increased diameter of both vessels beyond points of narrowing.

onstration of the shunt may be accomplished during the period of left heart opacification after the media have passed through the pulmonary circulation (Fig. 7*a*). Whenever possible, however, this type of shunt at the ventricular level is best shown by selective injections directly into the left atrium or ventricle (Fig. 7*b* and 12).

Demonstration of coexisting, separate, left-to-right shunts, defects in the a-v cushion, and the relationship of the aortic and pulmonary valve rings to the plane of the ventricular septum has usually been unsatisfactory or impossible when attempted by conventional right heart catheterization or venous angiocardiography. Fortunately, in the majority of patients who present one or another of these problems, it is a simple matter to catheterize the left atrium by way of an atrial septal defect or a patent foramen ovale, if the inferior caval approach is used. In more than 80% of this group it has been possible to catheterize the left ventricle by way of the mitral valve when the possibility of separate atrial and ventricular defects, a common a-v canal, or mitral regurgitation in combination with an atrial septal defect was suspected (2).

When the communication across which the catheter tip is passed at the atrial level is a patent foramen ovale with an adequate valve to prevent a left-to-right shunt, contrast media injected into the left atrium do not cross the atrial septum, and excellent selective opacification of the left heart and aorta is obtained (Fig. 8). If the primary objective of an injection into the left atrium is to demonstrate the plane of the ventricular septum and the root of the aorta, it should be made with the patient rotated from sixty degrees to eighty degrees into the left anterior oblique position.

When a communication at the atrial level is a true atrial septal defect or a large foramen ovale with an incompetant valve, selective left atrial injection will demonstrate the location and size of the defect (Fig. 9). For this purpose the patient should be rotated only fifteen to twenty degrees into the left anterior oblique position, as this projection separates the planes of the atrial and ventricular septa, but has the disadvantage of partially obscuring the membranous portion of the ventricular septum and the aortic valve annulus.

If selective left atrial opacification reveals a large left-to-right shunt at the atrial level, an additional injection is made into the left ven-

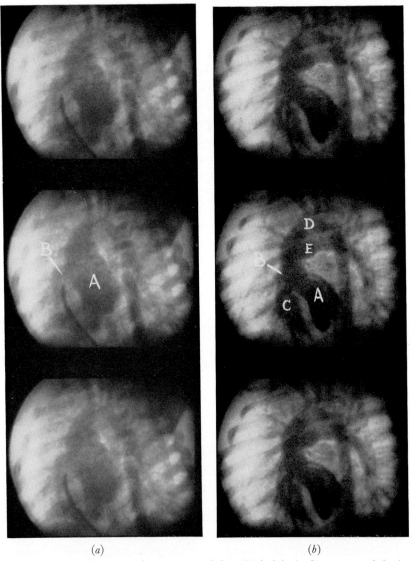

(a)   (b)

Fig. 7. (*a*) An interventricular septal defect (B) is faintly demonstrated during the phase of left heart opacification after media injected into the right ventricle have traversed the pulmonary circulation. The large left atrium (A) is superimposed on the left ventricular outflow tract and obscures detail. (*b*) A cardioangiogram made into the left ventricle (A) of the same patient by using an equal quantity of contrast media provides a better demonstration of the area being studied. The ventricular septal defect is actually smaller than it appeared to be in (*a*). It lies in the membranous portion of the septum and does not extend as high as the plane of the aortic annulus (B). The right ventricle (C) is outlined better. The muscular portion of the ventricular septum is intact. The aorta (D) and pulmonary artery (E) are seen more distinctly. Note the absence of mitral regurgitation.

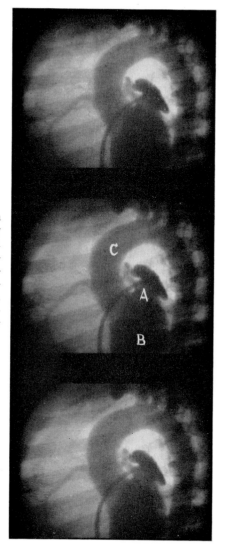

Fig. 8.   Selective cardioangiogram
into the left atrium entered by way
of a patent foramen ovale. No media
crosses the atrial septum. This technique provides better demonstration of the left atrium (A), left ventricle (B), and thoracic aorta (C),
than can be accomplished by injections into the systemic veins or
right heart.

tricle with the patient rotated sixty to eighty degrees in the left anterior oblique projection. Mitral regurgitation due to an associated defect in a mitral leaflet, or to severe dilatation of the valve annulus, is
easily demonstrated by selective left ventricular cardioangiograms
(Fig. 10). This type of regurgitation may be absolutely ruled out if no
media cross the plane of the valve back into the left atrium (Figs. 11

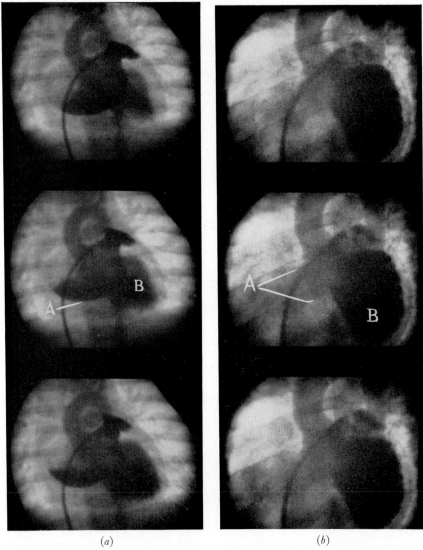

(a)   (b)

Fig. 9. (a) Injection into the left atrium with the patient rotated fifteen degrees toward left anterior oblique position reveals no shunt at the atrial level. The plane of the atrial septum (A) is well defined. The left ventricle (B) is shown in the period of early diastolic filling. The ventricular septum is intact. (b) Selective left atrial opacification provides demonstration of a large atrial septal defect (A). Left ventricular opacification (B) shows the lower portion of the ventricular septum. The membranous portion of the ventricular septum is obscured by the left atrium.

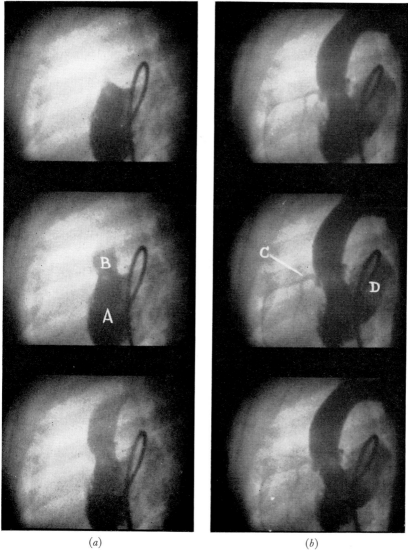

(a)   (b)

Fig. 10. (a) Selective opacification of the left ventricle (A) in patient with atrial septal defect demonstrates the plane of the aortic valve annulus and early filling of the ascending aorta (B). (b) Mitral regurgitation, with heavy opacification of left atrium (D) is shown late in systole. Incidental opacification of the right coronary artery (C) is demonstrated. The origin of the left coronary artery is visualized, but its major branches cannot be seen because of left heart opacification.

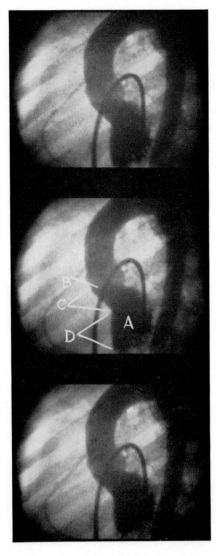

Fig. 11. Selective left ventricular (A) opacification demonstrates an intact ventricular septum and no evidence of mitral regurgitation. The plane of the aortic valve annulus is seen at B. Note the sharp anterior curve of the membranous (C) portion of the ventricular septum above its muscular portion (D).

and 12). In about 20% of such injections slight artifactual regurgitation is seen across normal valves due to valve cusp displacement by the catheter. The minimal quantity of such regurgitation usually permits it to be disregarded, but occasionally this type of artifact has led to the false positive diagnosis of mitral regurgitation in association with an atrial septal defect.

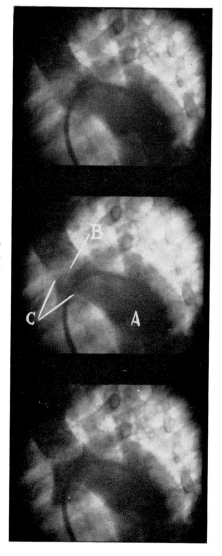

Fig. 12. Selective injection into the left ventricle (A) demonstrates a defect in the upper membranous portion of the ventricular septum which extends up to the plane of the aortic valve annulus (B).

Selective left ventricular opacification allows the best possible demonstration of the size and location of ventricular septal defects. Their relationship to the aortic valve annulus in the vertical plane is easily recognized (Fig. 12). Agenesis of the ventricular septum or multiple coexisting ventricular defects have been repeatedly demonstrated (1).

The scope of this communication does not permit detailed recapitulation of all the diagnostic problems that have been encountered and solved by the technique described. Instead, an attempt has been made to sketch the broad potential application and versatility inherent in this diagnostic approach to cardiovascular malformations. It has been used effectively in demonstrating a wide variety of lesions including tricuspid atresia, mitral atresia, Ebstein's malformation of the tricuspid valve, truncus arteriosus, transposition of the great vessels, valvular and subvalvular forms of aortic stenosis, aneurysm of the sinus of Valsalva, anomalies of the coronary arteries, aortic pulmonary window, atypical forms of patent ductus arteriosus, several varieties of aortic ring, anomalies of systemic and pulmonary venous drainage, and a bewildering number of anatomic variants falling into the general classification of "tetralogy of Fallot."

The recent development of larger image amplifiers with effective screen diameters of 8, 9, and 11 in. has simplified the practical application of cinecardioangiography to the study of adult patients with congenital heart disease, and has provided a stimulus to the development of similar techniques for the study of acquired valvular and degenerative lesions.

With progressive experience and refinement of technical methods it is anticipated that high-speed x-ray motion picture photography will facilitate the establishment of a more exacting basic standard of diagnosis in the field of cardiovascular disease. If this is accomplished and effectively duplicated at a practical clinical level, we shall, with increasing diagnostic frequency, generalize less and specify more for the ultimate benefit of patients entrusted to our care.

REFERENCES

1. Sones, F. M. Cine-cardioangiography. *Pediat. Clin. North Am.* 945, November 1958.
2. Sones, F. M. Diagnosis of septal defects by the combined use of heart catheterization and selective cine-cardioangiography. *Am. J. Cardiol.* 2:724 (1958).

The Present Status of Intracardiac Phonocardiography*

DAVID H. LEWIS,† ABDOL-NABI MOGHADAM, GEORGE W. DEITZ, JOHN D. WALLACE, JAMES R. BROWN, JR., and SAMI A. KHALIL

Division of Cardiology, Philadelphia General Hospital, Philadelphia, and the U. S. Naval Air Development Center, Johnsville, Pennsylvania

It is perhaps trite to say, yet nonetheless true, that within the clinical lifetime of the various members of this symposium congenital heart disease has been transformed from a medical curiosity into a field of prime importance. As this gathering indicates, advances in therapy have given the impetus for improved methods of diagnosis and these, in turn, have stimulated further refinements in therapy, and so on. The purpose of this presentation is to indicate the present contributions and future prospects of a relatively new and, as yet, incompletely explored diagnostic technique, the recording of heart sounds and murmurs from within the heart.

Auscultation and Phonocardiography in Congenital Heart Disease

One area that has received great stimulus from the improvements in diagnosis and therapy is cardiac auscultation, along with its graphic representation, phonocardiography. Several recent reviews discuss this area in great detail, and no attempt will be made here to review the field (1–4). The most important advance in the field of cardiac auscultation has come from the appreciation of the physiological basis of heart sounds and murmurs. The various auscultatory phenomena are based of necessity on certain mechanical events. This is as true for dis-

*Supported by research grants from the National Heart Institute of the National Institutes of Health (H-2559) and from the American Heart Association.

† This work was done during the tenure of an Established Investigatorship of the American Heart Association.

ease as it is for the normal. It follows from this that a consideration of the alterations in the sounds and murmurs in disease should lead to an understanding of the altered physiology of the circulation and from here to an anatomical as well as a physiological diagnosis. There have been many recent important contributions in this area. The English workers have been most active in this field and one might cite, as one example, the studies of Leatham and his associates (5). It is in this area of physiologic correlation that intracardiac phonocardiography shows promise of making important contributions. By virtue of its ability to localize precisely the origin of heart sounds and murmurs, this phonocardiographic technique provides a unique opportunity for correlation of sounds and murmurs at their point of origin with any other phenomena.

Techniques of Intracardiac Phonocardiography

Several types of techniques have been used for the determination of sounds and murmurs from within the heart. In 1954 Yamakawa and his associates (6) reported in English the results of their investigations both in animals and man by using a condenser microphone with the body as one pole. Both sounds and murmurs are recorded by this method, but it has certain problems as have been pointed out (7). In 1958 Yamakawa (8) reviewed in detail his pioneering work in this field and concluded that intracardiac phonocardiography is of diagnostic value in congenital heart disease.

In 1954 Soulié and his associates (9), using the Allard-Laurens micromanometer, reported on studies of intracardiac phonocardiography in man. This device, mounted at the tip of a Cournand catheter, employs an inductance type transducer designed originally for pressure registration. The frequency response of the pickup is sufficiently good so that when the frequencies below 20 cycles per second are cut off, one records the intracardiac sounds. Their experiences to date with this technique have convinced them that it is a valuable addition to the diagnostic methods in congenital heart disease (10, 11).

In 1956 our group (12) adapted to phonocardiography the undersea warfare techniques developed by the United States Navy. In this method a barium titanate ceramic, an underwater microphone, is mounted at the tip of a specially designed cardiac catheter (Fig. 1), and

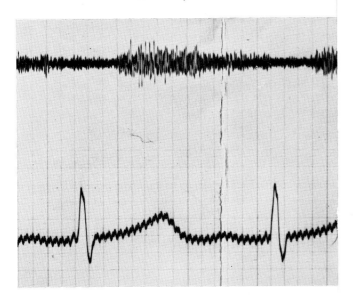

Fig. 2. IJ 7 female. Patent ductus arteriosus. Intracardiac (top) from the pulmonary artery and Lead II of the electrocar Description in text.

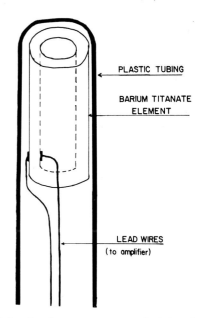

Fig. 1. Schematic diagram of phonocatheter. The barium titanate element is in the form of a hollow circular cylinder and is coated inside and out with silver. The lead wires are soldered to the ceramic as shown and are in the form of a coaxial cable. The whole is within a plastic tube sealed at the end shown and with a connection at the opposite end to the amplifier.

PLASTIC TUBING

BARIUM TITANATE ELEMENT

LEAD WIRES (to amplifier)

or a questionable shunt, we have observed in the puln the ductus a systolic murmur and a short, faint diastoli diastolic murmur has been present in the intracardia gram even when not present in the chest phonocardic no observations at this time in cases with a wholly rig through a ductus. On theoretical grounds and from defects at the ventricular level, we would expect no ductus type in the pulmonary artery.

Observations postoperatively in cases that have ha shunt indicate that the ductus murmur is replaced by ; systolic murmur in no way different from that seen It is present in the pulmonary artery, as in the normal, it is audible on the chest.

Pulmonic Stenosis. In valvular pulmonic stenosis a high-pitched, diamond-shaped systolic murmur in artery with a diminished second sound. The murmur l the first sound but shortly after it, with the onset of fl(monary artery, and it ends before the second sound. '

the sounds and murmurs from within the heart are recorded in the same manner that one records chest phonocardiograms. This transducer has been shown to have a linear response in the frequency range necessary for heart sounds and murmurs, but it cuts off sharply below 10 cycles per second, and since it does not go down to DC, it will not record the intracardiac pressures (13). Our experiences to date have convinced us, too, that intracardiac phonocardiography is a valuable addition to the diagnostic methods in congenital heart disease (14).

In 1957 Luisada and Liu (15) reported on sound tracings taken by using the column of fluid within the catheter (Cournand for the right heart and polyethylene for the left heart) as the carrier of the sound waves. The catheter is attached to a strain gage, and the electric output of this manometer is differentiated, amplified, filtered, and recorded by a phonocardiograph. The advantage of this technique is that it does not require special transducers. It has limitations in its frequency response, (16) but important information has been obtained with this method (17). This group, too, considers intracardiac phonocardiography an important contribution to diagnosis in congenital heart disease (18, 19).

In addition to these studies, Moscovitz and his associates (20) have

reported studies on intracardiac phonocardiog
titanate transducer somewhat different from th
This transducer is designed in such a way that t
of the sounds and murmurs deflect a diaphrag
by a pointer to one end of a barium titanate ce
ceramic is bent and thus generates the voltage
(21). They have reported results of investigatic
perimentally produced lesions in animals simil
tients with congenital heart disease, and agree,
will prove helpful in localizing cardiac defects

Results in Congenital Heart Disease

We have now made observations of the intr
gram in some 80 cases of congenital heart dise
illustrate the type of results obtained in murm
discussion of the areas that deserve further inv
tailed discussion of our results is available in a r

SINGLE LESIONS

Patent Ductus Arteriosus.   In patent ductus
a normal pulmonary artery pressure, there is a c
the type described by Gibson (23), which is local
artery. It is not present in the aorta but seems
ductus and reaches its fullest extent in the pu
opening of the ductus. Depending apparently c
it may, with a small shunt, be localized to that
artery at the ductus or, with a large shunt, it ma
out the pulmonary tree. If the latter is the case,
ductus. In any event it is not audible in either
atrium. We have found this murmur to be suf
so that a positive diagnosis can be made even th
blood samples are equivocal. We have suggested
have shown that the precise localization of th
means of differentiating patent ductus arterios
nary septal defect.

In the presence of pulmonary hypertension w

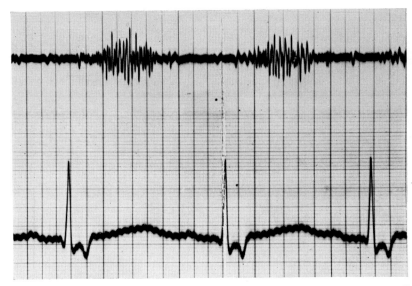

Fig. 3.   WH 3-month-old female. Pulmonic stenosis, valvular. Intracardiac phonocardiogram (top) from the pulmonary artery and Lead II of the electrocardiogram (bottom). Description in text.

best seen just beyond the valve in the main pulmonary artery but is also present, to a lesser degree, throughout the pulmonary tree. The shape of the murmur may be no different from that seen in the normal, but the frequency characteristics and the second sound are different, as will be discussed in more detail later. This murmur, too, is not present in the ventricle or in the atrium. In those cases in which the catheter has passed through a patent foramen ovale it has been possible to record this murmur in both the pulmonary vein and in the left atrium. This has been helpful when entry into the pulmonary artery has been unsuccessful.

Figure 4 shows records taken at the time of operation in a patient with valvular pulmonic stenosis. Before transventricular dilation one notes the harsh murmur and the diminished second sound. In this patient, because of the large size of the pulmonary artery, complete dilation was not possible. There was a decrease in the systolic gradient across the valve as measured at the operating table, and it was felt that some enlargement of the opening had been made. However, repeat sound tracings just before the chest was closed revealed no change in the murmur or the second sound and in addition the presence of a

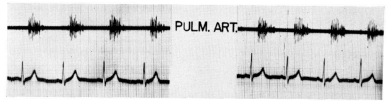

Fig. 4. GLaC 30 male. Pulmonic stenosis, valvular. Intracardiac phonocardiogram (top) from the pulmonary artery and Lead II of the electrocardiogram
(bottom), taken at the time of operation (transventricular valvulotomy). On the
left before dilation and on the right after dilation. Description in text.

short, faint diastolic murmur. This evidence would suggest little or no
change in the patient. Wells (24) has recently pointed out that from a
phonocardiographic standpoint one can evaluate better the effects of
valvotomy if consideration is given to the frequency characteristics of
the murmur and the time to peak intensity rather than just simply
the overall intensity of the murmur. Our observations are in keeping
with this and we would concur in this opinion.

We have studied and reported one case of isolated infundibular pulmonic stenosis. In this case the murmur was loudest just distal to the
stenosis. It was systolic in time and began with the first heart sound.
The murmur was present in the pulmonary artery but not in the main
body of the ventricle proximal to the region of stenosis. Baculard (11)
has made similar observations and has studied extensively the intracardiac sounds and murmurs in valvular stenosis, in infundibular
stenosis, and in combined stenosis. He also has compared the intracardiac murmurs with those on the chest and has shown, as we have,
the transmission to the chest wall of the typical murmur in the two
types of stenosis. Of greater interest from a diagnostic standpoint is
his observation that, in combined stenosis, the murmur on the chest
has characteristics of both lesions but resembles more closely the dominant lesion.

Ventricular Septal Defect. In ventricular septal defect (Fig. 5) with
a left-to-right shunt, the intracardiac phonocardiogram shows a characteristic systolic murmur loudest in intensity in the ventricle opposite
the defect. This murmur begins with the first sound and extends into
the second sound. The second sound may be split, but the pulmonic
component is not delayed. The murmur may also be present in the
pulmonary artery but with different frequency characteristics, as will
be discussed below. Depending apparently on the size of the defect

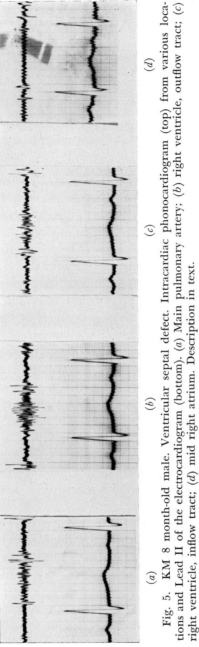

Fig. 5.   KM 8 month-old male. Ventricular septal defect. Intracardiac phonocardiogram (top) from various locations and Lead II of the electrocardiogram (bottom). (*a*) Main pulmonary artery; (*b*) right ventricle, outflow tract; (*c*) right ventricle, inflow tract; (*d*) mid right atrium. Description in text.

and on the streaming of the jet into the right ventricle, the murmur may be isolated to the region just opposite the lesion or may be present throughout the ventricle. In those cases in which the catheter has gone through the defect there has been no murmur noted in the left ventricle. Upon withdrawal of the catheter the murmur is noted at the point that the catheter enters the right ventricle. Upon further withdrawal the murmur again disappears at the point that the catheter enters the right atrium. In ventricular septal defect, as in patent ductus arteriosus, the intracardiac phonocardiogram has been sufficiently characteristic to permit a positive diagnosis even when the blood samples are equivocal. Our observations indicate that so long as there is a left-to-right shunt there is a murmur in the right ventricle but that with only a right-to-left shunt there is no murmur in the right ventricle.

Atrial Septal Defect. In atrial septal defect the intracardiac phonocardiogram is less striking than in the above-mentioned lesions. However, it does have important diagnostic features. As noted in Fig. 6 there is a systolic murmur in the pulmonary artery. Simultaneous comparison of intracardiac and chest phonocardiograms shows that this is the site of origin of the systolic murmur heard in this lesion. There may also be, as noted here, a systolic murmur in the right ventricle. The second sound in the pulmonary artery is often exaggerated, and this appears to be related to the amount of shunt. There is in this case, but not in all, a tricuspid opening sound followed by a short, decrescendo diastolic murmur. Here, too, comparison of simultaneous intracardiac and chest phonocardiograms indicates that this is the site of origin of the diastolic murmur heard on the chest. This murmur also appears to be related to the degree of shunt. In addition to these findings there is also a diastolic murmur in the right atrium which is apparently the murmur due to the shunt itself, but it is not audible on the chest wall.

In this case the patient was studied postoperatively. Here there was noted a decrease in the systolic murmur in the pulmonary artery but no change in the second sound. The tricuspid opening sound is still noted in the ventricle. There is a decrease, not a disappearance, of both the ventricular and atrial diastolic murmurs. These findings indicate reduction but not obliteration of the shunt. The blood samples indicated the same thing.

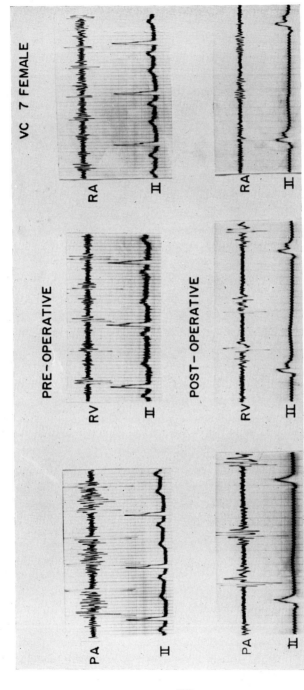

Fig. 6. VC 7 female. Atrial septal defect. Intracardiac phonocardiograms and Lead II of the electrocardiogram. (Left) pulmonary artery (PA); (middle) right ventricle (RV); (right) right atrium (RA). (Top row) before operation (hypothermia, closure of defect with sutures under direct vision); (bottom row) after operation. Description in text.

OTHER SINGLE LESIONS STUDIED

Aortic Stenosis. In congenital aortic stenosis we have observed the characteristic diamond-shaped murmur and diminished second sound localized to the aorta and not heard in the pulmonary artery or in the right heart.

Coarctation of Aorta. In coarctation of the aorta we have observed a systolic and a diastolic murmur in the aorta in the region of the lesion. There is also a different systolic murmur in the ascending aorta. Simultaneous comparison of intracardiac and chest phonocardiograms indicates that the basal systolic murmur often heard in this lesion resembles more closely the latter murmur and would appear to be an ejection type murmur due to flow into a dilated ascending aorta, when it is not due to coexistent aortic stenosis. From a phonocardiographic standpoint the recent very beautiful observations of Spencer and his associates (25) on the correlation of the murmurs in coarctation of the aorta with the pathologic physiology are of great interest.

COMBINED LESIONS

We have made observations of the intracardiac phonocardiogram in a number of combined congenital lesions. Results in most of these are too few at present to reach any overall conclusions. However, there have been sufficient observations made in the combination of pulmonic stenosis and ventricular septal defect to reach some tentative conclusions, and these will be discussed as an example of what intracardiac phonocardiography can yield.

Pulmonic Stenosis and Ventricular Septal Defect. In the presence of both pulmonic stenosis and ventricular septal defect our observations indicate that there is the murmur of pulmonic stenosis in the pulmonary artery and the murmur of ventricular septal defect in the ventricle. Most of our observations have been in patients in whom the shunt was left to right. As noted above when the shunt is wholly right to left, we have not observed a murmur of ventricular septal defect in the right ventricle.

The question arises as to the site of origin of the murmur heard on the chest wall. In the situation in which the shunt is wholly right to left we feel that this important problem remains unsettled. When the shunt is left to right our observations indicate that there are apparently two murmurs on the chest, one from the ventricular septal defect

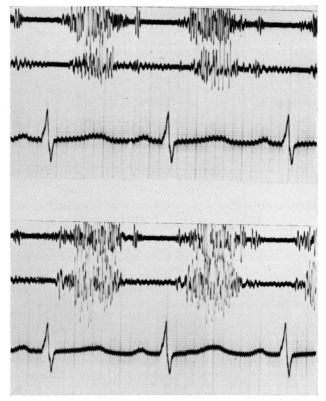

Fig. 7. AC 4 female. Pulmonic stenosis and ventricular septal defect, left-to-right shunt. Upper tracing, from above downward: chest phonocardiogram from the second intercostal space at the left sternal border (2 ics LSB), intracardiac phonocardiogram from the main pulmonary artery, and Lead II of the electrocardiogram. Lower tracing, from above downward: chest phonocardiogram from the second intercostal space at the left sternal border (2 ics LSB), intracardiac phonocardiogram from the right ventricle, and Lead II of the electrocardiogram. Description in text.

and one from the pulmonic stenosis. This would appear to be the case when the stenosis is wholly or predominantly valvular, for when it is infundibular the similarity of the two intracardiac murmurs makes differentiation difficult. Figure 7 shows records taken on a patient with pulmonic stenosis and ventricular septal defect with a left-to-right shunt. At the pulmonic area on the chest (2 ics LSB) there is a murmur which has characteristics of both the pulmonary artery murmur and the right ventricular murmur. However, as seen in Fig. 8, if

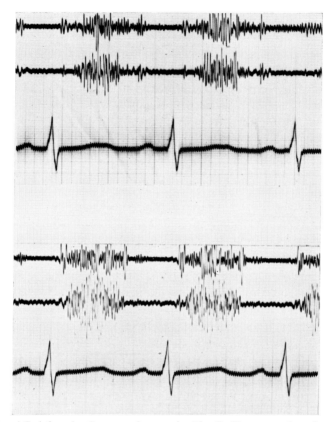

Fig. 8. AC 4 female. Same patient as in Fig. 7. Upper tracing, from above downward: chest phonocardiogram from the left infraclavicular area, intracardiac phonocardiogram from the main pulmonary artery, and Lead II of the electrocardiogram. Lower tracing, from above downward: chest phonocardiogram from the fourth intercostal space at the left sternal border (4 ics LSB), intracardiac phonocardiogram from the right ventricle, and Lead II of the electrocardiogram.

the recording on the chest is moved away from this area to the left infraclavicular region, the murmur here resembles more closely that seen in the pulmonary artery. And if the chest recording is moved down lower along the left sternal border (4 ics LSB), it resembles more closely the murmur seen in the right ventricle.

Prospects for Intracardiac Phonocardiography

The prospects for intracardiac phonocardiography revolve mainly about its usefulness as a correlative technique. It has been demonstrated that it is possible to use this method to correlate the sounds and murmurs at their point of origin with these same phenomena as heard on the chest wall. A further step in this type of investigation is a correlation of these findings with the physiological data of cardiac catheterization. We feel that this type of investigation by many groups will eventually answer the question, "How much physiological information can be obtained from a phonocardiogram?"

Our observations are just now beginning to reveal to us some of the fruitful avenues of study. We might take as one example the problem of pulmonic stenosis and ventricular septal defect. It is common knowledge that this combination presents a broad spectrum. From the point of view of the ventricular septal defect with left-to-right shunt, one might then investigate the effect of pulmonic stenosis on the dynamics of the lesion especially as regards the shunting and the obstruction to right ventricular outflow. Figure 9 shows records taken in four patients with ventricular septal defect and compares the tracings taken at the pulmonic area on the chest with those taken from within the pulmonary artery. Not shown here, but discussed above, are the recordings from the ventricle and from other areas on the chest. In the first case there is no pulmonic stenosis. There is (not shown here) the murmur of ventricular septal defect within the heart and on the chest. The sound of pulmonic closure is accentuated, but its relationship to aortic closure is normal. In the next case there is a gradient across the pulmonic valve which is small, and here the pulmonic component of the second sound is reduced in amplitude as compared with the aortic component, and it is delayed. With a larger gradient, as seen in the third case, there is a greater delay in the pulmonic component of the second sound. Finally, with a large gradient which reverses the shunt, pulmonic closure is not seen. It would appear then that this type of information which has been applied in pulmonic stenosis without ventricular septal defect may also be applicable in the presence of the combined lesion. With regard to the combined lesion, Wood (27) has studied the mechanism of syncope in tetralogy of Fallot and indicated that it is most likely due to overactivity of the infundibular portion of the right ventricle. These attacks are associated with changes in the murmurs, and one would expect that there are also changes in the second sound. Study of the phonocardiogram then during attempts

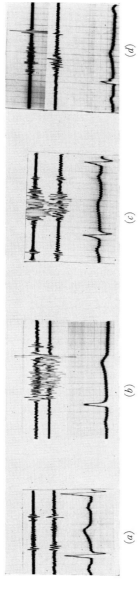

Fig. 9. Four cases of ventricular septal defect. (*a*) Without pulmonic stenosis and with a left-to-right shunt; (*b*) and (*c*) with pulmonic stenosis and with a left-to-right shunt (acyanotic tetralogy of Fallot); (*d*) with pulmonic stenosis and with a right-to-left shunt (cyanotic tetralogy of Fallot). In each tracing, from above downward: chest phonocardiogram from the second intercostal space at the left sternal border (2 ics LSB), intracardiac phonocardiogram from the main pulmonary artery (in case 4 this particular tracing is from the pulmonary vein), and Lead II of the electrocardiogram. RV-PA (gradient across the pulmonic valve in mm Hg): (*a*) 0, (*b*) 15, (*c*) 30, and (*d*) 70. A2-P2 (interval from the aortic component of the second sound to the pulmonic component of the second sound in seconds): (*a*) 0.02, (*b*) 0.06, (*c*) 0.07, (*d*) none.

at altering infundibular activity might enable one to decide on the exact nature of the obstruction to ventricular outflow.

We have also been interested in the frequency characteristics of the murmurs observed and suggest that here, too, analysis will provide valuable physiological data. Figure 10 shows spectral phonocardiograms taken on four patients with the apparatus described by McKusick and his associates (28). These are recordings taken from within the pulmonary artery. In each the arrow points to the systolic murmur. The first case is a child without heart disease and without a murmur on the chest. No doubt more sensitive recording apparatus would have recorded this murmur on the chest as Groom (29) has pointed out. Note that the frequencies recorded lie below 300 cycles per second. In the second case, also without heart disease but with an audible systolic murmur at the pulmonic area, the frequency characteristics of the murmur are similar. In the third case, a patient with an atrial septal defect, again the frequency characteristics of the murmur are the same as those seen in the patients without heart disease. Certainly this is added documentation to the well-established belief that this is indeed a "functional" murmur due to the increased flow. In contradistinction in the fourth case, a patient with valvular pulmonic stenosis, there are frequencies as high as 700 cycles per second. On this basis we feel that a more detailed analysis of the frequency components of murmurs will yield valuable information as to their exact nature.

In this figure note also the frequency characteristics of the second sound. In the case of the atrial septal defect, here without pulmonary hypertension, there are higher frequency components than in the normal. In the case of pulmonic stenosis, as previously noted by McKusick and associates (30), the lowest frequencies are not recorded, and in this regard the sound resembles more closely a snap.

We are also investigating the part that frequency analysis of murmurs can play in revealing the nature of their production and transmission. Baculard (11) has studied this problem in pulmonic stenosis both in patients and in circulation models and has reached important conclusions about the genesis and transmission of the various frequency components within the pulmonary vascular tree. He has observed a very rapid dissipation of the high frequency as one moves away from the lesion. We have made similar observations in ventricular septal defect. Figure 11 shows spectral phonocardiograms taken in the

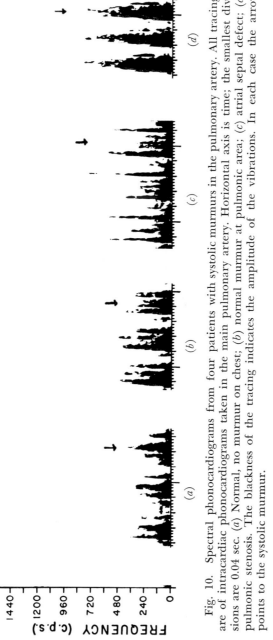

Fig. 10. Spectral phonocardiograms from four patients with systolic murmurs in the pulmonary artery. All tracings are of intracardiac phonocardiograms taken in the main pulmonary artery. Horizontal axis is time; the smallest divisions are 0.04 sec. (*a*) Normal, no murmur on chest; (*b*) normal murmur at pulmonic area; (*c*) atrial septal defect; (*d*) pulmonic stenosis. The blackness of the tracing indicates the amplitude of the vibrations. In each case the arrow points to the systolic murmur.

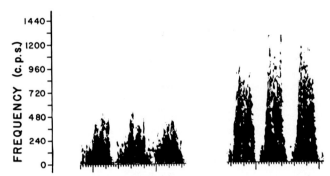

Fig. 11.   Spectral phonocardiograms from a patient with a ventricular septal defect with a left-to-right shunt. On the left, the intracardiac recording from the main pulmonary artery. On the right, the intracardiac recording from the outflow tract of the right ventricle opposite the defect. Frequency, time, and amplitude as in Fig. 10.

outflow tract of the right ventricle opposite the defect (as seen on the right) and from the main pulmonary artery just beyond the valve (as seen on the left). At the lesion there are very high frequencies well above 1000 cycles per second, but a short distance away they are completely dissipated. This is also well brought out on the tape recordings from which these spectral analyses were made.

Summary

1. We would like to reemphasize the point that the phonocardiogram is an important tool in the diagnosis of congenital heart disease and should not be neglected. The evidence of many workers indicates that it will yield information of a physiological nature as well as anatomical.

2. A complete description of the relationship between the pathologic physiology of the various congenital lesions and the phonocardiogram awaits further data. In this regard the intracardiac phonocardiogram promises to be an important aid.

3. As a diagnostic tool, the intracardiac phonocardiogram, by virtue of its ability to localize precisely the origin of heart sounds and murmurs, has proved to be of great value in congenital heart disease. This technique has added another dimension of information to be obtained at the time of cardiac catheterization. In the majority of cases studied thus far it has provided additional confirming data on the nature of

the lesion and its physiology. In a significant number of cases it has provided the sole means of positive diagnosis, and in another group of cases it has enabled us to rule out certain suspected lesions.

4. We feel that it should be made a part of the routine data obtained at the time of cardiac catheterization in congenital heart disease.

ACKNOWLEDGMENT

The authors are indebted to Dr. Byongsok Min for his translation of Dr. Yamakawa's paper published in Japanese.

REFERENCES

1. Kjellberg, S. R., Mannheimer, E., Rudhe, U., and Jönsson, B. *Diagnosis of Congenital Heart Disease.* Year Book Publishers, Inc., Chicago, Ill., 1955.
2. Mannheimer, E. Phonocardiography in children. *Advances in Pediat.* **7**:171, (1955).
3. Holldack, K., and Wolf, D. *Atlas und Kurzgefasstes Lehrbuch der Phonokardiographie.* Georg Thieme, Stuttgart, 1958.
4. McKusick, V. A. *Cardiovascular Sound in Health and Disease.* Williams and Wilkins, Baltimore, Md., 1958.
5. Leatham, A. Auscultation of the heart. *Lancet* **2**:703,757 (1958).
6. Yamakawa, K., Shionoya, Y., Kitamura, K., Nagai, T., Yamamoto, T., and Ohta, S. Intracardiac phonocardiography. *Am. Heart J.* **47**:424 (1954).
7. Lewis, D. H., Deitz, G. W., Wallace, J. D., and Brown, J. R., Jr. Intracardiac phonocardiography in man. *Circulation* **16**:764 (1957).
8. Yamakawa, K. Progress in intracardiac phonocardiography (in Japanese). *Japan. Clin.* **16**:1005 (1958).
9. Soulié, P., Laurens, P., Allard, E., Bouchard, F., and Cornu, C. The Allard-Laurens intracardiac micro-manometer. *Proc. 2nd World Congress of Cardiology*, Washington, D. C., 1954.
10. Laurens, P., Bouchard, F., Brial, E., Cornu, C., Baculard, P., and Soulié, P. The recording *in situ* of the murmurs or sounds and of the pressures of the vessels and of the heart due to a micromanometer. *Abstracts of Communications, 3rd World Congress of Cardiology*, Brussels, Belgium, 1958, p. 445.
11. Baculard, P. Étude phonocardiographique extra et intra cardiaque des stenoses de l'artère pulmonaire. Dactylo-Sorbonne, Paris, 1958.
12. Wallace, J. D., Brown, J. R., Jr., Lewis, D. H., and Deitz, G. W. Acoustic mapping within the heart. *Proc. 2nd International Congress on Acoustics*, Cambridge, Mass., 1956.
13. Wallace, J. D., Brown, J. R., Jr., Lewis, D. H., and Deitz, G. W. Acoustic mapping within the heart. *J. Acoust. Soc. Am.* **29**:9 (1957).
14. Lewis, D. H., Ertugrul, A., Deitz, G. W., Wallace, J. D., Brown, J. R.,

Jr., and Moghadam, A. N. Intracardiac phonocardiography in the diagnosis of congenital heart disease. *Pediatrics* (in press).

15. Luisada, A. A., and Liu, C. K. Simple methods for recording intracardiac electrocardiograms and phonocardiograms during left or right heart catheterization. *Am. Heart J.* **54:**531 (1957).

16. Lewis, D. H., Deitz, G. W., Wallace, J. D., Brown, J. R., and Ertugrul, A. Intracardiac phonocardiography in man. *Abstracts of Communications, 3rd World Congress of Cardiography,* Brussels, Belgium, 1958, p. 439.

17. Luisada, A. A. Mechanism of the heart sounds and intracardiac phonocardiogram. *Abstracts of Round Table Discussions, 3rd World Congress of Cardiology,* Brussels, Belgium, 1958, p. 275.

18. Luisada, A. A., and Liu, C. K. *Intracardiac Phenomena. Grune and Stratton,* New York, 1958.

19. Liu, C. K., and Jacono, A. Phonocardiography in atrial septal defect: External and intracardiac phonocardiograms. *Am. J. Cardiol.* **2:**714 (1958).

20. Moscovitz, H. L., Donoso, E., and Gelb, I. J. The demonstration of flow murmurs by intracardiac phonocardiography. *Clin. Research* **5:**162 (1957).

21. Welkowitz, W., and Traite, M. Intracardiac catheter microphone. *Rev. Sci. Inst.* **29**(3) (March 1958).

22. Moscovitz, H. L., Donoso, E., Gelb, I. J., and Welkowitz, W. Intracardiac phonocardiography. Correlation of mechanical, acoustic, and electric events of the cardiac cycle. *Circulation* **18:**983 (1958).

23. Gibson, G. A. Persistence of the arterial duct and its diagnosis. *Edinburgh Med. J.* **8:**1 (1900).

24. Wells, B. The effect of valvotomy on the murmurs of pulmonary and aortic stenosis. *Brit. Heart J.* **20:**523 (1958).

25. Spencer, M. P., Johnston, F. R., and Meredith, J. H. The origin and interpretation of murmurs in coarctation of the aorta. *Am. Heart J.* **56:**722 (1958).

26. Laurens, P. Personal communication.

27. Wood, P. W. Attacks of deeper cyanosis and loss of consciousness (syncope) in Fallot's tetralogy in Symposium on Congenital Heart Disease. *Brit. Heart J.* **20:**282 (1958).

28. McKusick, V. A., Talbot, S. A., and Webb, G. N. Spectral phonocardiography. Problems and prospects in the application of the Bell sound spectrograph to phonocardiography. *Bull. Johns Hopkins Hosp.* **94:**187 (1954).

29. Groom, D. The "normal" systolic murmur. *Circulation* **18:**1044 (1958).

30. McKusick, V. A., Massengale, O. N., Jr., Wilgod, M., and Webb, G. N. Spectral phonocardiographic studies in congenital heart disease. *Brit. Heart J.* **18:**403 (1956).

Relative Roles of Various Technics in Diagnosis and in Selection of Cases for Surgical Treatment

HOWARD B. BURCHELL

Section of Medicine, Mayo Clinic and Mayo Foundation,* Rochester, Minnesota

My assigned task "to summarize the values of various methods of diagnosis in congenital heart disease and the selection of the proper ones for surgical therapy" is a prodigious one, and my approach will be that of giving personal experiences and not that of reviewing the published results of the many who have contributed to this field of endeavor. The problems might be placed in five interrelated categories: (*a*) the problem of the repeat reliability of the diagnostic method in question and the discriminatory function of the test; (*b*) the management of the problem case in relation to the weighting of results that are conflicting; (*c*) the problem of the additional lesions that must always be suspected as being associated with or complicating the primary, predominating and recognized defect; (*d*) the problem inherent in some specific congenital cardiac syndromes and their diagnosis; and (*e*) the problem of operability. In this communication I shall attempt to integrate the problems in these five areas by approaching them from the clinical viewpoint with emphasis on the clinical examination and by making pertinent reference to the aid derived from roentgenologic, electrocardiographic, and cardiocatheterization investigations.

Each discipline within biology and medicine has contributed significantly to the progress in the accurate diagnoses of congenital cardiac defects; one may emphasize that pathologic anatomy, in par-

* The Mayo Foundation, Rochester, Minnesota, is a part of the Graduate School of the University of Minnesota.

ticular, regarded by certain scientific contemporaries as a dead science, figuratively came to life in the field of congenital cardiac disease, and the term "functional pathology" is especially applicable to it. One may further emphasize that, in any discipline, as soon as concepts and opinions are crystallized, there is lack of progress. In any single case study, functional pathology and hemodynamic physiology can go hand in hand, and can illustrate where either the anatomic observation or the physiologic record may take precedence in directing the observer to a proper appraisal of the whole problem. As examples, if a marked systolic pressure gradient were demonstrated between a ventricular chamber and the great vessel connecting to it, it is obvious that stenosis of the outflow area is present, whether the pathologist can readily demonstrate it or not. On the other hand, if the catheterization data have been interpreted as showing a ventricular septal defect and the pathologic anatomist can find only a single ventricle, then the latter is just as obviously the correct diagnosis. The pathologist has given the clinician a knowledge of the structural anomalies that are likely to be encountered in any age group.

Clinical Examination

The history as taken from the parents or the patient remains important. The age when murmur or cyanosis was first noticed may give a clue to the lesion present. The literature is replete with the significance of poor growth and nutrition in children with severe congenital cardiac defects. In cyanotic children with pulmonary stenosis, the assumption of the squatting position with fatigue is a well-known feature. In a severely cyanotic baby a blood smear may reveal Howell-Jolly bodies, an index of asplenia and the probability of a severe intracardiac defect (1). In respect to general appearance, one should be constantly aware of any sign suggesting Marfan's trait, Turner's syndrome (when coarctation is present), varied skeletal deformities, and mongolism. It is of curious coincidence that many of our early cases of endocardial cushion defect, the common atrioventricular-canal anomaly, were associated with mongolism, but in the large number of cases, approximately 100 including the incomplete form, that have been studied more recently there are very few mongoloids; however, if a mongoloid has congenital heart disease, it is proper to suspect an atrioventricular-canal defect.

One must always be alert to the presence of differential cyanosis. In the infant, when this occurs with the feet being redder than the upper part of the body, the diagnosis of transposition with an open ductus is practically assured. In older patients, cyanosis of the feet, and perhaps of the left hand, may be the clue to a "reversing ductus." Mattingly (2) has emphasized that in some children with large left-to-right shunts there is redness of the ends of the digits. In the old records of an adult patient with ventricular septal defect who was operated upon recently it was of interest to find a water-color painting of the hands that had been made when she was at the Mayo Clinic in 1924, at 4 years of age, and that showed this feature of redness of the digits, which had engaged the interest of the attending pediatrician, Dr. Helmholz, at that time.

In respect to the practice of auscultation, I would like to make a strong plea for the continued use of descriptive terms, not categorically conceptual ones. The originator of catch phrases may know what he means, but his disciples may not use the term to mean the same thing. When analyzing charts years hence a research student may not have any reliable evidence as to what actual sound complexes were present when, for instance, he might read of "ejection," "diamond-shaped," or "flow" murmurs. The phonocardiogram has added immeasurably to the appreciation of the frequency components, intensity and timing of sounds produced by the heart, but the ear can still delineate much in the way of pitch and quality which the routine phonocardiographic recording will not portray. Attention to the nature of the second sound has added greatly to the refinement of clinical diagnosis, and historically the fixed wide splitting (greater than 0.04 sec) occurring with atrial septal defect scarcely needs mention. In certain instances of pulmonary atresia, severe pulmonary stenosis, and truncus arteriosus, the second sound is clear and single, and even as an isolated finding it may strongly direct one to the correct diagnosis. Sharp early systolic sounds ("ejection clicks") in the traditional auscultatory aortic and pulmonary areas need further analysis, and in some instances of pulmonary valvular stenosis there is good evidence from angiocardiograms that the source of the sound is related to reversal of the curvature of the dome-shaped valve (3).

The absence of murmur in an infant who is deeply cyanotic would suggest a single ventricle with pulmonary atresia, or transposition of the great vessels. In a cyanotic adult, absence of murmur is most likely to be related to a ventricular septal defect with pulmonary hypertension. Exceptions, of course, are to be expected, but these are valid working guides. One encountered exception was a cyanotic patient with severe pulmonary valvular stenosis, an intact ventricular septum, and a small atrial septal defect, who, despite a gradient of more than 100 mm Hg across the pulmonary valve, exhibited no murmur. The explanation may be in part related to the fact that the patient had a low cardiac output and heart failure. I would also like to call attention to a characteristic prolonged discontinuous murmur that may be associated with a patent ductus in complicated severe pulmonary hypertension in adult patients. This murmur, located in the left infraclavicular space and heard well down toward the left side of the sternum by clinical auscultation and phonographic recording, begins and rapidly increases its intensity in late systole, and persists throughout diastole. Pulmonary incompetence may be a factor, but it is suspected that there is a higher ductus flow in diastole in these cases in contradistinction to what may occur in the infant with a patent ductus who exhibits only a systolic murmur.

When a continuous bruit is heard over the precordium, the differential diagnosis lies between patent ductus arteriosus, aortic-pulmonary communication above the semilunar valves, rupture of an aortic-sinus aneurysm, truncus arteriosus, and ventricular septal defect associated with aortic insufficiency. To make the list more nearly complete, one should mention systemic arteriovenous fistula in the mediastinum and coronary artery-coronary sinus communication, that is, arteriovenous fistula in the coronary circulation. In addition, it may be emphasized that communications between a normal coronary artery arising from the aorta and a coronary artery anomalously connected to the pulmonary artery may in some instances act as an arteriovenous fistula (4). Even when one has all these anatomic defects mentally displayed for perusal in an individual case, it is not always easy to determine the existing fault from auscultation. If one compares the hemodynamic situation in an individual who has a ventricular septal defect and aortic insufficiency with that in an individual who has a ruptured aortic-sinus aneurysm, it can be recognized that the same pressure gradients and transients could exist in both. In the rare individual case, with these competing diagnoses in mind, one would be hard pushed to state with confidence, from auscultation alone, which lesion was present. In such a problem case, however, there would be real discriminatory value in utilizing the pulse-pressure findings and the vascularity of the lungs. If there is a very wide pulse pressure associated with marked left ventricular enlargement, and if the pulmonary vasculature is not greatly accentuated, the findings would jointly point to a type of rapid aortic runoff, not runoff into the right ventricle to recirculate through the lungs, but rather regurgitation back into the left ventricle. Thus, in such a case the diagnosis of ventricular septal defect and aortic insufficiency would be reached.

Edwards and I (5) have discussed the pathologic anatomy of the aortic-root and aortic-sinus areas and have pointed out how the clinical findings in association with the catheterization data could lead not only to a diagnosis of aortic-sinus aneurysm with rupture but also to the ready prediction of which aortic sinus is involved and the likelihood of any associated ventricular septal defect. Our laboratories (6) have demonstrated the value of dye-dilution technics, utilizing multiple sampling sites and injection sites to demonstrate and differentiate the various defects at the aortic root. It is of some interest that after these refinements have been so developed as to render one proud of the advanced state of the art, the surgeon may no longer be interested in a detailed, minute diagnosis, being content to have the main problem outlined and to plan to take care of such complications or associated defects at the time that he can visualize the whole area.

Many years have passed since clinicians equated cyanosis simply with a right-to-left shunt, it being universally recognized in the present era that cyanosis is present only with a moderate-to-large shunt, and in particular when a large shunt is composed of markedly desaturated venous blood. Minor venous-arterial (or right-to-left) shunts are often present without cyanosis; for example, our group (7) has demonstrated the frequent slight shunting of venous blood, particularly from the inferior vena cava, in individuals with the usual type of atrial septal defect. Most patients displaying a clinical picture of mild cyanosis and prominence of the main pulmonary arteries are inoperable. It is important, however, to separate those patients who have cyanosis because of pulmonary vascular obstruction and a right-to-left shunt from those who have cyanosis, perhaps of mild degree, that is related to complete mixing of the pulmonary venous and systemic venous blood before it is partitioned between the systemic and pulmonary circuits. If the pulmonary vascular resistance is low in the presence of complete venous admixture, no cyanosis will be present. One can actually predict the approximate pulmonary flow by means of the systemic arterial saturation alone (8). If the pulmonary flow is high, the condition will be cured by surgical measures, if the technical aspects of the surgical repair are possible.

Roentgenologic Aids to Diagnosis

Routine x-ray examination of the thorax is of greatest help in showing (*a*) the pulmonary vasculature and (*b*) the size and shape of the heart and great vessels. As a general rule, one should not attempt from the x-ray appearance to draw rigid conclusions concerning which chamber is the predominant one in contributing to the enlargement. However, in some instances clues are offered as to the type of defect that may be present if the left atrium is enlarged, as it may be in instances in which the basic defect (for instance, a ventricular septal defect) is associated with mitral insufficiency. In many cases, one's attention will be focused mainly on the pulmonary vasculature and on whether this is exaggerated or the reverse, that is, on whether the lungs are oligemic. Many traps are laid for the unwary in this field. In infants it may be particularly difficult to judge the degree of pulmonary engorgement if the lungs are not fully expanded, and even in some adults there may be a very large pulmonary flow, but the relatively normal appearance of the vasculature may belie the true situation. The reverse of this does not hold, however, in that if the vasculature is prominent out into the midlung field and beyond and the lung is well expanded, one can be confident that pulmonary flow is increased.

The specialized forms of x-ray diagnosis have reached their highest development in those centers that have depended to a considerable extent upon x-ray technics for diagnosis. I may mention that as one sees difficult, complicated cases when visiting clinics where angiocardiographic work is carried on most competently, it is not infrequently the opinion of the consultants, in agreement with my assessment, that the angiocardiographic method has not always delineated the defects that exist in the particular cases presented for discussion. It seems an inconvertible fact that cases should be selected intelligently and that central injections, into either the right or the left side of the heart, are necessary if one is to be rewarded by having angiocardiograms or cineroentgenograms that are of discriminatory value. Our interest in the development of dye-injection technics in the elucidation of intracardiac shunts largely supplanted the need for angiocardiographic technics and has had the result of limiting angiocardiographic experience and collateral investigations.

Electrocardiographic Aids to Diagnosis

From the electrocardiogram one can usually recognize hypertrophy and enlargement of either ventricle when one ventricle is predominantly overloaded. This may not be possible when two ventricles are not developed, or both are hypertrophied, and when the heart is markedly displaced within the thorax. At this point it seems proper to refer to those electrocardiographic changes attributed to dynamic alterations, particularly since Cabrera and Monroy's (9) terms of expressing "systolic and diastolic overloading" are now frequently encountered in discussion groups and in the literature (10). To understand the development in this field one must have the concept that physiologic factors unrelated to hypertrophy may affect the electrocardiogram and, hence, produce electrocardiographic changes that might reflect pressure in either ventricle or in both. Originally Barnes (11) used the term "strain," and pointed out that while the QRS complex could mirror hypertrophy, the T-wave inversion appeared to be a dynamic effect, either in relation to left ventricular systolic hypertension or right ventricular systolic hypertension. The recently further developed concept contrasting cardiac output (or stroke volume) and the systolic pressure, and the expression "systolic and diastolic overloading," introduced by the Mexican school, have become popular in some clinics.

While acknowledging the usefulness of the contribution made, I believe that some of the disciples of this system have used it in an absolute and categorical way and have overrated its superiority over other methods. If such expressions related to ventricular loading are to be used, modifications in the terminology, necessitated by scientific clarity, are to be demanded; and instead of "systolic and diastolic overloading" it would be better to use the terms "pressure loading" and "volume loading." Simplicity, however, defies ready achievement because what is important additionally is the tension in the wall. If one thinks of "tension loading," this factor is dependent upon the size of the chamber; with enlargement of the heart, the systolic intraventricular pressure remaining the same, the tension will increase according to LaPlace's law $(P = kT/r)(12, 13)$. If one assumes that hypertrophy might be related primarily to the tension developed in the wall and to the duration of systole, then the degree of hypertrophy might be expected to vary with the product of the systolic pressure, the radius of curvature of the ventricle, and the systolic time. The shapes of the two ventricles are different, and with acquired loads the right ventricle can increase its stroke volume at a smaller percentage increase in its wall tension than can the left.

In general, the angle of the mean axis, particularly as determined from scalar leads, may not be particularly meaningful when the vector swings through a wide arc, when the standard leads show biphasic or multiphasic complexes and the frontal vector cardiogram shows a double loop variably disposed about the isoelectric point.

It is my belief that hypertrophy is well reflected in the height of the R wave in the right and left precordial leads respectively, when the R wave occurs as the initial deflection or is preceded by a Q wave. The duration of the R wave in these precordial leads contributes also to the diagnosis. When the right precordial leads show an rsR configuration, simulating partial right bundle-branch block and suggesting excess right ventricular volume loading (or "diastolic overload"), it may be impossible to assess the degree of hypertrophy with accuracy. A high upright T wave, emphasized by Cabrera and Monroy (9) as characteristic of left ventricular volume loading, is a useful sign but is not invariably present.

During the past five years in our studies of increasing numbers of patients with ventricular septal defects and pulmonary hypertension, it early became apparent that certain cases were characterized by electrocardiograms indicating left ventricular hypertrophy, whereas others were characterized by the pure picture of right ventricular hypertrophy. In the former instance the heart was bounding, overactive, and enlarged, and the vascular shadows in the lungs were increased. In the latter instance, in which the electrocardiogram showed right ventricular hypertrophy, the heart was quiet and usually only slightly enlarged, and the pulmonary vascular shadows were normal or decreased, although the proximal part of the pulmonary artery was sometimes prominent. The electrocardiogram often was a reliable clue as to the existing hemodynamic situation, and the possibility was suggested that, in young children, it might reflect the usual or average hemodynamic state from day to day more accurately than would the data obtained at the time of cardiac catheterization (14).

While the two extremes of the electrocardiographic picture may be readily recognized, it is now my personal opinion that there is a significant intermediate group of patients wherein the electrocardiographic record does not discriminate particularly well between the relative stroke volumes of the two ventricles and wherein the record, although an important feature in the assessment of the case, is not in itself an index of operability or inoperability. Details of our early experience are given in the paper of Agustsson and co-workers (14). A report of the experience of the Minneapolis group (15) indicates that they did not find a good correlation between various items in the electrocardiogram and either hemodynamic data or surgical survival. The cases were all surgical, so that part of the spectrum of clinical states associated with a ventricular septal defect, namely cyanotic ones, would be excluded from their study.

One must be alert to the possibility that patients who have ventricular septal defects with electrocardiographic evidence of left ventricular hypertrophy may have an associated ductus, a complicating mitral insufficiency, aortic incompetence, or coarctation of the aorta.

A few conditions are associated with very characteristic, at times almost diagnostic, electrocardiograms. One of these is Ebstein's disease (16), wherein a picture of right bundle-branch block may be present, and if the R wave in the right precordial lead is of low voltage and multiphasic, the condition is practically definitely Ebstein's. Also, in this condition auscultation may be diagnostic. Other conditions associated with near-diagnostic electrocardiograms are tricuspid atresia (which is historically a lesion, to be early associated with a characteristic left ventricular hypertrophy type of electrocardiogram), atrioventricular cushion defect (or common atrioventricular canal) (17), and transposition of the great vessels (wherein the late vector associated with right ventricular hypertrophy may be oriented to the right and forward, but not upward toward the right shoulder, resulting in the picture of right ventricular hypertrophy but with a very small or no R wave in VR). The last type of electrocardiogram showing evidence of right ventricular hypertrophy without a high R in VR may also be seen in some cases of infundibular stenosis, wherein the infundibular chamber is thin walled. In some cases of corrected transposition, heart block is a particularly characteristic finding, and, when it is associated with the signs of ventricular septal defect and mitral insufficiency, it constitutes a syndrome in its own right, as described by Walker (18), Anderson and co-workers (19), and our group (20).

Cardiac Catheterization as Aid to Diagnosis

In the problem case, cardiac catheterization remains the essential keystone of our diagnostic efforts in the laboratory. This would appear to be true not only now but also in the foreseeable future; it is combined universally with dye-injection methods and is supplemented occasionally by selective angiocardiographic procedures. With the extensive experience that has been built up in our laboratory as well as that represented in the published work of others, the cardiac-catheterization data, which are related primarily to (*a*) the position of the catheter, (*b*) the saturation of the blood at various intracardiac and great-vessel sites, (*c*) the pressures therein, and (*d*) the contour of dye-dilution curves, can generally be related to a structural or anatomic diagnosis. In addition to deriving the anatomic diagnosis, one makes a hemodynamic diagnosis, and these usually, but not always, correlate well with the structural and physiologic diagnosis arrived at by clinical means.

Discrepancy between a high pulmonary flow and rather minor increases in the roentgenologic vascular shadows within the lungs has already been alluded to, as well as the difficulties inherent in the electrocardiographic interpretation relating to the amount of hypertrophy and the size of the two ventricles.

When pulmonary obstruction is present either at the level of the main pulmonary artery or in its terminal ramifications, resulting in severe right ventricular systolic hypertension, the potentials engendered by hypertrophied ventricle will dominate the electrocardiographic picture as a rule, whether one utilizes routine scalar leads or vector analysis. Correlations of right ventricular systolic pressure in cases of pulmonary stenosis and intact ventricular septum with the electrocardiographic findings are quite inexact. In a young adult the electrocardiogram may be normal even when the right ventricular systolic pressure is as high as 75 mm Hg. In these cases the diagnosis may be suggested by the observation of a prominent *a* wave in the neck. If the right ventricular systolic pressure is more than 100, one may expect to see a characteristic electrocardiographic picture of right ventricular hypertrophy as portrayed in a qR deflection in the right precordial lead with a negative *T* wave, though occasionally the picture may be obscured by evidence of partial right bundle-branch block as exhibited by an rsR pattern, and not occasionally in children the *T* wave may be upright or diphasic rather than inverted. In infants, particularly, the upright *T* wave may be quite characteristic of right ventricular systolic hypertension.

At one time we added an electrocardiographic lead to the end of the catheter, but this was discontinued because of the extra cost of the catheters, because their larger size did not allow them to be introduced through a needle and because of the limited information that was forthcoming from the routine recordings of the intracardiac potentials. Their value in helping to determine the zone of localized obstruction at the pulmonary valve or in the infundibulum is acknowledged, as well as their characteristic form in Ebstein's malformation of the tricuspid valve (21, 22).

In past years a number of generalities regarding the importance of positions of the catheter in diagnosis have been advanced, but basic truths remain; for example, the easy and repeated entrance of the catheter from the right atrium into the left ventricle is consistent with the presence of an atrial septal defect of the common atrioventricular canal type, or continued difficulty or failure to enter the pulmonary artery should suggest severe pulmonary stenosis or transposition of the great vessels. Ready accessibility of the aorta from the right ventricle, while quite characteristic of cases of tetralogy of Fallot, may also suggest transposition of the vessels.

My position in respect to difficulties in the diagnosis of the site of obstruction to the right ventricular outflow has undergone no change recently, being that, when severe *valvular* stenosis exists, it may be impossible on withdrawal of the catheter to recognize an associated infundibular stenosis. On the other hand, if there is severe infundibular stenosis at a considerable or at any reasonable distance from the valve and the latter is normal or moderately stenosed, the infundibular site of the obstruction can be so designated.

When right-to-left shunts are present, the site of the shunt can be accurately ascertained by the injection of dye at various sites and sampling at the radial artery (23). By use of the new green dye which oximetric instruments can readily quantitate in venous blood and the use of multiple sampling sites on the right side of the heart, one can now readily determine by dye-dilution technics the site of left-to-right shunts and quantitate their magnitude (24).

In our clinic the need of the surgeon to have a diagnosis of the structural nature of the outflow tract of the right ventricle has been obviated to a large extent by the nearly universal application of direct-vision surgery. In certain cases, however, on clinical grounds there would seem to be a real need for laboratory appraisal of the outflow tract of the right ventricle and the pulmonary artery, and herein lies one of the indications for selective angiocardiographic procedures. In some instances in which there exists a high pulmonary flow with a single ventricle, catheterization data may suggest a ventricular septal defect, and when there is close approximation, even if not identity, of the oxygen content of the pulmonary artery with that of the radial artery, a selective angiocardiogram made with medium injected into the ventricle should contribute greatly to one's understanding of the problem.

In one's approach to the diagnosis one may ask, "What types of problem are the most challenging and baffling?" Of a number of overlapping categories in this field, three may be mentioned: (*a*) the category of isolated levocardia or isolated dextrocardia, (*b*) the general category of heart failure in the newborn characterized by enlarged heart with or without congested lung fields, and (*c*) the category of hearts with multiple defects. In the infant the syndrome of heart failure related to severe pulmonary stenosis or to stenosis of the pulmonary veins should be kept in mind as well as the more commonly encountered heart failure that is seen with patent ductus arteriosus, ventricular septal defect, or coarctation of the aorta. The problems of recognizing fibroelastosis in association with the last condition may be particularly trying. I have already referred to the syndrome of corrected transposition of the great vessels with ventricular septal defect and heart block; this syndrome may be associated with insufficiency of the left atrioventricular valve, as this structure partakes of the configuration of the tricuspid type of valve rather than the more soundly engineered mitral type of valve.

Many of you in this audience will remember Abbott's classic monograph (25) on congenital heart disease and will recall the frequency with which the various defects, as categorized, were associated with complicating lesions. Experience in the decade from 1940 to 1950, when active advance in diagnosis was taking place, seemed to refute the generalization that associated defects were common in cardiologic practice in the field of congenital defects, and one wondered at that time whether the specimens sent to Dr. Abbott were selected because of their curiosity value and whether the conclusions were thus subject to a natural bias. The classic text of Taussig (26) with the clear descriptions of clinical diagnostic entities would, I believe, support the hypothesis that the lesions are single rather than multiple. Experiences gained in the past five years or so would indicate that single defects may be too often diagnosed and that the profession should be alerted to the frequency with which associated defects may be present. While patients selected for cardiac catheterization represent specialized problems and perhaps are more likely eventually to come to postmortem examination, it is nevertheless of interest that in the period of more than ten years that we have utilized this technic, 33% of the 130 patients who did come to post-mortem examination (27) had either a partially inaccurate or incomplete diagnosis, though many of the errors or missed lesions were clinically and hemodynamically inconsequential. The conclusion that such inaccuracy or incompleteness prevails today would be erroneous, since some of the failures in diagnosis date back to the period when physiologic studies were less extensive than they are today. However, it would now be an anachronistic thought that a simple catheterization procedure would always reveal the accurate diagnosis, if ever such a thought had been held.

Contribution of Pulmonary Vascular Histologic-Physiologic Correlation

Pulmonary hypertension related to vascular obstruction in the small vessels in the lungs constitutes the main block to the complete success of surgical correction of many defects (28). In essence, the technical problems of the closure of a ventricular septal defect have faded into the background, with the spotlight remaining on the cause and the control of the pulmonary hypertension associated with left-to-right shunt. This problem has been investigated by many with rather meager practical rewards. When pulmonary vascular resistance is so greatly increased as to exceed systemic resistance, one may expect the underlying structural components in the vessels or alterations in the vessels to prevent return of the pulmonary circuit to normal. The decrease in resistance of the pulmonary vasculature with the breathing of a high concentration of oxygen or with the infusion of acetylcholine, or with both, has been considered a favorable omen in regard to reversibility, but completely adequate data to substantiate this are not existent as yet. At the present time in the difficult cases with pulmonary vascular obstruction, the decision for surgical treatment lies primarily with the surgeon in respect to the risk that he will take to ameliorate a condition though not cure it completely. Cases in which pulmonary flow is less than systemic flow are inoperable.

Regression in the pulmonary vascular obstruction might be expected to be more likely to occur in young children, but we have no proof that this is necessarily the case. In so far as one can interpret trends at the present time, it would appear that regression in pulmonary vascular changes and in pulmonary hypertension would be akin to that which has been observed following closure of a patent ductus when this has been associated with severe pulmonary hypertension (29), namely, that if the pulmonary vascular resistance has been high prior to closure, the peripheral vascular bed in the lung will not return completely to normal and in the majority of instances it apparently will stay at a static level. One must emphasize that conclusions such as this give one cause for some optimism because there may be no progression of the pulmonary vascular obstruction with the continuing hypertension.

In addition, it would seem likely that a certain, although unknown, percentage of individuals would have actual regression of the pulmonary vascular changes and that the large majority might be able to live normal lives for many years without significant disability. One case has been recently studied in which there is a possibility that the pulmonary hypertension continued to progress after complete closure of the ventricular septal defect, but the data are not adequate for a definite conclusion. Although recent work (30) has indicated that the histologic state of the pulmonary vasculature correlates fairly well with fixed pulmonary resistance, particularly with the presence of the "dilatation lesion," it would not seem possible to decide operability on the basis of pulmonary biopsy.

It may be reemphasized that there must be considerable variation in the reactions of the pulmonary vasculature in cases of ventricular septal defect in the neonatal period. The fact that we have not yet seen a heart with a large ventricular septal defect in a child or adult in whom the pulmonary artery was not larger than the aorta would indicate that universally there has been a phase of excess pulmonary flow. However, the time that this has persisted may be relatively short, and the work of Heath and Edwards (31) on the structure of the great vessels indicates that in a considerable number of cases the main pulmonary artery retains a histologic appearance similar to that of the aorta, which supports the view that in such cases pressure in the pulmonary artery has always been high and equivalent to the aortic pressure. Studies on the size of the ventricular septal defect in relation to the pulmonary-artery and systemic pressures have indicated that once the ventricular septal defect exceeds a diameter of 1 cm per square meter of body area the pressures equalize, but pulmonary flows vary tremendously.

Associated Defects and Complicating Lesions

The importance of always suspecting complicating lesions, once the apparent main defect is recognized, needs constant reemphasis. The not uncommon defects or acquired complications that have been encountered and often clinically recognized are given in Table I.

TABLE I.   Some associated defects and complicating lesions

Common Recognized Lesion	Lesions to Be Suspected	
	Associated	Complicating
Valvular pulmonary stenosis	Infundibular stenosis	Foramen ovale
Subvalvular pulmonary stenosis	Small ventricular septal defect	
Coarctation of aorta	Subaortic stenosis Bicuspid aortic valve Double aortic arch	Aortic insufficiency Fibroelastosis
Aortic stenosis	Supravalvular aortic stenosis Infravalvular aortic stenosis Pulmonary stenosis	Functional or dynamic outflow stenosis Aortic insufficiency
Ventricular septal defect	Infundibular pulmonary stenosis (noncyanotic tetralogy) Ductus arteriosus "Corrected transposition"	Pulmonary vascular disease Mitral insufficiency Aortic insufficiency Tricuspid insufficiency
Atrial septal defect	Anomalously connected pulmonary veins Ventricular septal defect AV commune—mitral incompetence	Tricuspid incompetence Pulmonary incompetence Pulmonary vascular disease
Patent ductus arteriosus	Ventricular septal defect Coarctation	Pulmonary vascular disease Pulmonary insufficiency

Indications for Surgical Treatment

The general problems that may be favorably treated by surgical means have been pertinently mentioned in the foregoing paragraphs on diagnosis. The indications for surgical treatment have not changed in their essentials in the past two years, and these have been discussed in detail in previous communications (32, 33). With the establishment of operations utilizing extracorporeal pump-oxygenators as routine, relatively safe procedures, it has been justifiable for the surgeon to accept higher medical risks than in the early years of this type of surgery. However, the salvage value and immediate operative mortality rate in severely ill children with complicated defects still have to be determined.

Conclusion

It may be stated that the blueprint for diagnosis is to recognize a "fit" of the available data but not to force a "fit." When everything available falls into place one's diagnosis is close to perfect. When it does not, one is alerted to the possibility of an associated or complicating defect. When the initial clinical data constitute an inadequate scaffolding with which to build a strong diagnosis, more data, that is, extra tests, are needed.

ADDENDUM

Since the presentation of this paper in December, 1958, there have been no developments to force any gross change in the basic opinions expressed and generalizations made. Cineangiocardiography has been further developed and established as a diagnostic method, and the indications for selective angiocardiograms have been more definitely formalized. The references have been modified to mention published articles in certain instances wherein originally the reference was a personal communication to the author. A recent article from the Mayo Clinic deserves mention: J. W. DuShane and J. W. Kirklin. Selection for surgery of patients with ventricular septal defect and pulmonary hypertension. *Circulation* **21**:13–20 (1960).

REFERENCES

1. Lyons, W. S., Hanlon, D. G., Helmholz, H. F., Jr., DuShane, J. W., and Edwards, J. E. Cardiac clinics. CXLVIII. Congenital cardiac disease and asplenia. Report of seven cases. *Proc. Staff Meetings Mayo Clin.* **32**:277–286 (1957).
2. Mattingly, Thomas. Personal communication to the author.
3. Hay, John. Personal communication to the author.

4. Edwards, J. E. Anomalous coronary arteries with special reference to arteriovenous-like communications (Editorial). *Circulation* **17:***1001*–1006 (1958).

5. Edwards, J. E., and Burchell, H. B. The pathologic anatomy of deficiencies between the aortic root and the heart, including aortic sinus aneurysms. *Thorax* **12:**125–139 (1957).

6. Semler, H. J., and Brandenburg, R. O. Demonstration of site of rupture of aortic-sinus aneurysms. *Proc. Staff Meetings Mayo Clin.* **33:**604–608 (1958).

7. Swan, H. J. C., Burchell, H. B., and Wood, E. H. The presence of venoarterial shunts in patients with interatrial communications. *Circulation* **10:**705–713 (1954).

8. Burchell, H. B. Total anomalous pulmonary venous drainage: clinical and physiologic patterns. *Proc. Staff Meetings Mayo Clin.* **31:**161–167 (1956).

9. Cabrera, C. E., and Monroy, J. R.: Systolic and diastolic loading of the heart. II. Electrocardiographic data. *Am. Heart J.* **43:**669–686 (1952).

10. Sodi-Pallares, Demetrio, and Marsico, Federico. The importance of electrocardiographic patterns in congenital heart disease. *Am. Heart J.* **49:**202–217 (1955).

11. Barnes, A. R. *Electrocardiographic Patterns: Their Diagnostic and Clinical Significance.* Charles C Thomas, Springfield, Ill., 1940.

12. Burton, A. C. The importance of the size and shape of the heart (Editorial). *Am. Heart J.* **54:**801–810 (1957).

13. Rushmer, R. F. Work of the heart. *Mod. Concepts Cardiovascular Disease* **27:**473–477 (1958).

14. Agustsson, M. H., DuShane, J. W., and Swan, H. J. C. Ventricular septal defect in infancy and childhood: Clinical and physiologic study of 19 cases. *Pediatrics* **20:**848–864 (1957).

15. Char, F., Adams, P., Jr., and Anderson, R. C. Electrocardiographic findings in one hundred modified cases of ventricular septal defect. *A.M.A. J. Diseases Children* **97:**48–60 (1959).

16. Kilby, R. A., DuShane, J. W., Wood, E. H., and Burchell, H. B. Ebstein's malformation: A clinical and laboratory study. *Medicine* **35:**161–185 (1956).

17. Toscano-Barboza, Ely, Brandenburg, R. O., and Burchell, H. B. Electrocardiographic studies of cases with intracardiac malformations of the atrioventricular canal. *Proc. Staff Meetings, Mayo Clin.* **31:**513–523 (1956).

18. Walker, W. J., Cooley, D. A., McNamara, D. G., and Moser, R. H. Corrected transposition of the great vessels, atrioventricular heart block, and ventricular septal defect: A clinical triad. *Circulation* **17:**249–254 (1958).

19. Anderson, R. C., Lillehei, C. W., and Lester, R. G. Corrected transposition of the great vessels of the heart: A review of 17 cases. *Pediatrics* **20:**626–646 (1957).

20. Helmholz, H. F., Daugherty, G. W., and Edwards, J. E. Cardiac clinics. CXLV. Congenital "mitral" insufficiency in association with corrected transposition of the great vessels: Report of probable clinical case and review of six cases studied pathologically. *Proc. Staff Meetings Mayo Clin.* **31:**82–91 (1956).

21. Hernandez, F. A., Rochkind, Reuben, and Cooper, H. R. The intracavitary electrocardiogram in the diagnosis of Ebstein's anomaly. *Am. J. Cardiol.* **1:**181–190 (1958).

22. Yim, B. J. B., and Yu, P. N. Value of an electrode catheter in diagnosis of Ebstein's disease. *Circulation* **17:**543–548 (1958).

23. Swan, H. J. C., Zapata-Diaz, J., and Wood, E. H. Dye dilution curves in cyanotic congenital heart disease. *Circulation* **8:**70–81 (1953).

24. David, André, Birkhead, N. C., Swan, H. J. C., and Wood, E. H. Venous dilution curves and their application to the localization and quantitation of left-to-right shunts in man. *Proc. Staff Meetings Mayo Clin.* **33:**562–568 (1958).

25. Abbott, Maude E. *Atlas of Congenital Cardiac Disease.* American Heart Association, New York, 1936.

26. Taussig, Helen B. *Congenital Malformations of the Heart.* Oxford University Press, London, 1947.

27. Ledbetter, M. K., Helmholz, H. F., Jr., and Edwards, J. E. Unpublished data.

28. Burchell, H. B.: Studies in pulmonary hypertension in congenital heart disease. *Brit. Heart J.* **21:**255–262 (1959).

29. Limon Lason, Rodolfo. Pulmonary hypertension in patent ductus arteriosus. *Pulmonary Circulation,* W. R. Adams and Ilza Veith, Editors. Grune & Stratton, New York, 1959, pp. 216–219.

30. (*a*) Heath, Donald, and Edwards, J. E. The pathology of hypertensive pulmonary vascular disease: A description of six grades of structural changes in the pulmonary arteries with special reference to congenital cardiac septal defects. *Circulation* **18:**533–547 (1958).

    (*b*) Heath, Donald, Helmholz, H. F., Jr., Burchell, H. B., DuShane, J. W., Kirklin, J. W., and Edwards, J. E. Relation between structural changes in the small pulmonary arteries and the immediate reversibility of pulmonary hypertension following closure of ventricular and atrial septal defects. *Circulation* **18:**1167–1174 (1958).

31. Heath, Donald, Wood, E. H., DuShane, J. W., and Edwards, J. E. The structure of the pulmonary trunk at different ages and in cases of pulmonary hypertension and pulmonary stenosis. *J. Pathol. Bacteriol.* **77:**443–456 (1959).

32. Burchell, H. B. Physiologic considerations and clinical indications for cardiac surgery. *Bull. N. Y. Acad. Med.* **33**:263–281 (1957).
33. Burchell, H. B. Clinical problems related to the surgical repair of intracardiac defects with the aid of an extracorporeal pump-oxygenator. *Circulation* **16**:976–987 (1957).

IV

SURGICAL THERAPY

Surgical Treatment of Pulmonary Valvular Stenosis and Atrial Septal Defects Using Hypothermia

HENRY SWAN

Department of Surgery, University of Colorado School of Medicine, Denver, Colorado

The successful development within a few years of two different techniques for performing operative manipulations under direct vision within the open heart has been a surgical achievement of real magnitude. Both hypothermia and cardiopulmonary bypass can now be said to be clinical techniques of proven merit. Both have advantages and disadvantages, and both have clearly definable limitations. It would appear, at the present time, that any team doing cardiac surgery should be thoroughly familiar with both techniques in order to offer operation to each patient at the lowest possible risk, selecting one method or the other for the specific cardiac lesion to be repaired. Both methods are in frequent use in our own clinic.

Since hypothermia was used clinically with success several years before cardiopulmonary bypass, it is not surprising that familiarity has brought to this modality a degree of safety which the latter technique has yet to achieve. At the present time, in our hands, by utilizing the precautions which we have come to regard as important, circulatory arrest during hypothermia is essentially without risk. However, the limitation in available time (which must be strictly observed) is the primary limiting factor in the use of this technique. Only those procedures which can be comfortably done in less than 12 min of operating time are suitable for current day hypothermia. All those requiring a longer period should be done with the pump-oxygenator, even though the cost, the complexity, and the risk of the method is somewhat greater. The two techniques, therefore, we consider as being complementary rather than conflicting.

Hypothermia

At the University of Colorado, experience with over three hundred and fifty patients undergoing general hypothermia has led us into a fairly standardized technique. No longer are ventricular fibrillation or bleeding dyscrasias dreaded complications. We believe that the following precautions and limitations are important factors in achieving this safety for the method.

1. The temperature range employed is 30° to 32° C, rectally. This is the lowest level reached after drift. Every effort, including use of diathermy, is made to prevent the temperature from falling below 30° C (1).

2. Cooling is external, by immersion in ice water. The patient, premedicated by Demerol (meperidine) or barbiturate and small doses of scopolamine (not morphine or atropine), is anesthetized to the second surgical plane with ether. He is then immersed in a tub containing lukewarm water. When all vital signs appear stable, cubes of ice (about 50 to 75 lb for an adult) are added to the tub. The water is constantly stirred. An adult may take 30 to 45 min, a small child 8 to 12 min, to cool to 34° C (rectal), at which temperature he is removed to the operating table. The end temperature will usually be about 30 to 30.5° C with this method (2).

3. Throughout the induction, the course of cooling, the operation, and the recovery period, deliberate respiratory alkalosis is maintained by hyperventilation (3).

4. Throughout the entire course of the procedure, a constant drip of 5 to 10% dextrose is maintained at 30 to 40 drops a minute. A deliberate hyperglycemia is thus achieved. A beneficial effect of intravenous nutrients on the myocardium during hypothermia now appears to be confirmed (4).

5. The first two pints of blood used for transfusion are freshly drawn, heparinized in plastic bags. The presence of platelets, fibrinogen, and other enzyme elements of the clotting mechanism, together with absence of citrate, are considered to be helpful in avoiding the bleeding diathesis formerly seen in hypothermia (5). A low blood

volume is scrupulously avoided as hypovolemia is poorly tolerated by the hypothermic individual (6).

6. The patient is warmed by internal heating, i.e., diathermy, applied to the pelvis. He is breathing spontaneously and beginning to respond before being returned to the recovery room. Careful drying and padding, and intermittent use of the diathermy are essential to avoid skin burns of the sacral area.

For those patients undergoing cardiac surgery the following precautions also are taken.

1. The patient is very carefully positioned so that the cardiotomy will be at the most superior aspect of the heart (7). Thus, for auricular defect the patient is tipped to the left with head elevated; for pulmonary valve to the right with head markedly elevated, etc. The air may thus escape from all chambers of the heart through the cardiotomy at the time of retreat from the heart.

2. At the onset of the circulatory occlusion period, the heart is slowed by the injection of 1:4000 neostigmine given by coronary perfusion. From 1–2 cc of this solution will slow but not stop the hypertrophied hypothermic heart. The heart should stay pink almost throughout the occlusion period. It will resume its beat readily once coronary circulation is allowed (8–10).

3. The root of the aorta is always clamped (except with aortic stenosis) in order to prevent coronary blood flow during occlusion. This helps prevent coronary air embolism, maintains the bradycardia, and in diminishing the coronary return to the heart insures a dry operative field (11).

4. The period of circulatory occlusion should not exceed 6 min, and *must* not exceed 8 min. If it is apparent that the complete operation cannot be accomplished in this period of time, the procedure should be stopped and escape from the heart effected, bringing out any unfinished sutures. Circulation is restored. After 10 or 15 min to allow reestablishment of normal myocardial metabolism, the occlusion may be repeated. At least 10 to 12 safe minutes of intracardiac time may thus be achieved (12).

5. Postoperative anticoagulants are given to patients who have gross enlargement of the pulmonary vascular bed (atrial septal defect). It is realized that marked slowing of the circulation through the lungs occurs immediately after the closure of a septal defect and the

TABLE I.   Progressive mortality in 250 patients undergoing open procedures during hypothermia

	Died	Rate, %
First 100	16	16
Second 100	6	6
Last 50	1	2

obliteration of the shunt. The volume flow is suddenly diminished, the enlarged vascular bed remains unchanged, so the rate is markedly reduced. No doubt pooling of blood in some areas also occurs. The stage is set for postoperative intravascular thrombosis. Antiprothrombin agents, therefore, are continued for at least three weeks, then tapered to discontinuance (13).

As a result of the application of these principles, the risk of open-heart surgery during hypothermia has fallen progressively. This is illustrated by the data on our first 250 such patients presented in Table I. At the present time, we believe that hypothermia is the method of choice for pulmonary stenosis, auricular septal defect, and the combination of the two lesions (trilogy of Fallot). For example, we have operated on 50 patients with pulmonic stenosis, and 77 consecutive patients with secundum type atrial septal defect without a single death. Since almost all the procedures were curative and the mortality was zero in this group of 127 patients, we see no reason to change from hypothermia to the pump-oxygenator for these particular lesions.

Pulmonary Stenosis

Obstruction to the outflow tract of the right ventricle occurs in a variety of congenital lesions. Our total open-heart operative experience with this problem is presented in Table II. Although the risk was low in tetralogy of Fallot and the clinical results were good, we are currently attempting the more nearly complete repair, both resecting the pulmonic obstruction and closing the septal defect. Since this requires the use of the pump-oxygenator, our experience with the latter technique is not the concern of this report. However, a glance at the table will indicate that all other forms of pulmonic stenosis can be readily treated at a low risk and with eminent success by means of

TABLE II.   Results of direct vision surgery in 95 patients with pulmonic stenosis during hypothermia

	Patients	Improved or Cured	Deaths
With intact septa			
Valvular stenosis	50	50	0
Infundibular stenosis	5	5	0
With ventricular septal defect (tetralogy)			
Valvular stenosis	7	7	0
Infundibular stenosis	11	8	3
With atrial septal defect (trilogy)	21	17	4
With aortic stenosis	1	1	0
Total	*95*	*88*	*7*

the simpler technique of hypothermia. We recommend this method, therefore, in all patients in whom the ventricular septum is intact.

Our experience to date with pulmonic stenosis occurring as a single or isolated defect has been particularly gratifying. The technique for the open transarterial approach and plastic revision of the stenotic valve was applied clinically for the first time in February 1953, and was reported in November of the same year (14). Since that time, 54 more patients with isolated pulmonic stenosis have been treated by the open approach without mortality.

The operation on the valvular lesions consists of a plastic revision by the placement of three incisions in the lines of the primitive commissures. These incisions extend all the way to the valve ring. Essentially total relief of the obstruction follows this maneuver in the vast majority of cases (15), as demonstrated by postoperative pressure tracings obtained by catheterization. Therefore, it is not necessary, in our opinion, to resect any of the hypertrophied muscle in the outflow tract of the right ventricle as an additional procedure. If the commissures are quite rudimentary, a soft murmur in diastole, suggesting some degree of pulmonary valvular insufficiency, may be heard postoperatively in some patients. In the five-year followup period now available on our early patients, this occurrence has apparently had no ill effect upon the circulatory dynamics. The patients are asymptomatic, normally active, and growing in accordance with expected norms. The early increase in the size of the heart, which one expects with the increased blood flow through it, has not progressed as time has passed, and any strain pattern present in the electrocardiogram preoperatively has disappeared.

The results in the few patients who have infundibular stenosis with intact ventricular septum have been equally satisfying. It is surprising that there apparently exists a widespread opinion that incision into the right ventricle in man during hypothermia is particularly dangerous and productive of ventricular fibrillation in many instances. Our experience is not in accord with this opinion. Although right ventriculotomy in the dog at 25° C rectal temperature will regularly initiate ventricular fibrillation, in man at 28° to 32° C it apparently will rarely do so. We have incised the right ventricle to operate on infundibular stenosis in 16 patients (Table III), and in no instance has the placing of stay sutures, the actual incision of the muscle, or the suturing of the wound incited ventricular fibrillation. We have no reason, therefore, to expect this particular complication.

The operative procedure consists of opening the ventricle, observing the fibrous ring of tissue constricting the outflow tract, and excising as much fibrous and muscular tissue as appears to be desirable in order to relieve the obstruction and give an anatomically adequate outflow tract. To date, no interference with coronary circulation or the conduction system has accompanied this maneuver in these patients, although both have occurred during the operative repair of tetralogy during cardiopulmonary bypass. The incision in the ventricle is temporarily closed by big traction sutures as circulation is resumed. Mattress sutures can be rapidly placed to close the incision as the heart action is resuming. The results of this operation have been studied by postoperative catheterization. Obstruction to the outflow tract has been completely relieved.

On the basis of this experience, therefore, we are of the opinion that these two simpler forms of visual intracardiac operations are ideally suited for the use of the hypothermic technique. With the ventricular septum intact, it really makes no difference if infundibular stenosis is not distinguished from valvular in the preoperative

TABLE III. Direct vision repair of atrial septal defect (ASD) secundum in 133 hypothermic patients

	Patients	Cured or Improved	Deaths
1. ASD as only lesion present	98	91	7
2. ASD with aberrant pulmonary veins	20	18	2
3. ASD with patent ductus arteriosus	2	2	0
4. ASD with pulmonic stenosis (trilogy of Fallot)	13	10	3
Total	*133*	*121*	*12*

evaluation, since either lesion can be readily relieved at operation during hypothermia with very little risk to the patient.

The second large group of patients who seem well suited for repair during hypothermia are those with atrial septal defects of the so-called secundum type. Our experience with these lesions in the first 250 patients undergoing open-heart surgery is shown in Table III. These defects may be associated with other abnormal developments such as patent ductus arteriosus, aberrant pulmonary venous drainage, or pulmonary valvular stenosis. Such associated anomalies, however, can be treated effectively at the time of repair of the defect by using multiple short (6 min) occlusion periods if necessary. Precision in the preoperative recognition of such variants, therefore, need not be perfect, although it is obviously helpful to the surgeon to be aware of the possibility of aberrant venous return before surgery.

Of much more importance, however, is the distinction between the secundum type lesion and the primum defect, which include clefts in the mitral valve, and also atrioventricularis, with its much more complicated anatomy. These last two anomalies require a longer period of intracardiac operating time than is provided by hypothermia, and, therefore, they are more suited to repair by use of cardiopulmonary bypass. The preoperative distinction between these various entities can, in fact, be made. In our series of 133 patients as presented in Table III, each patient was correctly diagnosed as having secundum lesions preoperatively; also, there were no other patients explored with a preoperative diagnosis of secundum, who proved at surgery to have a primum defect. Since the secundum type lesion can be identified with such a degree of reliability by those skilled in this diagnosis (16), the surgeon can approach the problem by cooling the patient, fully confident that a lesion will be found which will be amenable to repair by this technique.

The details of the surgical procedures employed to meet the various technical problems posed by variations in the anatomy have been recently published (17), and need not be reviewed in detail here. In general, after exploring the heart through a unilateral thoracotomy in the fourth interspace on the right and transecting the sternum to allow very rapid extension of the incision, if it should prove necessary, tapes are placed about the superior and inferior vena cavae, and about any accessory vena cava that may be found. An incision is made into right auricle over a noncrushing clamp. After inflow occlusion is established, the auricle is opened, the blood is removed by suction, and the defect is observed. After palpation of the mitral valve, the defect is closed by a running suture of silk, and all air is allowed to escape the left auricle before the final bite of the suture is tightened and tied. The right auricle is filled with blood by releasing the superior cava as the clamp is applied to the auricular incision. Blood flow is resumed. If aberrant veins are present, the anterior edge of the defect in the septum is sewed to the right wall of the auricle in front of the veins in such a fashion that the mouths of the veins debauch through the defect into the left auricle. Occasionally, the septal defect must be enlarged upward or downward in order to accomplish this. Occasionally also, special maneuvers on the superior vena cava are necessary. Attention must also be paid to be sure that a residual valve of the inferior vena cava does not mislead the operator into transposing the entrance of the inferior cava into the left auricle. With these precautions in mind, however, all the variants of secundum defect, either occurring alone or in association with aberrant pulmonary venous drainage to the right auricle, can be successfully repaired by this technique, usually in no more than two periods of inflow occlusion.

The results in these patients have been increasingly gratifying. All seven deaths occurred in the first 43 patients. Since that time, 77 consecutive patients were operated upon without a single operative or hospital mortality as we learned better to apply the safeguards described in the opening section of this report. Two patients have subsequently died weeks or months after returning home. Thus, of these 120 patients, 111 are alive and well, and essentially cured of their disease.

Trilogy of Fallot

Of particular interest are those patients who have the combination of these two major anomalies, namely, pulmonary stenosis and atrial septal defect. This anomaly has been termed the trilogy of Fallot. The pulmonary obstruction is almost invariably valvular; the atrial defect is usually of the foramen ovale type, wherein the defect is small or medium sized and lies in the center of the septum. We have not seen the situation in which pulmonic stenosis is associated with either a high secundum lesion or a low primum defect.

The abnormal physiology in most instances consists of a large right-to-left shunt at atrial level and a high right ventricular pressure. Thus, the patients are usually very cyanotic, and clubbing may be a prominent feature of the disease. Clinically, the mistaken impression may be held that the patient has tetrology of Fallot, and it is known that some patients have been sent to surgery with this incorrect diagnosis. Fortunately, in our clinic, this error in diagnosis has not occurred,* but the point again should be noted that the use of hypothermia imposes the need for accurate preoperative diagnosis in order to avoid cooling patients who should be operated upon with cardiopulmonary bypass and vice versa.

There is one rare variant of the disease which presents an entirely different clinical picture, namely, left-to-right shunt even in the face of the high right ventricular pressure. Why this occurs is not easily understood. In a group of 21 patients, however, whom we have subjected to surgery for this disease, only one was acyanotic.

Our opinion of the proper form of treatment for this disease has undergone considerable modification as our experience has increased. At first we thought that relief of the pulmonic stenosis would suffice, and that with the change in ventricular pressures, the shunt would

---

* All these patients were carefully evaluated pre- and postoperatively by Dr. S. Gilbert Blount, Jr., of the Department of Medicine, University of Colorado School of Medicine, Denver.

decrease and the valve of the foramen ovale might close (18). This, however, has not been our experience. The shunts have continued (the left-to-right patient became much worse), and although most patients were improved, they remained cyanotic. For this reason we reoperated on two of these nine patients to close the septal defect (including the noncyanotic one). The second operation was well tolerated in each instance, and these patients are now cured.

As our experience with multiple periods of circulatory occlusions increased, and we learned more of the safety of the method, we have changed our operative plan to one which contemplates complete cure in a single sitting. The incision is a bilateral sternal-cutting thoracotomy in the fourth interspace on the right and the third on the left. The pulmonary valve is first visualized by using the transarterial approach, as described earlier. After repairing the valve, the circulation is allowed to return to an essentially normal state while the arterial incision is being sutured. When all seems quite satisfactory and the patient is repositioned to place the right auricle more superiorly, a second period of occlusion is taken to enter the auricle and suture the atrial septal defect. This usually can be done easily in 4 or 5 min because of the simple nature of these ovale defects. The auricles are allowed to fill with blood as the clamp is reapplied to the auricular incision. Circulation is then resumed, and the auricle is closed at leisure.

By using this concept, our last nine patients have undergone curative single stage procedures. One died postoperatively of an unrecognized concommitant brain tumor; another died very suddenly and unexpectedly the night of the surgery. The remaining seven have done very well and are now cured. It is a dramatic sight to see these previously very cyanotic patients come off the operating table looking as pink as any normal individual. Clubbed fingers which have a bright pink appearance are indeed a curious sight. Interestingly, the clubbing tends to recede rapidly in the months following operation.

Summary

1. Currently, hypothermia of 30° to 32° C rectal temperature has achieved a degree of safety which approaches that of ether anesthesia.

Approximately 10 to 12 min of safe open-heart operating time are made available by this technique.

2. Pulmonary stenosis, atrial septal defect of the secundum type, and the combination of the two lesions can be readily repaired within this time limit, even when one of the more complex variants are present.

3. Since these lesions can be recognized with precision preoperatively, inaccurate diagnosis need not be a reason for employment of more dangerous and complicated operative techniques.

4. Hypothermia, because of its safety, remains the technique of choice for the repair of these specific anomalies.

REFERENCES

1. Swan, H. Relationship between hypothermia and operative risk. *Bull. Soc. Nat. Chir.* 14:64–67 (1955).
2. Blair, E., Swan, H., and Virtue, R. Clinical hypothermia: a study of the ice-water surface immersion and short-wave diathermy rewarming techniques. *Am. Surgeon* 22(9):869 (1956).
3. Swan, H., Zeavin, I., Holmes, J. H., and Montgomery, V. Cessation of circulation in general hypothermia. I. Physiologic changes and their control. *Ann. Surg.* 138(3):360 (1953).
4. Caranna, L., Telmosse, F. J. P., and Swan, H. The effect of intravenous nutrient solutions on ventricular fibrillation in the hypothermic dog. *Arch. Surg.* 76:394–397 (March 1958).
5. Swan, H., Virtue, R., Blount, S. G., Jr., and Kircher, L. W. Hypothermia in surgery. Analysis of 100 clinical cases. *Ann. Surg.* 142(3):382 (1955).
6. Wilson, J. N., Marshall, S. B., Beresford, V., Montgomery, V., Jenkins, D., and Swan, H. Experimental hemorrhage: the deleterious effect of hypothermia on survival and a comparative evaluation of plasma volume changes. *Ann. Surg.* 144(4):696 (1956).
7. Swan, H. Hypothermia of general and cardiac surgery. *Surg. Clin. North Am.* 36(4):1009 (1956).
8. Prevedel, A. E., Montgomery, V., and Swan, H. Effect of coronary perfusion of prostigmine on ventricular fibrillation in the hypothermic dog. *Proc. Soc. Exptl. Biol. Med.* 85:596 (1954).
9. Montgomery, V., Prevedel, A. E., and Swan, H. Prostigmine inhibition of ventricullar fibrillation in the hypothermic dog. *Circulation* 10(5):721 (1954).
10. Baer, S. B., Montgomery, V., Blair, E., and Swan, H. The relation of

coronary blood flow to prevention of ventricular fibrillation in the cold canine heart. *Surg. Forum* **6:**200 (1955).

11. Swan, H., and Zeavin, I. Cessation of circulation in general hypothermia. III. Technics of intracardiac surgery under direct vision. *Ann. Surg.* **139**(4):385 (1954).

12. Blair, E., Austin, R. R., Blount, S. G., Jr., and Swan, H. A study of the cardiovascular changes during cooling and rewarming in human subjects undergoing total circulatory occlusion. *J. Thoracic Surg.* **33**(6):707–718 (1957).

13. Swan, H., Blount, S. G., Jr., and Virtue, R. Direct vision suture of interatrial septal defect during hypothermia. *Surgery* **38**(5):858 (1955).

14. Swan, H. Surgical closure of interauricular septal defects. *J. Am. Med. Assoc.* **151:**792–794 (1953).

15. Blount, S. G., Jr., van Elk, J., Balchum, O. J., and Swan, H. Valvular pulmonary stenosis with intact ventricular septum. *Circulation* **15:**814 (1957).

16. Blount, S. G., Jr., Davies, D. Hywel, and Swan, H. Atrial septal defect. Results of surgical correction in 100 consecutive patients. *J. Am. Med. Assoc.* **169:**210–13 (1959).

17. Swan, H., Kortz, A. B., Davies, D. H., and Blount, S. G., Jr. Atrial septal defect, secundum. An analysis of one hundred patients undergoing open surgical repair. *J. Thoracic Surg.* **37:**52–80 (1959).

18. Swan, H., and Blount, S. G., Jr. Visual intracardiac surgery in a series of 111 patients. *J. Am. Med. Assoc.* **162:**941–946 (1956).

Surgical Correction of Ventricular Septal Defects and Aneurysms of Sinus of Valsalva*

C. WALTON LILLEHEI

Department of Surgery and Variety Club Heart Hospital, University of Minnesota Medical School, Minneapolis, Minnesota

Less than five years ago there was no patient alive who had been cured of the common congenital cardiac malformation of ventricular septal defect, not to mention the less frequently encountered condition of ruptured aneurysm of a sinus of Valsalva.

The development and introduction into routine clinical use of effective methods of extracorporeal circulation which have allowed safe bypass of the heart and lungs for temporary intervals has removed this barrier and opened a new era in the treatment of cardiovascular disease of both congenital and acquired origins (1).

From 1954 until the present date, 257 patients have had ventricular septal defects closed under direct vision by utilizing extracorporeal circulation at the University of Minnesota Variety Club Heart Hospital. Today, upon the basis of this experience, there is little question about the desirability of surgically closing all ventricular septal defects associated with any significant degree of shunt and particularly with pulmonary hypertension.

Moreover, ventricular septal defects are common congenital malformations, probably ranking first in incidence and exceeding even patent ductus arteriosus in prevalence.

Prior to the availability of a surgical cure, the malformation has

* Research supported by grants from: Graduate School, University of Minnesota; Minnesota Heart Association; American Heart Association; Life Insurance Medical Research Fund; United States Public Health Service Grant #830; Minnesota Cardiovascular Research Fund.

been a lethal one. Less than one child in ten born with a ventricular septal defect survived beyond the pediatric age range (15 years).

The lethal element of ventricular defects has been, primarily, the early rapid and progressive development of pulmonary hypertension associated with pulmonary arteriosclerosis. Other contributing factors are cardiac decompensation, increased susceptibility to pneumonia, and blood stream infections.

As a result, the indications for closing a ventricular defect have been progressively broadened to include both the asymptomatic individuals (with evidence of a significant shunt) as well as the frequently encountered patients with far advanced pulmonary hypertension.

Previously (2), we analyzed the results of surgical correction of ventricular septal defects in 154 patients operated upon from the time treatment began in 1954 until 1957. In that initial series there were 109 successful cases or an overall mortality of 29%. Subsequently, an additional 103 have had ventricular defects closed at this center with 10 deaths to give a mortality rate of 9.7%. Moreover, in the last fifty patients operated upon, there have been only two deaths despite the fact that eleven of the fifty had very severe pulmonary hypertension (pulmonary artery systolic pressures 100 mm Hg or above). These results are summarized in Table I.

This favorable combination of a substantial reduction in the operative risk combined at the same time with the progressive extension of surgical correction to those patients with the most advanced conditions, often considered inoperable, has come about as the result of a number of factors. Refinements in the perfusion apparatus and of the surgical techniques for its use have contributed. Important in this regard has been abandonment of the widely used elective potassium

TABLE I.   Closure of ventricular defects at University of Minnesota Heart Hospital

No. Patients	Period	Mortality
154	1954–56	45 (29%)
53	1957	8 (15%)
50[a]	1958	2 (4%)
257		

[a] Eleven patients had severe pulmonary hypertension (systolic pressures 100 mm Hg or above).

citrate arrest of the heart because of the deleterious effects of potassium and hypoxia upon the myocardium especially manifest in the patient who preoperatively is recognized as a poorer risk. Where elective arrest is deemed helpful, it is obtained by use of selective cardiac hypothermia (7, 8). In addition to these, a principal factor that may be mentioned is the better understanding of the pathologic physiology and management of pulmonary hypertension. Tracheotomy (1), done preoperatively in children with severe pulmonary hypertension to permit smoother and more uniform adjustment, with routinely assisted respiration postoperatively for several days or more, has contributed importantly to this reduction of operative risk in patients with septal defects and advanced degrees of pulmonary hypertension. The use of delayed closure by means of a perforated ventricular patch (8) has been lifesaving in certain individuals, where at the time of operation, with the chest open and the patient breathing a high concentration of oxygen, the pulmonary artery pressure is found to be equal to the aortic pressure by direct measurement. Another important agent contributing to lowered risk, especially for the more advanced patients with larger defects, has been the more positive control of the complication of complete heart block made possible by insertion of a wire into the myocardium to control the heart rate by use of repetitive electric stimuli from an external (hearing-aid size, transistorized) pacemaker (3–5).

Space permits only a brief reference to the late recatheterization studies that now have been carried out in 57 patients and which indicate by physiologic measurements that 93% of these patients operated upon have been significantly benefited (Table II).

Prior to our successful cases in 1956, a ruptured aneurysm of the

TABLE II. Ventricular septal defects: Postoperative recatheterization results, 57 patients

	Pulmonary Arterial Pressure Normal	Pulmonary Hypertension Present	Total
No shunt	41	6[a]	47
Residual	6	4	10

[a] One is symptomatic. Thus, 47 + 6 = 53 patients (93%) are cured or significantly improved.

sinus of Valsalva remained an incurable condition. Although relatively uncommon compared to a number of other cardiac conditions, it has remained important because of the extremely serious effects upon life expectancy, most patients succumbing within a year of onset.

Since 1956, we have operated upon eight such individuals by utilizing extracorporeal circulation. Three of these patients had an isolated lesion and all survived corrective surgery (6). Three others have had a ruptured aneurysm of the sinus of Valsalva together with a ventricular septal defect, tetralogy of Fallot, and infundibular pulmonic stenosis respectively. One patient in this group died later of complete heart block. Two other patients had an unruptured aneurysm of a sinus of Valsalva corrected successfully at the time ventricular septal defects were closed.

In conclusion, it is evident that the development of safe and reproducible techniques for working within the open heart has completely altered the grim prognosis often associated with the presence of a sizable ventricular septal defect or a ruptured aneurysm of a sinus of Valsalva.

REFERENCES

1. Lillehei, C. W. Contributions of open cardiotomy to the correction of congenital and acquired cardiac disease. *New Engl. J. Med.* **258**:1044–1049, 1090–1095 (1958).
2. Lillehei, C. W., Warden, H. E., DeWall, R. A., Stanley, P., and Varco, R. L. Cardiopulmonary bypass in surgical treatment of 305 patients with congenital or acquired cardiac disease. *Arch. Surg.* **75**:928–945 (1957).
3. Weirich, W. L., Gott, V. L., and Lillehei, C. W. Treatment of complete heart block by the combined use of a myocardial electrode and an artificial pacemaker. *Surg. Forum* **8**:360–363 (1958).
4. Weirich, W. L., Gott, V. L., Paneth, M., Stirling, G., Sellers, R. D., and Lillehei, C. W. The control of complete heart block by the use of an artificial pacemaker and a myocardial electrode. *Circulation Research* **6**:410–415 (1958).
5. Thevenet, A., Hodges, P. C., and Lillehei, C. W. The use of a myocardial electrode inserted percutaneously for control of complete atrioventricular block by an artificial pacemaker. *Diseases of Chest* **34**:621–631 (1958).

6. Lillehei, C. W., Stanley, P., and Varco, R. L. Surgical treatment of ruptured aneurysms of the sinus of Valsalva. *Ann. Surg.* **146**:459–472 (1957).
7. Gott, V. L., Long, D. M., Johnson, J. A., Bartlett, M. M., and Lillehei, C. W. Glycogen, lactic acid, and high energy phosphate levels during hypothermic arrest of the human heart. *Circulation* **20**:703 (1959).
8. Gott, V. L., Bartlett, M., Johnson, J. A., Long, D. M., and Lillehei, C. W. High energy phosphate levels in the human heart during potassium titrate arrest and selective hypothermic arrest. *Surg. Forum* **10**:544–547 (1960).

Corrective Surgical Treatment for Cyanotic Congenital Heart Disease

JOHN W. KIRKLIN

Section of Surgery, Mayo Clinic and Mayo Foundation,* Rochester, Minnesota

This discussion is concerned with the surgical treatment of cyanotic patients who have congenital heart disease. Ordinarily, this implies patients with an arterial-blood oxygen saturation of 85% or less.

Cyanosis develops in congenital heart disease as a result of right-to-left shunt at atrial, ventricular, or aortic level. In cyanotic patients with the primary and only intracardiac lesion being a defect in the atrial or ventricular septum or between the great vessels, right ventricular systolic hypertension exists. Clinical experience has indicated that under these circumstances the hypertension results from obstruction to right ventricular emptying, posed by high pulmonary vascular resistance. Pulmonary blood flow is essentially the same as or less than systemic blood flow. Correction of the shunt without relief of obstruction results in either no immediate change in right ventricular systolic pressure or, if pulmonary flow was less than systemic flow prior to repair, an increase in pressure. In these types of anatomic defects, this has resulted in a high immediate and late mortality, and lack of significant clinical improvement in surviving patients. Therefore, my colleagues and I do not recommend surgical treatment at present for cyanotic patients with isolated atrial or ventricular septal defects, or aortic-pulmonary communications.

When relief of the obstruction to right ventricular emptying can be achieved at the time of correction of a venoarterial shunt, at atrial or ventricular level, increased pulmonary flow is accommodated at a

---

* The Mayo Foundation, Rochester, Minnesota, is a part of the Graduate School of the University of Minnesota.

lower right ventricular pressure than was present prior to operation. When cyanosis results from ventricular septal defect and pulmonary stenosis, that is, from the tetralogy of Fallot, or from pulmonary stenosis and atrial septal defect, closure of the shunt and relief of pulmonary stenosis can both be accomplished. Thus the results are then excellent. Surgical treatment is advisable for cyanotic patients with these defects.

In malformations with a common mixing chamber, into which enters the entire systemic and pulmonary venous return such as occurs in total anomalous pulmonary venous connection, common atrium and single ventricle cyanosis can exist without *severe* obstruction to right ventricular emptying. The oxygen saturation of the arterial blood is essentially the same as that of pulmonary-artery blood, both being that of blood in the common mixing chamber. This saturation is determined by the relative contributions of systemic and pulmonary venous blood to the common pool. Under certain circumstances streamlining of flow through the pool occurs, and allows differences to exist between the saturation of pulmonary arterial and that of systemic arterial blood.

In patients with a common mixing chamber, the degree of cyanosis is related to the magnitude of pulmonary blood flow. The larger this is, relative to systemic blood flow, the higher is the arterial oxygen saturation and the less the cyanosis. Indeed, if pulmonary blood flow is very large, cyanosis may be absent. When pulmonary and systemic blood flows are approximately the same in these malformations, cyanosis is marked. It is associated with severe elevation of pressure in the pulmonary artery on the basis of high pulmonary vascular resistance. Repair of the anatomic malformation relieves cyanosis under all circumstances, but the best results are obtained when operation results also in lowering of pressure in the pulmonary artery and right ventricle. In our experience this can be expected to occur only when pulmonary flow has been greater than systemic flow prior to operation.

Total Anomalous Pulmonary Venous Connection

ANATOMY

When all the pulmonary veins are abnormally connected so that they drain into the right atrium, either directly or via a systemic vein, the condition is designated "total anomalous pulmonary venous connection." The right atrium is the common mixing chamber. For survival, there must be a communication between the right and left sides of the circulation. This is most commonly through an atrial septal defect, and has always been so in our patients treated by operation.

In approximately 90% of the recorded cases (1, 2) the patient exhibits a common pulmonary venous sinus into which drain all the pulmonary veins and which connects with a persistent vertical vein along the left mediastinum, the superior vena cava, the coronary sinus, or the right atrium directly. Cases are recorded in which all pulmonary veins drained into the inferior vena cava, the portal vein, or the ductus venosus, but apparently in none was the anomaly treated surgically.

HEMODYNAMICS

Blood gains access to the left side of the heart through the atrial septal defect when this anomaly is present. If the defect is small, high right atrial and systemic venous pressure is present.

The magnitude of the pulmonary and systemic blood flows is related to the distensibility of the right and left ventricles. In some patients, pulmonary vascular resistance is low, pressure in the pulmonary artery is only mildly increased, and right ventricular hypertrophy is not marked. Under these circumstances pulmonary blood flow is greatly in excess of systemic blood flow. The saturation of blood in the common mixing chamber is maintained relatively high by the predominant contribution to it of pulmonary rather than systemic venous blood. Blood entering the systemic circulation from the common mixing chamber is only slightly desaturated when the patient is at rest, and cyanosis is minimal or absent.

When pulmonary resistance is somewhat higher, pressure in the pulmonary artery is increased, and there is some right ventricular hypertrophy. Pulmonary flow is still increased, but not to the extent seen in the previous example. There is a corresponding reduction in arterial oxygen saturation. Under conditions of still higher pulmonary vascular resistance and pulmonary hypertension, pulmonary flow is no longer increased and may in fact be less than systemic flow. The patient is considered inoperable under these circumstances, for the reasons previously enumerated.

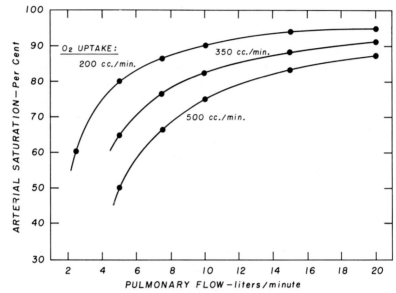

Fig. 1.   Calculations of arterial oxygen saturation in total anomalous pulmonary venous connection, assuming different values for pulmonary blood flow. Certain assumptions were made in establishing these theoretic curves. The upper curve is based on a resting oxygen uptake of 200 cc per minute, the lower curve (500 cc per minute) on an uptake such as might occur with mild exercise. (Reproduced with permission from reference 3.)

The relation between magnitude of pulmonary blood flow and arterial oxygen saturation has been expressed by Burchell[3] (Fig. 1).

INDICATIONS FOR SURGICAL TREATMENT

Operation is advised in all cases of total anomalous pulmonary venous connection in which pulmonary blood flow is in excess of systemic blood flow. Cyanosis and pulmonary hypertension are often present, but do not contraindicate surgical treatment as long as pulmonary flow exceeds systemic flow.

TECHNIC

An open complete repair, utilizing whole-body perfusion by means of a pump-oxygenator, is felt to be the method of choice. Lewis and associates (4) and Ehrenhaft and associates (5), utilizing hypothermia, have each reported complete correction in a case, and Senning (6), utilizing a closed technic, has reported a complete correction. Mustard and Dolan (7) have expressed doubt that complete repair by a one-stage procedure is advisable. In spite of this the experience in this clinic has been that an open, complete repair, utilizing whole-body perfusion by means of a pump-oxygenator, is the technic of choice. Bahnson and associates (8), Lillehei and associates (9), and Cooley and Ochsner (10) have expressed a similar view.

The safety of this, as well as other open intracardiac procedures, is best assured by accurate preoperative evaluation, use of completely adequate whole-body perfusion, precise surgical technic, and good postoperative care. This particular operation may be lengthy, at times requiring up to 2 hours of extracorporeal circulation. This is well tolerated by the patient if all aspects of the perfusion and operation are carefully and properly managed.

Important technical steps in the operation, no matter what the exact anatomy of the total anomalous pulmonary venous connection, are: (*a*) provision for an adequately sized left atrium, (*b*) connection of the common pulmonary venous sinus to the left atrium, (*c*) closure of the communication between the sinus and the right atrium or tributary to which it attaches, and (*d*) complete separation of the right and left atria.

The method for accomplishing this in the patients operated on at this clinic is indicated in Fig. 2. Details of technic have been described previously (8, 10, 11).

RESULTS

Nine patients with total anomalous pulmonary connection have been operated upon on this service. Six of these have survived operation and are considered cured. Their cyanosis has been completely abolished, they have no symptoms, and objective data on them indicate an excellent result in each.

Common Atrium

ANATOMY

In comon atrium (cor triloculare biventriculare) there is complete absence of the atrial septum. In all cases there is no remnant of atrial

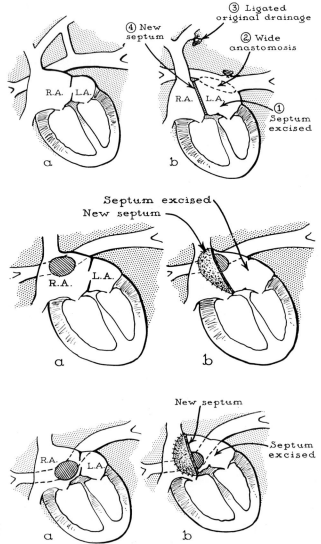

Fig. 2.   (Top) Schematic representation of important steps in the repair of total anomalous pulmonary venous connection to the left innominate vein. (Center and bottom.) The same is depicted for instances in which the total anomalous connection is directly into the right atrium or into the coronary sinus respectively. It is important to note that the basic maneuvers are the same no matter what the exact site of the connection is. (*a* and *b* represent appearance before and after correction respectively.)

septum above the atrioventricular valves. The anterior leaflet of the mitral valve is usually cleft, or both the mitral and the tricuspid valve may have cleft leaflets. In examples of the latter, there is usually an interventricular communication as well. These features suggest that common atrium is, in part, an endocardial cushion defect.

All pulmonary veins and the systemic veins attach to the common atrium.

HEMODYNAMICS

The single atrium serves as a common mixing chamber, and in general the oxygen saturation of blood in the aorta is nearly identical with that in the pulmonary artery. However, streamlining of flow through the chamber may be sufficient at times to cause differences.

In this, as in other conditions in which there is a common mixing chamber, the degree of arterial oxygen desaturation and of cyanosis depends upon the relative contributions of pulmonary venous and systemic venous blood to the common pool, and thus upon the relative magnitudes of pulmonary and systemic blood flow. These are in turn related in part to pulmonary vascular resistance, as was discussed for total anomalous pulmonary venous connection. The presence of mitral-valve incompetence, tricuspid incompetence, or an associated interventricular communication contributes importantly to the relative magnitudes of pulmonary and systemic blood flow.

The relation of pulmonary blood flow to systemic arterial-blood oxygen saturation that pertains to total anomalous pulmonary venous connection also pertains here.

INDICATION FOR SURGICAL TREATMENT

All patients with this malformation and with pulmonary blood flow in excess of systemic blood flow are advised to have an operation. Cyanosis and pulmonary hypertension are not contraindications to operation as long as these criteria are met.

TECHNIC

Open intracardiac repair, with the aid of a mechanical pump-oxygenator, is required. The important technical steps in the operation

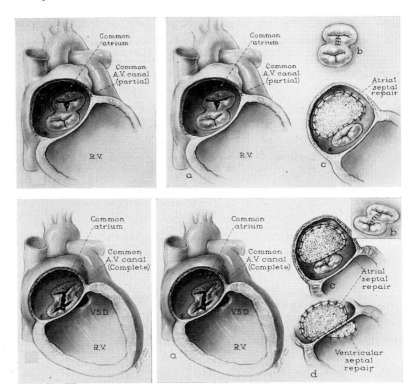

Fig. 3. (Upper left) Common atrium with cleft mitral valve. (Lower left) Common atrium with cleft mitral and tricuspid valves, and interventricular communication. (Upper and lower right) Steps in the repair of these malformations. (Reproduced with permission from reference 12.)

are: (*a*) repair of cleft in anterior leaflet of mitral valve and, when present, in septal leaflet of tricuspid valve; (*b*) insertion of atrial septum; and (*c*) repair of any interventricular communication that may be present.

Details of operative management were presented in a recent report by Ellis, Kirklin, and associates (12) from this clinic (Fig. 3).

RESULTS

Experience with this malformation is small. Ellis, Kirklin, and associates (12) reported operation in five cases, with four survivors. Cure, with complete relief of cyanosis and symptoms, can be anticipated in properly selected patients who survive complete repair.

Single Ventricle

Detailed discussion of the surgical treatment of cyanosed patients with a single ventricle that serves as a common mixing chamber is not warranted at present.

At the Mayo Clinic we have no cures of single ventricle. Only one surgically treated patient has survived operation, and he died suddenly 5 months after operation, presumably from a Stokes-Adams episode. He had complete atrioventricular dissociation after operation. No cures are reported in the literature.

Theoretically, this malformation could be corrected by insertion of a ventricular septum. However, the problem of maintenance of good ventricular function after insertion of an artificial septum has not yet been solved.

Pulmonary Stenosis and Atrial Septal Defect

ANATOMY

Cyanosis is usually present in patients with significant degrees of pulmonary stenosis associated with atrial septal defect or patent foramen ovale. In the great majority of instances, the stenosis is at the pulmonary valve. Many such patients have additionally a subvalvular narrowing that usually is associated with concentric hypertrophy of the outflow tract of the right ventricle (13). Rarely, a patient has localized infundibular pulmonary stenosis without valvular stenosis.

The interatrial communication may be through an atrial septal defect or through a patent foramen ovale that is either valvular competent or slightly valvular incompetent. Treatment by open intracardiac repair has revealed that more often than not the interatrial communication is a true atrial septal defect.

HEMODYNAMICS

Increase of systolic pressure in the right ventricle occurs because of the pulmonary stenosis. This increase may be moderate, with systolic pressure in the neighborhood of 100 mm Hg, or it may be severe, with pressure as high as 250 mm Hg during systole. Associated with the right ventricular hypertension and hypertrophy there is a venoarterial shunt at atrial level. Cyanosis and polycythemia secondary to this can be severe.

INDICATION FOR SURGICAL TREATMENT

All cyanotic patients with this malformation should be advised to have an operation.

TECHNIC

For reasons previously outlined, my colleagues and I believe that the proper treatment of this condition requires an attack on the pulmonary stenosis and closure of the interatrial communication (14). Although other technics have been used, it is our practice at present to employ open cardiotomy with extracorporeal circulation in these patients. It is felt that opportunity for complete repair of both is thereby enhanced and the operative risk minimized.

Details of technic in this operation are well understood and have been described previously (14). Suffice it to say that care must be taken to provide adequate relief of pulmonary stenosis. This may require in many cases not only pulmonary valvotomy but also resection of the hypertrophied muscle in the outflow tract as well. In very occasional instances, plastic reconstruction of this area may be necessary.

RESULTS

Twenty-four patients with pulmonary stenosis and intact ventricular septum have been operated upon with extracorporeal circulation at the Mayo Clinic. There has been one death. This series includes both cyanosed and noncyanosed patients with this malformation; 14 patients were cyanosed, and the one death was in such a patient.

Surviving patients are all well, without symptoms and without cyanosis.

Tetralogy of Fallot

The anatomy and hemodynamics of the tetralogy of Fallot have been discussed so repeatedly that it seems unnecessary to describe them herein. Since tetralogy is the commonest form of cyanotic congenital heart disease coming to open operation, certain aspects of its management should be emphasized. This discussion, then, will be limited to selection of operation, presentation of some important aspects of surgical technic, and review of results. Details of our experience with open operation for the tetralogy of Fallot are presented elsewhere (15).

SELECTION OF OPERATION

A little more than three years have elapsed since Lillehei and associates (16) first accomplished open intracardiac repair for the tetralogy of Fallot. The relatively small number of operations done by open technics and the short period of observation of the patients following operation render difficult a final evaluation of this technic.

It can be said that the operative mortality rate is acceptably low. The operation, although a demanding one, can be reproducibly accomplished except perhaps in the very small heart of the infant with this malformation. Infants in serious difficulty within the first year of life have usually had, in our experience, very narrow main pulmonary arteries and pulmonary valve rings, and have therefore seemed to require some form of plastic reconstruction. By present technics at least, efforts in this regard have seemed somewhat crude in this very small heart.

As will be detailed later, the subjective and objective evidences of improvement following open intracardiac repair are impressive. It has been our own experience that the results of this operation are truly magnificent.

Because of the reasonable mortality rate and the excellence of the end results in patients followed to date, it has been our practice to advise open intracardiac repair for all patients with the tetralogy of Fallot. In recent months, however, we have been concerned as to whether open operation is in fact the treatment of choice in the small infant 12 months of age or less who is in serious difficulty.

In the small infant with serious symptoms from the tetralogy of Fallot, complete relief of the pulmonary stenosis has been the major problem in open intracardiac repair. Our experience to date suggests that under these circumstances a prosthesis is usually required in the outflow tract of the right ventricle and in the pulmonary artery. The technical problems in the very small infant with the tetralogy of

Fallot are great in placing such a prosthesis in a manner that will not interfere with right ventricular function and will still relieve the pulmonary stenosis.

One must recall that a Blalock anastomosis in the small infant affords considerable palliation. Also the experience in our own institution has indicated clearly that a later open intracardiac repair can be done at an acceptably low risk in the patient who has had a previous anastomotic procedure.

For these reasons we are inclined at present to feel that intracardiac repair of the tetralogy of Fallot is the treatment of choice for all patients except the small infant. When these small patients are having serious symptoms, it is perhaps wise to perform a Blalock type of anastomosis, and plan to intervene again some years later by open intracardiac repair and disconnection of the previous anastomosis.

SOME IMPORTANT ASPECTS OF SURGICAL TECHNIC

The surgical technic employed in our institution for open intracardiac repair of the tetralogy of Fallot is described in detail elsewhere (15). Here, then, only the important principles involved will be reviewed.

Complete and accurate repair of the ventricular septal defect is obviously important. Of equal importance is the achievement of this repair without the production of complete permanent atrioventricular dissociation or heart block. The technic must then be directed toward insuring complete repair with a minimal incidence of heart block. Our experience suggests strongly that in nearly all cases of the tetralogy of Fallot this ideal can be most nearly approached by direct suture done in a specific and careful manner.

A low mortality rate and good results following open operation for the tetralogy of Fallot demand also good relief of the pulmonary stenosis. It is becoming increasingly apparent that this can be achieved in many cases by accurate excision of the infundibular obstruction, which usually implies complete removal of the crista supraventricularis. Pulmonary valvotomy must be done if valvular stenosis exists. There still remains a number of patients, perhaps 50% of the total group, in whom some sort of plastic reconstruction of the outflow tract or the pulmonary artery must be done. It is essential that the surgical pro-

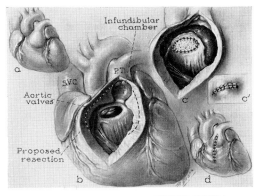

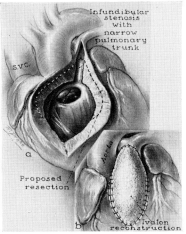

Fig. 4. (Top) Open intracardiac repair of the tetralogy of Fallot in cases in which pulmonary valvotomy and excision of the subvalvular narrowing result in the creation of an adequate pulmonary outflow tract. Although repair of the ventricular septal defect with ivalon sponge is depicted in this illustration, we usually have repaired the defect by direct suture. (Bottom) Reconstruction of the outflow tract with an Ivalon-Teflon prosthesis in patients in whom the pulmonary valve ring and the main pulmonary artery are very narrow.

cedure result in a right ventricular systolic pressure that is either normal or only moderately increased (Fig. 4).

RESULTS

We continue to have a significant operative mortality rate in the surgical treatment of the tetralogy of Fallot by the open technic. The overall mortality rate for our first 74 patients, reported on by us recently (15), was 28%. Between the time the last of these patients were treated and December 1, 1958, 32 additional patients have been operated on by open technic with five deaths, for a mortality of 15.6%.

Several late deaths were reported in the previous communication; these resulted clearly from incomplete relief of pulmonary stenosis or grossly incomplete repair of the ventricular septal defect. Excluding these, all patients have experienced significant improvement by operation. Cyanosis is absent in all save one in whom mild cyanosis develops with exertion. This patient is presumed to have a right-to-left shunt across a patent foramen ovale with exertion.

Objective evidence of cure has been obtained in many of these patients. The dramatic clinical improvement shown by patients with the tetralogy of Fallot who have been treated by open operation has led us to believe that this is indeed an effective mode of therapy. A continuing operative mortality rate of some 16% emphasizes the need for careful attention to methods of further reducing the surgical risk. In spite of this continuing mortality, the excellence of the results in surviving patients leads us to consider this the treatment of choice at present except in unusual circumstances.

Summary

Patients with cyanotic congenital heart disease present, in some ways, a greater challenge surgically than do patients without cyanosis. Progress has been made in understanding the circumstances under which cure can be hoped for and also in the manner of achieving complete surgical correction. Occasional disappointments occur, but the rewards that accrue to these patients from cure are so great that efforts to perfect methods of treatment must be continued.

REFERENCES

1. Edwards, J. E., and DuShane, J. W. Thoracic venous anomalies. I. Vascular connection of the left atrium and the left innominate vein (levoatriocardinal vein) associated with mitral atresia and premature

closure of the foramen ovale (Case 1). II. Pulmonary veins draining wholly into the ductus venosus (Case 2). *Arch. Pathol.* **49:**517–537 (1950).

2. Keith, J. D., Rowe, R. D., Vlad, Peter, and O'Hanley, J. H. Complete anomalous pulmonary venous drainage. *Am. J. Med.* **16:**23–38 (1954).

3. Burchell, H. B. Total anomalous pulmonary venous drainage: Clinical and physiologic patterns. *Proc. Staff Meetings Mayo Clin.* **31:**161–167 (1956).

4. Lewis, F. J., Varco, R. L., Taufic, Mansur, and Niazi, S. A. Direct vision repair of triatrial heart and total anomalous pulmonary venous drainage. *Surg. Gynecol. Obstet.* **102:**713–720 (1956).

5. Ehrenhaft, J. L., Theilen, E. O., and Lawrence, M. S. The surgical treatment of partial and total anomalous pulmonary venous connections. *Ann. Surg.* **148:**249–258 (1958).

6. Senning, Ake. Complete correction of total anomalous pulmonary venous return. *Ann. Surg.* **148:**99–103 (1958).

7. Mustard, W. T., and Dolan, F. G. The surgical treatment of total anomalous pulmonary venous drainage. *Ann. Surg.* **145:**379–387 (1957).

8. Bahnson, H. T., Spencer, F. C., and Neill, Catherine A. Surgical treatment of thirty-five cases of drainage of pulmonary veins to the right side of the heart. *J. Thoracic Surg.* **36:**777–799 (1958).

9. Gott, V. L., Lester, R. G., Lillehei, C. W., and Varco, R. L. Total anomalous pulmonary return: An analysis of thirty cases. *Circulation* **13:**543–552 (1956).

10. Cooley, D. A., and Ochsner, Alton, Jr. Correction of total anomalous pulmonary venous drainage: Technical considerations. *Surgery* **42:**1014–1021 (1957).

11. Burroughs, J. T., and Kirklin, J. W. Complete surgical correction of total anomalous pulmonary venous connection: Report of three cases. *Proc. Staff Meetings Mayo Clin.* **31:**182–188 (1956).

12. Ellis, F. H., Jr., Kirklin, J. W., Swan, H. J. C., DuShane, J. W., and Edwards, J. E. Diagnosis and surgical treatment of common atrium (cor triloculare-biventriculare). *Surgery* **45:**160–172 (1959).

13. Kirklin, J. W., Connolly, D. C., Ellis, F. H., Jr., Burchell, H. B., Edwards, J. E., and Wood, E. H. Problems in the diagnosis and surgical treatment of pulmonic stenosis with intact ventricular septum. *Circulation* **8:**849–863 (1953).

14. McGoon, D. C., and Kirklin, J. W. Pulmonic stenosis with intact ventricular septum: Treatment utilizing extracorporeal circulation. *Circulation* **17:**180–186 (1958).

15. Kirklin, J. W., Ellis, F. H., Jr., McGoon, D. C., DuShane, J. W., and

Swan, H. J. C. Surgical treatment for the tetralogy of Fallot by open intracardiac repair. *J. Thoracic Surg.* **37**:22–46 (1957).

16. Lillehei, C. W., Cohen, Morley, Warden, H. E., Read, R. C., Aust, J. B., DeWall, R. A., and Varco, R. L. Direct vision intracardiac surgical correction of the tetralogy of Fallot, pentalogy of Fallot, and pulmonary atresia defects: Report of first ten cases. *Ann. Surg.* **142**:418–445 (1955).

Surgical Therapy of Congenital Heart Disease: Present Status and Future Trends*

DENTON A. COOLEY

Cora and Webb Mading Department of Surgery, Baylor University College of Medicine, and Surgical Services Baylor Affiliated Hospitals, Houston, Texas

During the twenty years which have elapsed since Gross (8) performed the first successful operation for patent ductus arteriosus, a new field of surgical endeavor has been developed for treatment of congenital cardiovascular lesions. Particularly noteworthy were the contributions in 1944 of Blalock and Taussig (2) in treatment of tetralogy of Fallot and of Crafoord (7) and Gross (9) with coarctation of the aorta in providing additional stimuli to expansion of the field and the consideration of therapeutic possibilities for other congenital lesions. Subsequently Brock (4) and Sellors (17) performed valvotomy for pulmonic stenosis that demonstrated the feasibility of direct attack upon the heart itself in treatment of congenital cardiac lesions. This led the way for the ultimate development of technics for repair of cardiac septal defects first by closed or blind methods and more recently by the open technics of hypothermia and temporary cardiopulmonary bypass. Thus, the cardiac surgeon may now be called upon to treat the majority of congenital cardiac lesions. For some lesions the operative procedures may still be strictly palliative whereas for others, operation may be completely curative. Clinical diagnosis has reached a high degree of accuracy, and seldom is the surgeon expected to operate without a reasonable notion as to the exact nature of the

* Aided by grants from the Houston Heart Association, Junior League Clinic, the C. J. Thibodeaux Foundation, and the U.S. Public Health Service under Grant H-3137.

345

lesion. Nevertheless, surgical judgment is still a requirement since final decisions regarding technic are based upon recognition of anatomic abnormalities. Often after recognizing the lesion, the surgeon has difficulty in selecting the most satisfactory method of therapy, particularly when conflicting opinions of various authorities have been expressed. Decisions are based upon previous experience under these circumstances, and in instances in which the lesion is being treated for the first time, the problem may actually be enormous. Such problems must be solved in collaboration with the cardiologist, and many factors including the risk of attempted repair balanced against the prognosis without attempted repair must be considered.

Obviously the limited scope of this paper prevents a complete survey of the field of cardiac surgery of all congenital lesions. An attempt will therefore be made to present some of the methods of management of congenital cardiac lesions which are being utilized in Baylor Affiliated Hospitals since these concepts of therapy were selected by trial and error and observation of results over a period of years. Finally, an attempt will be made to propose possible future surgical trends which may further improve results.

Present Status

As already stated, certain congenital cardiac lesions are completely correctible by operative means, and in others indirect or palliative procedures produce the most satisfactory results. Repair of certain defects may be accomplished without interrupting cardiac function, whereas an increasing number are being treated by open cardiac technics. Opinions regarding choice of operation as expressed in Table I represent the general policy adopted in our own cases and have produced the most satisfactory results to date. Indications for and optimum technic of operation for several lesions are now more or less standardized and deserve only brief comment. Patent ductus arteriosus, coarctation of the aorta, and aortic vascular ring are examples of lesions with established technics of treatment.

Disagreement exists with regard to some of the methods recommended in Table I. For example, Lillehei (13) and Kirklin (11) would not agree with our attitude toward tetralogy of Fallot. Yet our operative mortality of 37% in 32 patients using a "curative" procedure

TABLE I. Operative procedures used for congenital cardiovascular lesions in Baylor Affiliated Hospitals

Lesion	Optimum Age (years)	Surgical Procedure of Choice
Patent ductus arteriosus	2–5	Division and suture
Coarctation of aorta	8–12	Excision with end-to-end anastomosis
Aortic vascular ring	0–2	Division of anomalous vascular trunks
Tetralogy of Fallot	0–2	Aorticopulmonary anastomosis (Potts) or subclavian-pulmonary anastomosis (Blalock)
Tetralogy of Fallot	2–10	Open repair with bypass
Valvular pulmonic stenosis with intact ventricular septum	2–10	Transventricular valvotomy with guillotine valvotome
Infundibular pulmonic stenosis	2–10	Open repair with bypass
Aortic stenosis, valvular and infundibular	2–10	Open repair with bypass
Ventricular septal defect	2–10	Open repair with bypass
Atrial septal defect includes ost. I & ost. II	5–15	Open repair with bypass
Aorticopulmonary septal defect	2–10	Open repair with bypass
Total anomalous pulmonary venous drainage	0–10	Open repair with bypass
Atrioventricularis communis	1–3	Open repair with bypass
Transposition of great vessels	0–2	Creation atrial septal defect
Transposition of great vessels	2–10	Baffes operation or attempted transposition of atrial septum with bypass

during cardiopulmonary bypass requires us to select patients with tetralogy of Fallot for open repair or for an anastomotic procedure. In our cases of tetralogy the highest mortality with open repair was in the severely cyanotic, polycythemic child with severe over-riding aorta and underdeveloped right ventricular outflow tract and pulmonary artery. Thus, in this type of patient we now employ an anastomotic procedure since the functional results are highly acceptable and operative mortality is less than 5%. Desperately ill newborn infants with severe anoxic spells and pulmonary atresia in our opinion are unsuitable for the open or complete repair, yet the response to an aorticopulmonary anastomosis may be dramatic (5) (Table II). Indeed, ultimate results of these so-called palliative operations in pa-

TABLE II.   Cardiovascular anomalies and survival in 140 infants less than one year of age treated surgically

Diagnosis	No. of Patients	Age Range	Survived, Improved	
Tetralogy of Fallot	35	3 wks–11 mos	29	82%
Ventricular septal defect	30	6 wks–12 mos	18	60%
Transposition of great vessels	19	1 wk–7 mos	12	63%
Coarctation of aorta	16	4 days–7 mos	11	68%
Tricuspid atresia	10	2 days–8 mos	7	70%
Patent ductus arteriosus	10	2 mos–11 mos	7	70%
Aortic stenosis	4	4 wks–6 mos	4	100%
Pulmonary stenosis	4	2 mos–5 mos	4	100%
Total anomalous pulmonary venous drainage	5	4 mos–6 mos	4	80%
Single ventricle with other anomalies	3	4 mos–7 mos	1	33%
Primary pulmonary hypertension	1	3 mos	0	0%
Aortic vascular ring	1	2 mos	1	100%
Miscellaneous lesions with high output failure[a]	2	5 wks–3 mos	1	50%
Total	*140*		*99*	*71%*

[a] Lesions for which banding of pulmonary artery for reduction of pulmonary flow is useful (14).

tients with tetralogy may be no less satisfactory than a corrective operation in which compressed polyvinyl sponges are placed in the ventricular septal defect and across the annulus in an anatomically destroyed pulmonary valve. Everyone agrees that in properly selected cases in which a satisfactory balance of circulation through right and left sides of the heart can be achieved without extensive reconstructions of the right ventricle, results of open operation are superior to anastomotic operations. Such a situation usually exists in the moderately cyanotic patient with an adequate-sized undivided pulmonary artery and moderate overriding of the aorta, and in these cases we employ open repair by choice.

Valvular pulmonic stenosis is another lesion in which multiple technics of surgical repair are available. Some surgeons such as Swan (18) and Lam (12) assert that valvotomy under direct vision is superior and should be employed in all such cases. Swan uses induced general body hypothermia with temporary inflow stasis whereas Lam employs extremely brief periods of temporary inflow stasis alone with-

out hypothermia. Both have had excellent results. Recently temporary cardiopulmonary bypass has been advocated by some as the procedure of choice in these cases. Our own technic in most cases consists
of a transventricular approach to the valve similar to the original
method employed by Brock and Sellors. An important modification
which has produced extremely satisfactory results has been the use of a
guillotine type instrument to cut the pulmonic valve back completely
to the annulus with subsequent complete dilatation. In these cases a
complete valvotomy is achieved with ultimate obliteration of the pressure gradient across the valvar zone. In some instances the gradient is
not eliminated immediately and may require six months to return
to normal, but this phenomenon has also been noted in cases operated
upon with direct vision of the valve. In contrast to the valvar stenosis,
little difference of opinion exists regarding operative technic in infundibular pulmonic stenosis. Direct vision of the infundibulum is
highly desirable because of the wide variation in anatomic location
and relationships to the ventricular septum and tricuspid valve which
may be present. Cardiopulmonary bypass is employed in all our cases
with infundibular or combined infundibular and valvular stenosis
since an adequate infundibulectomy may require more than 10 min
inside the heart. In instances of combined infundibular and valvar
stenosis and in some cases where exact preoperative diagnosis is not
possible, preparations for open-heart surgery are necessary.

Most surgeons including ourselves now endorse the technic of aortic
valvotomy under direct vision through an incision in the ascending
aorta. Since the procedures can usually be done in a few minutes, inflow occlusion under hypothermia may be satisfactory, but since cardiopulmonary bypass provides a somewhat wider margin of safety and
facilitates cardiac resuscitation when the distressed left ventricle fails
during operation, we employ it routinely. Moreover, if a subaortic
stenosis is present, a longer period of time inside the heart may be
necessary for accurate excision without damaging the aortic leaflet
and producing serious aortic valvular regurgitation. Using temporary
cardiopulmonary bypass we have operated upon 22 patients with congenital aortic stenosis, of which 11 were valvular, 8 subaortic, and 2
combined stenoses ranging in age from 4 weeks to 19 years (Table III).
Only one fatality occurred in these patients—in a 10-year-old boy with

TABLE III.   Congenital lesions operated upon using temporary cardio-pulmonary bypass

Lesion	No. Cases
Ventricular septal defect	181
Atrial septal defect (ostium II)	104
Atrial septal defect (ostium I)	22
Atrial septal defect (a-v communis)	15
Tetralogy of Fallot	32
Pulmonic stenosis	28
Aortic stenosis	22
Total anomalous pulmonary venous return	12
Sinus of Valsalva fistula	4
Transposition of great vessels	6
Aorticopulmonary septal defect	2
Miscellaneous congenital lesions	15
Total	*443[a]*

[a] Additional 82 cases of acquired heart disease operated upon giving total 525 cases of cardiopulmonary bypass.

supra-aortic stenosis in which an underdeveloped ascending aorta measuring 12 mm in diameter was encountered above a relatively normal aortic valve.

No question exists at present regarding the optimum method of treatment for ventricular septal defect since all are agreed upon direct vision technics, and temporary cardiopulmonary bypass is used by almost all surgeons. Selection of patients for operation remains somewhat controversial. The presence of increased pulmonary vascular resistance and pulmonary hypertension increases the risk of operation. Our own policy at present is to refuse operation in cases of isolated ventricular septal defect who have cyanosis and polycythemia, small hearts with predominant right ventricular hypertrophy and predominant right-to-left shunts. Such cases are examples of Eisenmenger's syndrome. Operation for ventricular septal defect in infants less than two years of age is attended by a high mortality, and only cases in which death from congestive heart failure seems imminent are selected for operation at such an early age (Tables IV and V).

Certain technical considerations are important in repair of ventricular septal defect and influence strongly the results of operation. Although induced cardiac arrest provides ideal conditions for repair in

TABLE IV. Results in ventricular septal defect according to age

Age (years)	No.	Deaths	Per Cent
Less than 2	41	16	39
2–15	111	8	7
More than 15	29	5	17
Total	*189*	*29*	*15*

TABLE V. Results in atrial septal defect (ostium II) according to age

Age (years)	No.	Deaths	Per Cent
0–25	76	0	0
26–55	31	7	22
Total	*107*	*7*	*6*

a quiet bloodless field, in our own cases arrest with potassium citrate increased the risk of operation. Results improved when this technic was abandoned more than one year ago. Method of closure of the defects is also important. In our opinion, large ventricular septal defects should be repaired with a patch of synthetic fiber cloth to avoid tension on the sutures placed in the myocardium. In smaller defects a rim of thickened fibrous endocardium usually surrounds the defect and direct suture gives a sturdy repair. Our experience with surgical repair of ventricular septal defect now includes 181 cases with an overall operative mortality of 15% (Table IV). It is significant that only one patient in the last 50 consecutive patients with ventricular septal defect was less than 2 years of age, whereas 16 patients in the first 50 were less than 2. Obviously the relative absence of these critically ill infants from the latter series partly accounts for the reduction of mortality from 18 to 8% in the most recent series. Particularly gratifying is the fact that in 111 patients between the ages of 2 and 15 years with ventricular septal defect undergoing surgical repair, the overall mortality was only 7% (Table IV).

Surgical treatment of atrial septal defect has recently been accomplished by various closed as well as open technics. Although good results were reported at one time for the closed methods, the trend even for the simpler defects has been toward use of direct vision repair of these defects. Among our 107 patients operated upon with cardiopulmonary bypass with ostium secundum type defects there were 7 deaths (6%) (Table V). All fatalities in our series occurred in 31 patients who were more than 25 years old, whereas in 76 patients less than 25 no deaths occurred. One concludes, therefore, that the method of repair using bypass is satisfactory and relatively safe, but patients should be operated upon before pulmonary vascular and myocardial changes become extreme.

Total anomalous drainage of pulmonary veins into the systemic veins is another example of the progress being made in expanding the field of cardiac surgery. Formerly this condition was considered to be extremely rare and almost incurable by closed technics. Yet we have operated upon 12 such patients with good results. Five patients had drainage of the pulmonary venous blood into the left innominate veins —a type known as the supracardiac drainage, and all recovered after complete correction using temporary cardiopulmonary bypass (6). Correction of total anomaly in which the drainage of pulmonary venous blood is into the right atrium directly is technically simpler than the repair of the supracardiac type, and results should be equally good. Thus, another lesion previously considered to be rare and for the most part incurable has become a more frequently recognized lesion, and surgical repair is being standardized.

Not all problems in surgery of congenital heart disease are solved even with the advent of direct vision technics, and some of the more challenging problems may continue to defy solution. Complete transposition of the great vessels is a good example of such a lesion. Palliative procedures such as creation of an interatrial septal defect or the partial cardiac venous transfer recently devised by Baffes (1) reduce the cyanosis but fall far short of correcting the basic anomaly. Attempts at complete repair by using the pump-oxygenator have uniformly met with failure regardless of whether the corrective procedure involved transfer of the atrial septum or attempts to transpose the great vessels themselves. Thus, at present it is not known whether total repair of this lesion is physiologically possible, and if it is feasible, which cases are operable. Other lesions may also be incurable even with the heart open. In our series of 525 patients undergoing temporary cardiopulmonary bypass for congenital lesions, 15 had complicated anomalies for which surgical correction was not feasible or resulted in failure

(Table III). Among these were cases of endocardial fibroelastosis, single ventricle with a rudimentary ventricular chamber, mitral atresia, and complicated anomalies of the systemic and pulmonary venous system draining into the atria. Many of these lesions are and will continue to be a problem no matter how far we progress in this field.

One aspect of congenital cardiac surgery deserves comment at present since it has become so important to the successful treatment of congenital cardiac disease, and this is need of surgical intervention in newborn and young infants. During the past four years we operated upon 140 infants less than one year of age who had various diagnoses before operation (Table V). Factors which influence the decision to operate in small infants included a history of frequent severe spells of cyanosis, intractable congestive heart failure with repeated respiratory infections and/or severe failure of growth and development. Tetralogy of Fallot and tricuspid atresia are lesions which may lead to death during a cyanotic attack, and creation of a small systemic to pulmonary shunt may be lifesaving (2, 5, 15). Surprisingly enough, such procedures employed during infancy may provide adequate relief of cyanosis and anoxic symptoms almost indefinitely. Since open repair of tricuspid atresia is not possible, the anastomosis must provide the only definitive treatment possible. Critically ill infants with complete transposition of the great vessels improve dramatically after creation of an interatrial septal defect (3) and this is the procedure of choice. Palliative therapy for infants with increased pulmonary flow associated with ventricular septal defect or more complicated anomalies may be obtained by partial constriction of the undivided pulmonary artery as advocated by Muller (14). This technic in some instances results in dramatic disappearance of pulmonary congestion and relief of myocardial strain. Early treatment of pulmonic or aortic valvular stenoses may lead to dramatic improvement in infants whose hearts are under great strain from the obstructed outflow. In contrast to some of these procedures already mentioned, the operation for correction of total anomalous pulmonary venous return is completely curative at this early age. This is true of patent ductus arteriosus and ventricular septal defect. If coarctation is repaired during infancy, it is conceivable that subsequent operation may be necessary after the child has grown larger, yet this should not deter one from operating on infants as a salvage procedure if the indications for surgery are strong. Frequently it is difficult to distinguish before thoracotomy whether the infant has a correctible type of coarctation of the aorta or not. Preductal or diffuse coarctations usually associated with severe anomalies in the left side of the heart were encountered in 4 patients among 16 operated upon with a diagnosis of coarctation. Thus, all but one of the 12 patients with correctible forms of the disease recovered from operation. In general, the results of operation in infants less than one year of age have been gratifying as evidenced by recovery of 71% of the patients (Table II).

Future Trends

The direction of some future trends and developments in the field of cardiovascular surgery seems evident at this time whereas other trends cannot be anticipated. Emphasis will undoubtedly continue to be placed upon adoption of corrective procedures in preference to indirect or palliative ones. Indications for surgery will be further broadened and liberalized. The changing attitude during the past twenty years toward the place of surgery in management of patients with patent ductus arteriosus is perhaps typical of the trends to be expected for lesions such as the small ventricular septal defect. During the first five years after the first successful surgical closure of a patent ductus arteriosus, operation was only recommended in the presence of strong indications such as cardiac decompensation, bacterial endocarditis, or serious failure of growth. As experience increased, the surgical mortality was finally reduced to such a low level that the risk of operation was considerably less than the risk of possible future complications and prophylactic repair of the patent ductus arteriosus was advocated. At present cardiologists are inclined to recommend surgical closure of a ductus in the presence of even the faintest machinery murmur. Indeed, the psychologic effect of the murmur on the patient and his parents may be the most important justification for operation. Closure of a small ventricular septal defect producing only mild physiologic disturbance should also be accepted more widely. Already the results of operation in septal defects justify this attitude. In approximately 30 of our cases of ventricular septal defect between 2 and 15 years of age in which pulmonary vascular changes were minimal and systolic pulmonary arterial pressure less than 50 mm Hg, no fatalities have occurred following operation. Thus, one can expect cardiologists to become more lenient in their willingness to recommend operation to these patients.

Open cardiac surgery will unquestionably replace certain technics which are still employed for correction of intracardiac lesions. Kirklin (10), for example, still utilizes the atrial well technic for repair of atrial septal defect, and we use closed valvotomy for pulmonic valvar stenosis. Admittedly, the results of these blind procedures have been satisfactory, otherwise these technics already would have been replaced. Certain factors are partly responsible for this somewhat confusing and paradoxical policy in these instances. An acute demand is being placed upon the schedules for bypass operations using the pump-oxygenator. The pressure of large numbers of patients awaiting open operation for other lesions in which cardiopulmonary bypass is an absolute necessity therefore accounts to some degree for continuation of older technics of treatment. Furthermore, the collection of blood for open surgery by present technics taxes the blood banking facilities to the point that it is necessary to continue to utilize some methods of cardiac surgery which, although proved to be satisfactory, are not altogether in keeping with changing attitudes and progress in this field. Presumably when the technics of cardiopulmonary bypass are further simplified, open cardiac surgery will be employed routinely for atrial septal defect and valvar pulmonic stenosis.

Until very recently most efforts in the technic of cardiopulmonary bypass were being exerted toward increasing the capacity of the extracorporeal system in an effort to maintain the entire body in completely homeostatic conditions during the period of bypass. Such heavy demands upon the extracorporeal apparatus tend to make the technic unnecessarily cumbersome and work unusual hardship upon blood banking facilities and technical personnel. Future success and expansion of open-heart surgery probably will depend upon reduction in the demands placed upon the pump-oxygenator system. Hypothermia could be used in conjunction with extracorporeal circulation. Sealy and Brown (16) have utilized a heat exchanger effectively in this manner and have induced general body hypothermia rapidly and safely. Low perfusion rates are then possible during the period of cardiopulmonary bypass which minimizes the blood loss and the need for a large volume pump-oxygenator system. Their efforts show real promise in providing a simpler and more compact method of perfusion. Induced local tissue hypothermia to protect vital organs of the body such as the central nervous system may be practical as utilized by Japanese surgeons. By this method the temperature of the blood stream would not be affected appreciably, and the cardiac complications of general body hypothermia could be avoided. Minimal perfusion rates could be made to suffice also if metabolic requirements of tissues were reduced by a metabolic blocking agent which had a reversible action on the oxidation processes in the cell. Such a drug should therefore have a temporary action, a dependable antidote, and should produce no permanent cellular damage.

Improved methods of blood collection and storage for open-heart surgery will assist in simplification of the open-heart project. Whereas at present it is necessary to collect fresh heparinized blood from donors in larger numbers, in the future blood may be collected and stored in a more practical manner. If blood were collected and stored routinely by blood banks utilizing a method of calcium extraction other than by citration, a ready source of blood for priming the pump-oxygenator and for use during bypass would be made available. Moreover, addition of blood fractions such as platelet suspension could be utilized to rejuvenate blood stored more than 72 hours so that it could be used satisfactorily. Solution of these and other problems will extend widely the application of open cardiac surgery in congenital heart disease.

Summary

Tremendous strides have been made in expansion of the field of surgery for congenital cardiovascular disease. Technics have been developed for complete anatomic and physiologic correction of some lesions and for partial or palliative relief for others. Recently the method of open-heart surgery has added tremendously to the scope of cardiac surgery. At present some lesions are treated without interruption of cardiac function, some during hypothermia or complete cardiopulmonary bypass, and in others a choice of technics is available depending upon several factors including age and severity of the anomaly. Operations have been successful in young infants and should be employed as salvage procedures even under the most critical circumstances. Future trends in surgery of congenital cardiac lesions should include liberalizing the indications for some lesions, greater emphasis upon use of curative procedures using extracorporeal circulation, reduction in volume of flow necessary to maintain life during bypass, and simplification of open-heart technics by improved methods of blood storage.

REFERENCES

1. Baffes, T. G. A new method for surgical correction of transposition of the aorta and pulmonary artery. *Surg. Gynecol. Obstet.* **102**:227–233 (1956).
2. Blalock, A., and Taussig, H. B. The surgical treatment of malformations of the heart in which there is pulmonary stenosis or pulmonary atresia. *J. Am. Med. Assoc.* **128**:189–202 (1945).
3. Blalock, A., and Hanlon, C. R. The surgical treatment of complete transposition of the aorta and the pulmonary artery. *Surg. Gynecol. Obstet.* **90**:1–15 (1950).
4. Brock, R. C. Pulmonary valvulotomy for the relief of congenital pulmonary stenosis: Report of three cases. *Brit. Med. J.* **1**:1121–1126 (1948).
5. Collins, H. A., Harberg, F. J., Soltero, L. R., McNamara, D. G., and Cooley, D. A. Cardiac surgery in the newborn and young infant: Experience with 120 patients under one year of age. *Surgery* **45**:506–519 (1959).
6. Cooley, D. A., and Ochsner, A., Jr. Correction of total anomalous pulmonary venous drainage. *Surgery* **42**:1014–1021 (1957).
7. Crafoord, C., and Nylin, G. Congenital coarctation of aorta and its surgical treatment. *J. Thoracic Surg.* **14**:347–361 (1945).
8. Gross, R. E., and Hubbard, J. P. Surgical ligation of patent ductus arteriosus: Report of first successful case. *J. Am. Med. Assoc.* **112**:729–731 (1939).
9. Gross, R. E., and Hufnagel, C. A. Coarctation of the aorta: Experimental studies regarding its surgical correction. *N. Engl. J. Med.* **233**:287–293 (1945).
10. Kirklin, J. W., Swan, H. J. C., Wood, E. H., Burchell, H. B., and Edwards, J. E. Anatomic, physiologic, and surgical considerations in repair of interatrial communications in man. *J. Thoracic Surg.* **29**:37–53 (1955).
11. Kirklin, J. W., and McGoon, D. C. Surgical technique for repair of high ventricular septal defects. *J. Thoracic Surg.* **35**:584–590 (1958).
12. Lam, Conrad R. Personal communication.
13. Lillehei, C. W., Cohen, M., Warden, H. E., Read, R. C., Aust, J.,

DeWall, R. A., and Varco, R. L. Direct vision intracardiac surgical correction of the tetralogy of Fallot, pentalogy of Fallot, and pulmonary atresia defects. *Ann. Surg.* **142:**418–445 (1955).

14. Muller, W. H., Jr., and Dammann, J. F., Jr. The treatment of certain congenital malformations of the heart by the creation of pulmonic stenosis to reduce pulmonary hypertension and excessive pulmonary blood flow. A preliminary report. *Surg. Gynecol. Obstet.* **95:**213–219 (1952).

15. Potts, W. J., Smith, S., and Gibson, S. Anastomosis of the aorta to a pulmonary artery. *J. Am. Med. Assoc.* **132:**627–631 (1946).

16. Sealy, W. C., Brown, I. W., Jr., Young, W. G., Jr., Stephen, C. R., Harris, J. S., and Merritt, D. Hypothermia, low flow extracorporeal circulation and controlled cardiac arrest for open heart surgery. *Surg. Gynecol. Obstet.* **104:**441–450 (1957).

17. Sellors, T. H., and Belcher, J. R. Surgical relief of congenital cyanotic heart disease: Late results in 72 cases. *Lancet* **2:**887–889 (1950).

18. Swan, H., Virtue, R. W., Blount, S. G., and Kircher, L. T. Hypothermia in surgery: Analysis of 100 clinical cases. *Ann. Surg.* **142:**382–400 (1955).

Index